Cochlear Implants
Principles & Practices

Cochlear Implants
Principles & Practices

Editors

John K. Niparko, M.D.

Director, Otology Neurotology
Professor, Department of Otolaryngology-Head and Neck Surgery
The Johns Hopkins University
Baltimore, Maryland

Karen Iler Kirk, PH.D.

Professor of Audiology, Department of Otolaryngo
Indiana University
Indianapolis, Indiana

Nancy K. Mellon, M.S.

Director, The River School
Washington, D.C.;
Clinical Coordinator, The Listening Center at Johns Hopkins
Department of Otolaryngology-Head and Neck Surgery
The Johns Hopkins University
Baltimore, Maryland

Amy McConkey Robbins, M.S.

Consulting Speech and Language Pathologist
Communication Consulting Services
Indianapolis, Indiana

Debara L. Tucci, M.D.

Assistant Professor, Department of Surgery
Duke University Medical Center
Durham, North Carolina

Blake S. Wilson, B.S.E.E.

Director, Center for Auditory Prosthesis Research
Research Triangle Institute
Research Triangle Park, North Carolina

Art Direction by
Robert F. Morreale

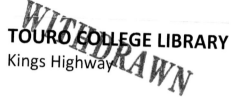

LIPPINCOTT WILLIAMS & WILKINS
A **Wolters Kluwer** Company
Philadelphia · Baltimore · New York · London
Buenos Aires · Hong Kong · Sydney · Tokyo

M W

Acquisitions Editor: Danette Knopp
Developmental Editor: Joyce A. Murphy
Production Editor: Brandy Mui
Manufacturing Manager: Kevin Watt
Compositor: The PRD Group
Printer: Edwards Brothers

© **2000 by LIPPINCOTT WILLIAMS & WILKINS**
227 East Washington Square
Philadelphia, PA 19106-3780 USA
LWW.com

Printed in the USA

Library of Congress Cataloging-in-Publication Data

ISBN: 0-7817-1782-5

Care has been taken to confirm the accuracy of the information presented and
to describe generally accepted practices. However, the authors, editors, and
publisher are not responsible for errors or omissions or for any consequences
from application of the information in this book and make no warranty,
expressed or implied, with respect to the currency, completeness, or accuracy of
the contents of the publication. Application of this information in a particular
situation remains the professional responsibility of the practitioner.

The authors, editors, and publisher have exerted every effort to ensure that
drug selection and dosage set forth in this text are in accordance with current
recommendations and practice at the time of publication. However, in view of
ongoing research, changes in government regulations, and the constant flow of
information relating to drug therapy and drug reactions, the reader is urged to
check the package insert for each drug for any change in indications and dosage
and for added warnings and precautions. This is particularly important when the
recommended agent is a new or infrequently employed drug.

Some drugs and medical devices presented in this publication have Food and
Drug Administration (FDA) clearance for limited use in restricted research
settings. It is the responsibility of the health care provider to ascertain the FDA
status of each drug or device planned for use in their clinical practice.

10 9 8 7 6 5 4 3 2 1

6/16/01

To

John L. Kemink, M.D.

His devotion to human achievement
through cochlear implantation was
one of many attributes that defined him
as a humane physician without peer

and

Karin E. Young, M.A., CCC-A

May life reciprocate in your recovery
the many gifts you gave to others

Contents

Contributing Authors xi

Preface xiii

Introduction 1

Section I: The Neurobiology of Hearing and Deafness

1.   Auditory Physiology and Perception 9
     Bradford J. May

Appendix 1A. Correlates of Sensorineural Hearing Loss and Their Effect
     on Hearing Aid Use: The Problem of Recruitment 28
     Ginger D. Grant

2.   Brain Plasticity: The Impact of the Environment on the
     Brain as It Relates to Hearing and Deafness 33
     David K. Ryugo, Charles J. Limb, and
     Elizabeth E. Redd

3.   Inner Ear Pathology in Severe to Profound Sensorineural
     Hearing Loss 57
     Matthew Ng, John K. Niparko, and
     George T. Nager

Appendix 3A. The Epidemiology of Hearing Loss: How Prevalent Is
     Hearing Loss? 88
     John K. Niparko

4.   Effects of Deafness on the Human Central Auditory
     System 93
     Jean K. Moore and John K. Niparko

Appendix 4A. Central Auditory System Effects of Cochlear Implantation:
     Animal Studies 97
     Debara L. Tucci

Section II: Cochlear Implant Technology

5.   History of Cochlear Implants 103
     John K. Niparko and Blake S. Wilson

6.   Cochlear Implant Technology 109
     Blake S. Wilson

Appendix 6A.   Microcircuitry in Cochlear Implants 119
                John K. Niparko

Appendix 6B.   Food and Drug Administration Approval Process for
                Cochlear Implants 122
                Harry R. Sauberman

7.   Strategies for Representing Speech Information with
                Cochlear Implants 129
                Blake S. Wilson

Section III: Assessment of Cochlear Implant Candidacy

8.   Assessment of Cochlear Implant Candidacy 173
                John K. Niparko

Appendix 8A.   Professional Roles in Multidisciplinary Assessment of
                Candidacy 178
                Betty Schopmeyer

Appendix 8B.   Parental Response to the Diagnosis of Hearing Loss 181
                Nancy K. Mellon

Appendix 8C.   Maternal Attachment and Adjustment: Impact on Child
                Outcomes 183
                Nancy K. Mellon

Section IV: Cochlear Implant Surgery

9.   Medical and Surgical Aspects of Cochlear Implantation 189
                Debara L. Tucci and John K. Niparko

Section V: Results and Outcomes of Cochlear Implantation

10.   Challenges in the Clinical Investigation of Cochlear Implant
                Outcomes 225
                Karen Iler Kirk

Appendix 10A.   Analyzing the Effects of Early Implantation and Results
                with Different Causes of Deafness: Meta-analysis of the
                Pediatric Cochlear Implant Literature 259
                André K. Cheng and John K. Niparko

Appendix 10B.   Music and Cochlear Implantation 265
                Charles J. Limb

11.   Outcomes of Cochlear Implantation: Assessment of Quality
                of Life Impact and Economic Evaluation of the Benefits of
                the Cochlear Implant in Relation to Costs 269
                John K. Niparko, André K. Cheng, and
                Howard W. Francis

Section VI: Language Learning and Cochlear Implant Rehabilitation

12.   Language Acquisition 291
Nancy K. Mellon

Appendix 12A.   Reading and Deafness 315
Betty Schopmeyer

Appendix 12B.   Psychosocial Development of Children in Deafness 319
Nancy K. Mellon

13.   Rehabilitation after Cochlear Implantation 323
Amy McConkey Robbins

Appendix 13A.   Rehabilitation for the Hearing Impaired: A Historical
Perspective 363
Mark Ross

Appendix 13B.   Motor Skills in Childhood Deafness 365
Betty Schopmeyer

Section VII: Cultural Aspects of Cochlear Implantation

14.   Culture and Cochlear Implants 371
John K. Niparko

Appendix 14A.   The Implications of Parental Choice of Communication
Mode: Understanding the Options 379
Nancy K. Mellon

Subject Index 385

Contributing Authors

André K. Cheng, M.D. *Research Fellow, Department of Otolaryngology—Head and Neck Surgery, The Johns Hopkins University, Baltimore, Maryland 21287-0910*

Howard W. Francis, M.D. *Assistant Chief of Services, Department of Otolaryngology—Head and Neck Surgery, The Johns Hopkins University, Baltimore, Maryland 21287-0910*

Ginger D. Grant, M.A. *Speech Pathologist, Department of Otolaryngology—Head and Neck Surgery, The Johns Hopkins University, Baltimore, Maryland 21287-0910*

Karen Iler Kirk, Ph.D. *Professor of Audiology, Department of Otolaryngology, Indiana University, Indianapolis, Indiana 46202*

Charles J. Limb, M.D. *Research Fellow, Department of Otolaryngology—Head and Neck Surgery, The Johns Hopkins University, Baltimore, Maryland 21287-0910*

Bradford J. May, Ph.D. *Associate Professor, Center for Hearing and Balance Sciences, Department of Otolaryngology—Head and Neck Surgery, The Johns Hopkins University, Baltimore, Maryland 21287-0910*

Nancy K. Mellon, M.S. *Clinical Coordinator, The Listening Center at Johns Hopkins, Department of Otolaryngology—Head and Neck Surgery, The Johns Hopkins University, Baltimore, Maryland 21287-0910*

Jean K. Moore, Ph.D. *Department of Neuroanatomy, House Ear Institute; Adjunct Faculty in the Department of Otolaryngology, University of Southern California, Los Angeles, California 90089*

George T. Nager, M.D. *Professor and Former Chairman, Department of Otolaryngology—Head and Neck Surgery, The Johns Hopkins University, Baltimore, Maryland 21287-0910*

Matthew Ng, M.D. *Department of Otolaryngology—Head and Neck Surgery, The Johns Hopkins University, Baltimore, Maryland 21287-0910*

John K. Niparko, M.D. *Director, Otology Neurotology, Professor, Department of Otolaryngology—Head and Neck Surgery, The Johns Hopkins University, Baltimore, Maryland 21205-2196*

Elizabeth E. Redd, M.D. *Research Fellow, Departments of Otolaryngology—Head and Neck Surgery, The Johns Hopkins University, Baltimore, Maryland 21287-0910*

Amy McConkey Robbins, M.S. *Consulting Speech and Language Pathologist, Communication Consulting Services, Indianapolis, Indiana 46260*

Mark Ross, Ph.D. *Adjunct Professor, University of Connecticut, Storrs, Connecticut 06269*

David K. Ryugo, Ph.D.   *Center for Hearing and Balance Sciences, Departments of Otolaryngology—Head and Neck Surgery, The Johns Hopkins University, Baltimore, Maryland 21287-0910*

Harry R. Sauberman, P.E., M.E.E.   *ENT Branch, Food and Drug Administration, Rockville, Maryland 20850*

Betty Schopmeyer, M.A.   *Coordinator of Cochlear Implant Rehabilitation, The Listening Center at Johns Hopkins, The Johns Hopkins University, Baltimore, Maryland 21287-0910*

Debara L. Tucci, M.D.   *Assistant Professor, Duke University Medical Center, Department of Surgery, Durham, North Carolina 27710*

Blake S. Wilson, B.S.E.E.   *Director, Center for Auditory Prosthesis Research, Research Triangle Institute, Research Triangle Park, North Carolina 27709*

Preface

The application of electrified implants to the auditory nerve marks a revolutionary step in the search for rehabilitative alternatives in deafness. This book describes the clinical practices related to cochlear implantation from selection of candidates to techniques of device placement, activation and use as a communicative tool. We have also attempted to provide both an orientation to basic concepts, both biological and technical, and an update of the many issues surrounding the communication change entailed by cochlear implantation.

As cochlear implants have gained wide notoriety and acceptance in many circles, our focus must begin to shift to consider the settings in which children with implants attain language competence, and adults with implants seek a broad and meaningful listening experience. Many factors impact success at home, in school, at work, and in the community. Thus, the technology brings with it a responsibility to support the process begun by the introduction of sound with the needed resources to allow an implant to be used to its greatest potential. This book seeks to identify those areas that require our continued attention, and to encourage development of innovative strategies for improving outcomes for individuals with cochlear implants.

Introduction

John K. Niparko

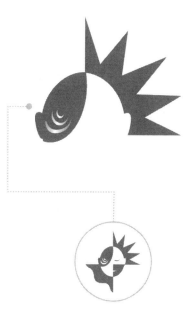

Throughout history, mankind has continually explored the possibilities of advancing the boundaries of communication. Celebrated historical events have marked attempts to bridge the gaps that exist between us. The development of language became a vital key that bonded people together. The Egyptians developed the first written communication in the form of a complex language of hieroglyphics. With this form of communication came the concepts of governance and edicts—concepts that enabled people to combine their efforts to achieve new heights. The Phoenicians developed the first alphabet, a powerful tool that facilitated lines of communication and commerce. In ancient Greece, the spoken word was elevated to a new art. Philosophers debated, and the theater was born. Later, all roads—North, South, East, and West—led to Rome. People, animals, and goods were not the only passengers; the roads became the fastest highways of information to that time. Over the ensuing centuries, Monks copied words

J. K. Niparko: Department of Otolaryngology—Head and Neck Surgery, The Listening Center at Johns Hopkins, The Johns Hopkins University, Baltimore, Maryland 21205-1809.

of wisdom, eventually giving way to the printing press with movable type. Ideas spread, and knowledge flourished. On the waves of digital circuitry and satellite communications of this century have come powerful ways of connecting with each other. The tools of communication continue to revolutionize the world.

This book examines the biology and technology that underlie one of the 20th century's most consequential developments in communication—the cochlear implant. The evolution of the cochlear implant is monumental for several reasons. Cochlear implants represent one of many innovative technologies that enable the rapid transfer of processed information. A unique feature of implant technology, however, is that it represents an alliance of strategies that use both manufactured and natural neural circuits. In terms of numbers of devices placed, the implant represents the most successful attempt to date to interface a prosthetic device with the human nervous system. For individuals with advanced hearing loss, the cochlear implant offers a reliable treatment alternative. This was a population with few options beyond visual (*e.g.*, sign) and tactile (*e.g.*, vibrotactile) modalities of communication before the 1970s. For many such patients, the cochlear implant has become the alternative of choice. In the 1990s, rates of cochlear implantation have increased by approximately 25% per year, and as of early 1999, more than 25,000 individuals had received a cochlear implant worldwide.

Understanding the process of cochlear implantation requires an appreciation of the intricacies of sensory function. The senses provide members of the animal kingdom with the ability to detect and interpret dynamic qualities of their environment. Aristotle asserted that human perception was rooted in the senses of touch, hearing, sight, taste, and smell; the ability to sense posture, balance, motion, pain, hunger, heat, and thirst are special senses. Each of these senses relies on receptor cells that are activated by the presence of a stimulus, with unique linkages to the brain.

The stimuli that we can perceive assumes a vast array of forms, and to be efficient, receptors are uniquely specialized to detect only a particular stimulus. The auditory pathway is composed of receptors and a preassigned neural pathway to sense and encode environmental and voiced sounds. Cochlear hair cells are unmatched in their ability to transduce the minute levels of vibratory energy in sound waves. Moreover, the process of transducing sound occurs during an extremely short time, and the signal is processed through a rich network of pathways in the central nervous system. This degree of specialization has served the evolution of humans well.

In Chapter 1, Brad May describes the physiology of hearing. The sense of hearing relies on a highly active circuit between receptors and neural pathways that effectively divides the labor of detecting, discriminating, storing, and retrieving an enormous range of acoustic signals. A network of integrated pathways links receptors within the ear to the brain to enable appreciation of the acoustic stimuli that comprise voiced and environmental sounds. Simulating the wide range and the complexity of the physiologic mechanisms of encoding sound represent substan-

tial obstacles. Biotechnology such as a cochlear implant that is used to simulate hearing must offer effective strategies that allow sound-based information to flow rapidly and faithfully.

In Chapter 2, David Ryugo, Charles Limb, and Beth Redd examine how changes in sensory input can manifest a range of modifications of the nervous system, from the whole pathways down to the subcellular level. Their review emphasizes that sensory experience throughout life activates and reinforces specific neural connections and may be required for the proper interactions between neurons, particularly those that subserve learning and memory. The plasticity required for neuronal systems to remain modifiable implies that sensory input can influence neuronal interactions. For example, strategies of encoding complex sound are presumably strengthened by experience. Continued exposure to selected acoustic patterns reinforces neural connections that encode speech features critical to comprehension of the spoken word. This process of neural reinforcement lends emphasis and salience to relevant acoustic cues over irrelevant, nonspeech sounds.

An important concept in sensory plasticity concerns periods when neuronal pathways are more susceptible to modification. Although some degree of malleability may exist within some pathways throughout life, other neuronal pathways require activity during periods when intrinsic neuronal factors dictate high degrees of responsivity for shaping connections.

The critical period hypothesis holds that neuronal modifiability in some pathways is subject to an early period of great sensitivity that is followed by a steady decline. Why do critical periods exist? Evolutionary explanations suggest that periods of modifiability exist to further highly specialized learning capabilities that are often specific to a given species. The critical period hypothesis is a focus for discussions of the early and specialized learning requirements for language acquisition. Plasticity may also be a characteristic of highly active circuits that carry high metabolic requirements, wherein plastic changes in neural connections may serve to balance metabolic budgets. The basic equation is simple: maintaining the sensory and regulatory machinery needed for plasticity has energetic costs, and plasticity is most economically applied to active systems under development. The basic logic of plasticity and critical period theory is compelling and underscores their relevance to intervention in deafness.

Just as cochlear hair cells represent the key point of reception in natural hearing, auditory nerve fibers form the basis for implant-mediated sound access. Probably because of their high degree of differentiation and their exquisite sensitivity, cochlear hair cells represent the most vulnerable of the structural links of the auditory pathway. Their damage and loss accounts for more than 85% of hearing loss and an even higher percentage of cases of functional deafness. Without hair cells, the synaptic activity that is normally triggered in auditory nerve fibers is lost, rendering the auditory periphery inactive. Despite this inactivity, nerve fibers with retained excitability remain in the auditory nerve. Along with Matthew Ng and George Nager, we describe patterns of nerve fiber distribution in the disorders that most commonly produce severe sensorineural hearing loss in Chapter 3.

Auditory nerve fibers are linked to a central pathway and to synaptic stations that maintain the structural features and functional capability of encoding complex patterns of activation. However, the work of Jean Moore and others described in Chapter 4 reminds us that because plasticity is reactive, it may produce maladaptive, as well as adaptive consequences. Consequently, not all individuals with profound deafness may have the same central apparatus, and patterns of degeneration may be more pronounced in cases of long-standing, early-onset deafness.

In addition to considering the biologic principles, this book examines the technol-

ogy that underlies cochlear implantation. We describe the strategies represented by the hardware and the processing strategies used in clinical devices. In Chapter 5, we trace the chronologic development of the cochlear implant. This historical record underscores the fact that numerous approaches to deafness have been advanced over centuries. The number of approaches attests to the challenge inherent in prosthetic alternatives to deafness.

The uniqueness of cochlear implantation is underscored by the distinctly different strategies of eliciting sound percepts relative to other strategies of auditory rehabilitation. For example, hearing aids filter, amplify, and compress the acoustic signal, delivering the processed signal to the ear for analysis and encoding. Cochlear implants receive, process, and transmit acoustic information by generating electrical fields. Electrode contacts implanted within the cochlea bypass nonfunctional cochlear transducers and directly depolarize auditory nerve fibers. Implant systems convey a further-processed electrical code that is based in those features of speech that are critical to phoneme and word understanding in normal listeners.

As Blake Wilson describes in Chapters 6 and 7, advances in microcircuitry have translated into new designs of cochlear implants. Acoustic signals can now be coded to convey information about the speech signal with dramatically faster and more flexible delivery of the electrical stimulus. Many technologic improvements in cochlear implantation mirror those associated with the development of information technologies in general.

The device approval process in the United States is recognized as the world's most stringent. Blind alleys may be encountered in getting a device to the marketplace. To the extent that harm and, more likely, no benefit are avoided, blind alleys are unavoidable in device development. After its initial manufacture, a device must endure premarket testing to satisfy requirements of safety and benefits. The device undergoes phases of human clinical trials in which it is tested to ascertain efficacy and reliability. If the findings are encouraging, the manufacturer assembles its data and files with the U.S. Food and Drug Administration (FDA). In Chapter 6, Harry Sauberman provides a comprehensive description of the approval process, underscoring the importance of communication among manufacturer, the clinician, the patient, and the FDA in ensuring a device's safety and efficacy for the marketplace.

We describe the numerous factors that influence outcome with an implant in Chapter 8. In some candidates, there is a risk of no or, more likely, limited capacity to comprehend the complex information contained in the speech signal. Patient and family understanding and expectations of cochlear implantation are likely to affect the perceived level of satisfaction with a cochlear implant. With clinical experience, however, has come recognition of the factors that help to predict the approximate gains in spoken communication. For properly selected candidates, the benefits of cochlear implantation are clearly recognized. Separate Consensus Conferences sponsored by the National Institutes of Health in 1988 and 1995 (NIH Consensus Statements of 1988 and 1995) concluded as much. Both conferences recommended that, given the success that had been observed, relaxed criteria for implant candidacy should be considered. Nonetheless, implant teams have an important responsibility to evaluate whether candidacy criteria are met and whether expectations are in line with the likely results. This determination requires a detailed understanding of a patient's otologic, audiologic, and psychosocial history before implantation is performed. Betty Schopmeyer discusses criteria for implantation and the role of the implant team in evaluating candidacy in this section.

Cochlear implantation is not without risks. There is potential morbidity inherent in the surgical exposure, the placement of a prosthesis, and wearing a prosthetic device in conducting the activities of daily living. The cochlear implantation procedure itself represents a composite dissection of the mastoid, facial recess, and cochlea, as well as placement of a prosthetic device using methods that ensure longevity through stability and avoidance of infection. The procedure is performed within close tolerances between neural and bony structures and major blood vessels. At virtually every step of the procedure, the need for exposure must be balanced with preservation of a critical nearby structure. Fortunately, the complication rate with this procedure is extremely low. In Chapter 9, Debara Tucci describes the concerted effort made by otologists to extend microsurgical techniques to their fullest potential in performing cochlear implantation.

What can a cochlear implant provide to a recipient? In Chapter 10, Karen Kirk provides information needed to understand implantation results and the challenges associated with measuring the effects of cochlear implantation. If the recent past serves as an indicator, many of the results attainable today will seem antiquated within 2 to 3 years. Accordingly, Dr. Kirk presents basic strategies in the clinical evaluation of results. Pooling of results across the many studies of cochlear implants potentially provides a broader perspective of the cochlear implant on large populations. André Cheng explores the insights and pitfalls inherent in such an approach in this section. Complex sound appreciation can be used to understand speech and listen to music. Charles Limb explores this aspect of implant listening in this section.

Restored hearing contributes to perceptual capabilities that can extend beyond speech recognition. We have examined the effects of cochlear implantation across domains and described what the introduction of sound means to those affected by deafness and to their families. Studies identifying quality of life changes in implanted children and adults have been well reported. Further assessment of the development of language competence in spoken and written forms, academic achievement, psychologic adjustment, and vocational achievement in individuals with implants is important for informing policy decisions related to cochlear implantation. Increasingly, measures of results are extended to assessment of practical, everyday experience such as schooling and employment and perceived effects on quality of life. These measures of outcome are discussed by André Cheng and Howard Francis in Chapter 11.

One of the most remarkable aspects of normal language acquisition in children is its fluid quality—most individuals are unaware of the crucial role of the listening process. The listener, immersed in the proper environments, enters almost unknowingly into the experience of learning language, rendering it an intuitive journey. Can hearing provided by a cochlear implant provide the exposure to language needed to develop linguistic competence naturally? In development and in maturity, there is an interplay between intrinsic and environmental cues in which the former specifies the general blueprint for neural circuitry and the latter sculpts refinements. This interplay is subject to a narrowing of developmental potential over time, although differentiation may continue well into adulthood. Nancy Mellon examines this interplay as it relates to hearing and language acquisition in Chapter 12, recognizing that the implant is one link in a chain that connects an array of cognitive and social processes.

Amy Robbins discusses the broad range of issues relevant to rehabilitation after implantation in Chapter 13. A cochlear implant produces a fundamental change in the perceptual experience of the recipient. Coping with this change through postimplantation rehabilitation can be important for some adult implant recipients, but it is critical for children to optimize the usefulness of an implant. The reasons for this are not always intuitive. It is often assumed that effective listening and language comprehension directly result from the sensitive hearing provided by an implant. However, hearing is not a sufficient condition for these higher skills. There is an increasingly a compelling rationale for a high priority to be placed on

postimplantation rehabilitation, particularly when the period of auditory deprivation has been lengthy. Equally compelling is the need for the professionals in related fields to comprehend the principles and practice of cochlear implantation to optimize outcomes.

The postactivation rehabilitative phases of cochlear implantation constitute an important subdiscipline of auditory rehabilitation. Whereas cochlear implant teams once comprised audiologists and otologists, they now routinely include psychologists, educators, rehabilitation therapists, speech-language pathologists, and developmental specialists from related fields such as neurology, pediatrics, and physical therapy. The evolution of the implant team mirrors the changing needs of this patient population and the greater appreciation of the services needed to nurture core capabilities after an implant is placed.

Effective cochlear implant rehabilitation is developed on the basis of the communication needs of the individual and the specific strategies needed to motivate a child or adult to develop auditory skills. Mary Koch provides practical suggestions for engaging an implant recipient in the listening process in this section.

The cultural impact of cochlear implantation is widely recognized. Controversy related to cochlear implants is further evidence that technology has had a profound effect on many established cultures; the high-velocity crisscross of development can be simultaneously exciting and bewildering. Cultural arguments surrounding cochlear implantation remind us that communication style is a very public behavior that carries with it a large personal stake in establishing identity. As noted by the linguist Leonard Bloomfield, an individual's response to language often involves deep-seated emotions that flare when one dares to question a basic view of language. Arguments over the linguistic implications of cochlear implantation can serve a useful purpose in informing approaches taken by clinicians and implant candidates, particularly by those with early-onset deafness. The passion that accompanies cultural arguments places a bright light on the validity of evidence presented on both sides of the issue. Nancy Mellon and I examine several concepts relevant to these discussions in Chapter 14. A true argument presents evidence for or against a proposition, and it is capable of being objectively tested by means that are agreed on. This requires common ground not yet found.

Cultural arguments also remind us that, although understanding the technologic innovation is key to understanding the effects of cochlear implantation, the story of cochlear implants emerges as a very human one. The potential for further development of cochlear implants is strongly motivated by many of mankind's most basic needs.

There is nothing quite like having someone say that he or she understands, that you have reached and affected them. . . . It is the feeling early humans must have experienced when the firelight first overcame the darkness of the cave. It is our need to know we are not alone.

—*Virginia Hamilton*

Cochlear Implants: Principles & Practices, edited by John K. Niparko, Karen Iler Kirk, Nancy K. Mellon, Amy McConkey Robbins, Debara L. Tucci, and Blake S. Wilson. Lippincott Williams & Wilkins, Philadelphia © 2000.

The Neurobiology of Hearing and Deafness

1

Auditory Physiology and Perception

Bradford J. May

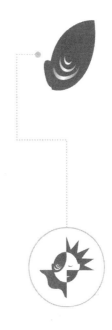

Auditory processing begins when an acoustic stimulus arrives at the external ear and is conducted by structures in the middle ear to the sensory organ in the inner ear, or cochlea. Within the cochlea, sound energy is transformed into a train of impulses in the auditory nerve, which carries a neural representation of acoustic events to the brain. Frequency tuning, dynamic range of function, and the cochlear nonlinearity that is known as two-tone suppression combine to create faithful representations of the spectral and temporal components of a sound as conveyed within the discharge rates of auditory nerve fibers.

As the representation ascends through the major auditory stations in the central nervous system, neurons with unique processing specializations work in parallel to extract biologically important acoustic information:

- Who made the sound?
- Where is it coming from?
- What does it mean?

This chapter explains the major properties

of auditory coding using data obtained with simple tones and the more natural steady-state vowels of human speech. Concluding remarks discuss how the representation of speech breaks down with sensorineural hearing loss (SNHL).

WHAT IS SOUND?

Sound is a pressure wave that is conducted to our ears by vibrations in the air that surrounds us. The remote movement of an object, perhaps the oscillations of a tuning fork, applies forces to nearby air molecules, which impact their neighboring molecules (Fig. 1.1). Although individual molecules suffer only small transient displacements, the resulting series of collisions can transmit the pressure wave over great distances.

Because the tuning fork resonates with a simple sinusoidal motion, the physical attributes that define its sound are straightforward. The frequency of the tone represents the rate at which individual molecules are first pushed forward and then pulled backward by the oscillations of the tuning fork. The intensity of the sound wave is determined by the magnitude of these displacements. In combination, frequency and intensity determine the velocity of movement for

B. J. May: Center for Hearing and Balance, Department of Otolaryngology—Head and Neck Surgery, The Johns Hopkins University, Baltimore, Maryland 21205.

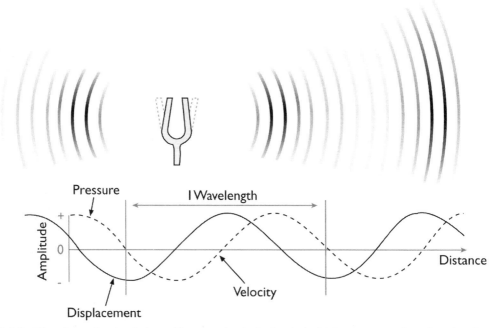

FIG. 1.1. Waveform of a simple tone. Movements of a tuning fork displace surrounding air molecules. The resulting sound pressure wave is usually characterized by its pressure (heard as loudness) and its frequency (heard as pitch). These properties of sound are determined by the magnitude of molecular displacements and how rapidly the tuning fork cycles though each series of sinusoidal movements. (Adapted from Pickles, 1988, with permission.)

air molecules. This velocity is not constant throughout the cycle of stimulus; rather, the molecules achieve their highest rate of movement near the midpoint of each positive and negative displacement and slow to a instantaneous velocity of zero as they reverse direction on reaching the point of maximum displacements. The velocity of air molecules is related to the pressure of a sound wave. Because direct measurement of molecular motions is not a simple task, the magnitude of a sound is usually described in units of sound pressure (dB SPL), which can be conveniently determined with microphones.

The levels of energy in natural sounds are distributed across a range frequencies and change with time. The spectral (pitch) and temporal (intermittency and duration) properties of this distribution are critical to the perceptual impact of complex acoustic signals. The vowels of human speech, like the amplitude spectrum shown in Fig. 1.2, are common natural stimuli in neurophysiologic experiments because they are spectrally complex but also steady state; the spectral shape of a vowel does not vary over the time course of stimulation. In contrast, the consonants of speech show dynamic changes in spectrum making it slightly harder to relate patterns of action potentials to specific stimulus features. Nevertheless, neural representations of consonants are fundamentally the same in principle as those for steady-state vowels.

A steady-state vowel has a discrete spectrum that can be approximated by a series of harmonically related tones. Relatively high levels of energy are seen in restricted frequency regions of the vowel's amplitude spectrum. These so-called formant peaks change in frequency to produce other vowel sounds and thereby impart meaning in the context of human language. The spacing of tones in the

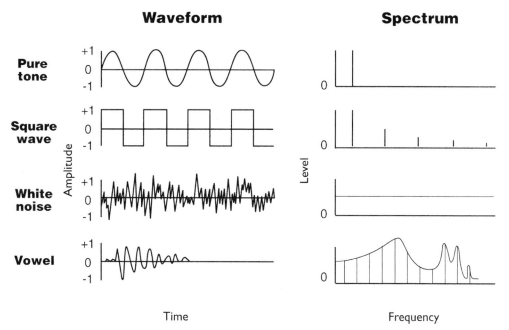

FIG. 1.2. Time waveforms and amplitude spectra of some complex sounds. White noise has a continuous spectrum, whereas the other sounds are composed of discrete frequencies. (Adapted from Pickles, 1988, with permission.)

vowel spectrum is related to the fundamental frequency of the harmonic series.

To understand these details from the perspective of normal speech production, the fundamental frequency of the vowel is created by the oscillations of the vocal folds as air is forced out of the glottis. The heavy vocal folds of a man move at relatively low fundamental frequencies, producing a low-voice pitch and close harmonic spacing in the speech spectrum; the lighter folds of a woman or child produce a higher pitch and widely separated harmonic spacing. Formant frequencies reflect resonances in the vocal tract that can be altered by movements of the tongue and lips to produce different vowels.

THE OUTER EAR: COLLECTING THE SOUND WAVE

The major anatomic features of the human ear are shown in Fig. 1.3. The structural framework of the outer ear is a complex system of cartilage. There are two major functional consequences of this system. The broad parabolic surface of the outer ear and its inherent resonances enhance auditory sensitivity by collecting and directing sound energy toward the relatively small surface of the ear drum. The effective pressure wave that reaches the ear drum may be amplified by as much as 20 dB at frequencies that are critical to human speech. The intricate convolutions of the outer ear create additional cavities with resonances that are capable of influencing sounds with much higher frequencies. These resonances produce directional filtering effects that can sharply increase or decrease the magnitude of frequency components within a complex sound, depending on the spatial location of the sound source. The resulting spectral cues are essential for the precise localization of sounds in space.

THE MIDDLE EAR: BRINGING SOUND TO THE COCHLEA

Although sound pressure waves are conducted to our ears by the movement of air

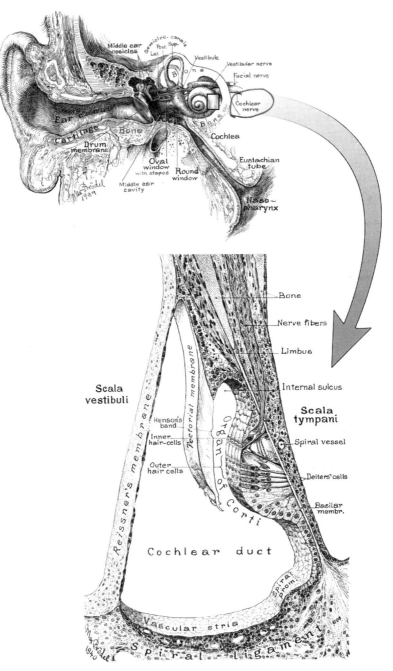

FIG. 1.3. Gross anatomy of the outer, middle, and inner ear. The cochlear duct (scala media) is shown in an enlarged cross-sectional view *(bottom)*. The organ of Corti contains the sensory hair cells that transduce sound energy to neural discharges in the auditory nerve. (Courtesy of Max Brödel Archives, The Johns Hopkins School of Medicine, Baltimore, MD.)

molecules, our perception of sound depends on the movement of fluids in the inner ear. Because cochlear fluids are less compressible than air, the same forces that set air molecules in motion can exert smaller displacements in a fluid medium. If the airborne pressure wave impinged directly on the cochlea, most of the energy would bounce off the fluid boundary. Instead, the auditory system has evolved an intricate impedance matching system in the middle ear.

Sound enters the middle ear space as a vibration of the ear drum and is conducted to the oval window of the inner ear by the ossicular bones that bridge the ear drum with fluids of the cochlea. The malleus (hammer) contacts the ear drum, the incus (anvil) serves as the intermediary, and the stapes (stirrup) inserts into the oval window of the cochlea.

Two major factors in the physical dimensions of the middle ear structures facilitate the change from an air-conducted sound wave to fluid movements. Of greatest importance, the surface area of the ear drum is large relative to that of the oval window membrane, and the pressure transmitted to the cochlear fluids is therefore greater. Because the long process of the malleus is longer than the incus, a movement of the ear drum produces a shorter but more forceful displacement of the stapes. Conductive hearing loss reflects a failure at some point in this sequence of impedance matching that can decrease auditory sensitivity by as much as 60 dB.

THE INNER EAR: TRANSFORMING SOUND TO A NEURAL CODE

The inner ear is a coiled spiral that contains three fluid-filled compartments: the scala vestibuli, scala media, and the scala tympani. Specialized ionic pumps in the highly vascularized stria vascularis concentrate levels of positively charged potassium ions in the endolymphatic fluids that fill the scala media. In contrast, perilymph in the scala vestibuli and scala tympani has a low potassium concentration that resembles the levels in normal extracellular fluids.

The auditory receptor cells, known as hair cells because their apical ends are covered with hairlike stereocilia, are arrayed along the organ of Corti within the scala media. The human ear contains about 15,000 hair cells at birth, but these numbers decline steadily with advancing age. The electrical potential of the hair cells is determined by the ionic environment in which they reside. The ciliary tufts on the apical ends of the cells contact the overlying tectorial membrane and are bathed in the potassium-enriched endolymph of the scala media. The bodies of the hair cells are situated on the basilar membrane in perilymph.

When a pressure wave propagates along the cochlear duct, the basilar membrane is set in motion relative to the tectorial membrane, and a sheering force is applied to the stereocilia. With each cycle of upward and downward movement of the basilar membrane, the ciliary tufts are splayed apart and then forced together. The tips of individual stereocilia are connected by microscopic filaments known as tip links. Convincing evidence has accumulated to suggest that the splaying of the tuft during movements of the basilar membrane stretches these links to open ion channels in the stereocilia. When potassium ions in the endolymphatic space pour through the channels, the hair cells are depolarized and release glutamate. Auditory nerve fibers innervating the depolarized hair cells respond to the release of excitatory neurotransmitter by firing action potentials. Because the receptor potential is established by the large reservoir of potassium ions in the scala media and modulated by the direct mechanical effects of the sound pressure wave, the peripheral auditory system can respond remarkably well to rapid fluctuations of sound pressure.

The basilar membrane changes in mass and stiffness along the cochlear partition. In the base of the cochlea, the membrane is relatively light and stiff as it stretches across the narrow gap between the bony processes of the internal modiolus and the outer cochlear wall. In the apex of the cochlea, the membrane becomes less stiff and heavier to accommodate the wide separation between its attachments to bone. This progressive change in mass and stiffness is similar to the strings of a musical instrument. When plucked by the musician's hand, heavy strings resonant at low frequencies and light, tight strings sound at high frequencies. Similar mechanical resonances can be observed in the response of the basilar membrane to acoustic stimulation. Low-frequency sounds exert their largest effects on the heavy apical portions of the membrane, and high-frequency sounds produce maximal displacements along the stiff basal membrane. The mechanical resonances that create this travelling wave phenomenon are sharply tuned so that at low sound pressure levels only a small portion of the membrane vibrates in response to a tone of a given frequency. The one-to-one mapping of stimulus frequencies to cochlear locations is known as tonotopy.

Major differences in structure and function are associated with the location of the auditory hair cells along the basilar membrane. The innermost row of hair cells, known as the inner hair cells, have flask-shaped cell bodies that are tightly joined to the surrounding supporting cells. Because these cells are innervated by the auditory nerve fibers, they are presumed to play the principal role in the conduction of sound information to the brain. Arrayed along the opposite side of the tunnel of Corti are three rows of outer hair cells. Although these rod-shaped cells are attached at base and apex to the basilar and tectorial membranes, their lateral walls are essentially free standing. An unusual physiologic property of the outer hair cells is that application of electrical currents can cause the cells to change in length. It has been hypothesized that the electromotile responses of outer hair cells can increase cochlear sensitivity and frequency tuning by applying energy to the traveling wave at a stimulus-dependent time and location along the basilar membrane. The importance of an active cochlear mechanism is supported by the elevated thresholds and poor frequency selectivity that follows the outer hair cell damage of loud sounds or ototoxic drugs.

AUDITORY NERVE: THE BRAIN'S INPUT

When auditory physiologists use the term auditory nerve, they are referring to the bundle of nerve fibers that connect the cochlea to the auditory brainstem. The auditory nerve is easily visualized by slight retraction of the cerebellum and has been the subject of extensive electrophysiologic investigation for several decades. The cell bodies that give rise to auditory nerve fibers can be found in the spiral ganglion of the cochlea.

The human cochlea contains approximately 30,000 spiral ganglion cells. Most of these neurons send peripheral projections to the base of a single nearby inner hair cell, with each inner hair cell receiving afferent terminals from about 10 spiral ganglion cells. These neurons are known as type I spiral ganglion cells. The remaining 5% to 10% of the spiral ganglion cells do not contact inner hair cells. These so-called type II neurons instead radiate across the tunnel of Corti and form synaptic contacts with several outer hair cells. In addition to the obvious differences in the site and manner of peripheral termination, type I spiral ganglion cells have large cell bodies and thick myelinated processes, whereas thin unmyelinated processes are characteristic features of the smaller type II neurons. The central processes of the spiral ganglion cells exit the cochlea by way of the internal auditory meatus and terminate in the cochlear nucleus of the central nervous system. Because it is extremely difficult to impale thin fibers with micropipette electrodes, our current understanding of auditory nerve physiology has been derived exclusively from studies of type I fibers. The functional role of the type II neurons remains one of the mysteries of cochlear physiology.

The basic response properties of two representative auditory nerve fibers are summarized in Fig. 1.4. The tuning curves in Fig.1.4A indicate the neurons' sensitivity to different tone frequencies. The stimulus intensity at each test frequency was adjusted to determine the sound pressure level at threshold, as defined as the level that consistently elicited a discharge rate 1 spike per second above spontaneous activity. Notice that the criterion for threshold is met at relatively low stimulus levels when 2-kHz tones are used as stimuli for one fiber and 8-kHz tones for the other. The sharp tips of the tuning curves identify these frequencies as each fiber's most sensitive frequency, or best frequency (BF). Presumably, one fiber is driven by an inner hair cell in an apical cochlear location where the basilar membrane resonance is tuned to 2 kHz; the other fiber innervates a more basal hair cell.

For both fibers, a tone must contain more energy to establish the threshold response as the test frequency moves from the BF. This filtering effect is particularly evident in the steeply sloped upper frequency limit of the tuning curves. When the auditory system is stimulated with a spectrally complex vowel sound, these fibers continue to respond preferentially to energy near their respective BFs. A large population of auditory nerve fibers arrayed along the basilar membrane and therefore tuned to different frequencies can be said to perform a frequency-to-place mapping of the vowel's complete energy spectrum.

The rate-level functions in Fig.1.4B plot the discharge rates of the representative auditory nerve fibers in relation to different levels of BF tone bursts. The lower left-most components of the resulting S-shaped functions reflect levels of spontaneous activity because the fibers are not responding at subthreshold tone levels. There is an upward transition of the functions at intermediate stimulus levels where changes in tone level produce concomitant changes in discharge rate. The lower limit of this transition is threshold; the upper limit represents the point at which the fibers' discharge rates reach saturation. The fibers cannot respond

to further increases in stimulus level with higher rates after they reach saturation; one stimulus level corresponds to one discharge rate only in the transitional component of the rate-level function. Because this unambiguous one-to-one relationship is the basis of neural representations that rely on discharge rates to encode auditory information, the dynamic range of rate encoding is implicit in the shape of the rate-level function. A function that rises more sharply than the response curves in Fig. 1.4B has a reduced dynamic range because the transition from threshold to saturation occurs over a narrow range of stimulus levels. A function with minimal slope provides a poor representation of the sound pressure level at BF because large differences in stimulus level produce small changes in discharge rate.

The synaptic contacts between inner hair cells and auditory nerve fibers are exclusively excitatory; however, the auditory nerve discharge rates evoked by one tone can be reduced by the simultaneous presentation of a second tone with different frequency. This cochlear nonlinearity resembles inhibition but is more correctly referred to as two-tone suppression. The filled regions flanking the excitatory tuning curves in Fig. 1.4A circumscribe the range of frequencies and levels that suppress the responsiveness of the representative fibers to BF tones. Although two-tone suppression was first described in the auditory nerve, subsequent experiments have demonstrated the phenomenon in inner hair cell receptor potentials and basilar membrane mechanics. The early site of this nonlinearity predicts a pervasive influence on auditory response patterns; virtually every auditory nerve fiber shows suppression effects when tested under appropriate stimulus conditions. These conditions are not restricted to two-tone paradigms. Sounds that contain many frequency components also produce suppression effects, and these nonlinearities have profound implications for the neural encoding of stimuli with prominent spectral features like vowels.

The most extensively studied form of com-

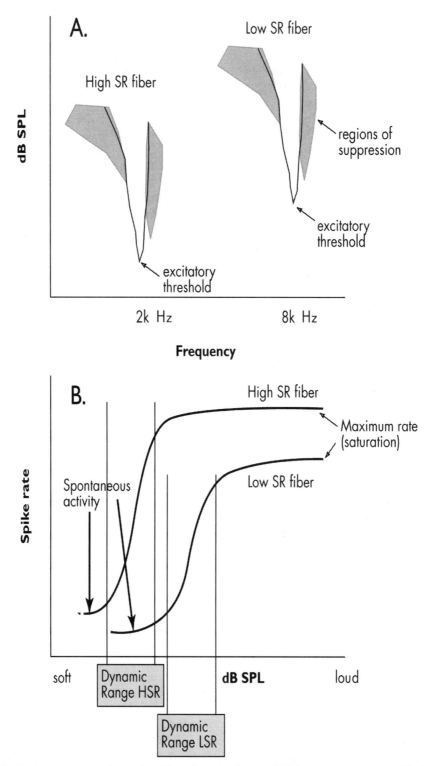

FIG. 1.4. Tuning curves and rate-level functions for low and high spontaneous rate (SR) auditory nerve fibers; the best frequencies are 2 And 8 kHz. In the idealized frequency tuning curves **(A)** and rate-level functions **(B)** for two auditory nerve fibers, the shaded regions surrounding the tuning curves indicate the combinations of frequency and level that suppress the fibers' excitatory responses. Vertical lines crossing the rate-level functions mark the range of stimulus levels that are unambiguously encoded by changes in the fibers' discharge rates (*i.e.*, the dynamic range of the excitatory response). Fibers with high spontaneous rates *(left)* tend to show lower excitatory thresholds, less suppression, and smaller dynamic ranges than fibers with low spontaneous rates *(right)*.

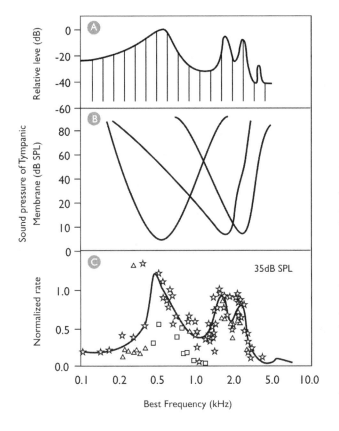

FIG. 1.5. Representation of vowels by the discharge rates of auditory nerve fibers. **A:** Formant structure of the vowel ε shows energy peaks at formant frequencies. **B:** Tuning curves of fibers with best frequencies near the vowel's major formant frequencies. **C:** The average population response of the auditory nerve exhibits maximum rates among fibers with best frequencies (BF) near formant features in the vowel's amplitude spectrum *(line)*. Each symbol is the response of one fiber plotted at its BF; different symbol types are used to distinguish fibers with high *(star)*, medium *(triangle)*, and low *(box)* spontaneous rates. (Adapted from Sachs *et al.*, 1988, with permission.)

plex sound representation is based on the distribution of vowel-driven discharge rates across a population of auditory nerve fibers. Peaks of activity within the neural population correspond to peaks of energy within vowels. The amplitude spectrum of the vowel ε [as in bet] is shown in Fig. 1.5A. Notice the relatively high levels of energy at the formant frequencies (512, 1792, and 2432 Hz) and the deep spectral trough that separates adjacent formant peaks. The frequency tuning curves of three auditory nerve fibers are plotted in Fig. 1.5B. Because the BFs of the fibers correspond to the formant frequencies where the vowel shows maximum energy, these neurons are likely to exhibit strong responses to a vowel sound. The vowel-driven discharge rates for a large sample of fibers are shown in Fig. 1.5C.

The magnitude of the rate response is ex-

pressed in terms of normalized rates, for which a normalized rate of 1 is equal to the fiber's maximum driven rate and a normalized rate of 0 indicates spontaneous activity. As expected, fibers that are tuned to the formant frequencies show high normalized rates, and fibers with BFs near spectral troughs have weaker responses. When other vowel sounds are produced by altering the frequency of formant peaks, differences in formant structure are reflected by changes in the distribution of fibers showing maximum discharge rates within the array of auditory nerve fibers.

The auditory nerve conducts a relatively homogeneous pattern of sound-driven activity to the cochlear nucleus; nevertheless, individual fibers vary in threshold, dynamic range, and sensitivity to suppression. These differences are strongly correlated with

spontaneous activity; the tendency to produce action potentials without sound stimulation. For this reason, spontaneous rate is
the most common method for classification
of responses in the auditory nerve. As shown
in Fig. 1.4, the fiber with a low spontaneous
rate (<1 spontaneous spike per second) has
a high threshold, large dynamic range, and
substantial suppression effects; the opposite
pattern of sensitivity, tuning, and nonlinearity is observed for the fiber with high spontaneous rate (>18 spikes per second). In Fig.
1.5C, the normalized rates of low versus high
spontaneous rate fibers are indicated by
squares and stars, respectively. Responses
for a third class of fibers with intermediate
(medium) spontaneous rates are marked
with triangles. The line in Fig. 1.5C follows
the moving average of the normalized discharge rates of the low-threshold, high–
spontaneous rate fibers. Rate differences
among this class of auditory nerve fibers provide an excellent representation of the vowel's formant frequencies at quiet vowel
levels.

A major limitation for auditory representations that are based on discharge rates is
the inability of any one class of auditory

nerve fibers to encode stimulus levels over
the extraordinary range of human hearing.
This dynamic range problem can be visualized by returning to the rate-level functions
in Fig. 1.4B. Consider a vowel level that corresponds perfectly to the dynamic range of
the representative high spontaneous rate fiber. The lowest trough feature would contain
energy near the fiber's threshold; the first
formant peak would exist near the saturation
point. The full dynamic range of the fiber's
discharge rates could be used to encode the
shape of the vowel's amplitude spectrum.
These ideal conditions are approximated
when high spontaneous rate fibers are tested
with quiet vowels, as shown in Fig. 1.5C.

In contrast, many of the fibers with low
and medium spontaneous rates are weakly
driven under the same stimulus conditions.
This lack of response also can be understood
by examining the rate-level functions in Fig.
1.4B. Many features in the amplitude spectrum of a quiet vowel are likely to fall on
the flat subthreshold component of the rate-
level function for low spontaneous rate fibers
because these neurons have relatively high
thresholds. Without the requisite modulation of discharge rates by spectral peaks and

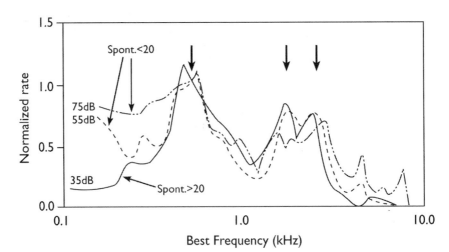

FIG. 1.6. Selective listening: effects of vowel level on the average rate profiles of auditory nerve fibers. Fibers with high spontaneous rates provide a good representation of the vowel's formant structure at low levels (35 dB), whereas the low spontaneous rate fibers encode the vowel at higher levels (55 and 75 dB). (Adapted from Sachs et al., 1988, with permission.)

troughs, the resulting rate profile cannot encode formant structure. Dynamic range limitations also pose problems when the amplitude spectrum of a loud vowel falls above the saturation point of the high spontaneous rate fibers. These stimulus conditions yield a featureless rate profile because formant peaks and troughs are capable of eliciting maximum driven rates (*i.e.*, normalized rates near 1). Nevertheless, as shown in Fig. 1.6, the less sensitive low– and medium–spontaneous rate fibers do convey an adequate representation at high vowel levels. Moreover, the rate-place representation changes very little as the stimulus level increases from 55 to 75 dB SPL, because because high levels of energy in the formant peaks suppress, or reduce, the normalized rates elicited by spectral troughs.

COCHLEAR NUCLEUS: ESTABLISHING CHANNELS OF INFORMATION PROCESSING

Auditory nerve fibers project from the cochlea to the auditory brain stem, where they form obligatory terminations on the principal cells of the cochlear nucleus. Synaptic specializations involving the nature of auditory nerve inputs and the descending inputs from both ears and a rich intrinsic innervation create diverse cell types in the cochlear nucleus that are uniquely sensitive to particular features of sound stimuli. Higher centers must rely on this system of parallel processing to communicate the information-bearing elements of acoustic stimuli because auditory nerve fibers do not project beyond the cochlear nucleus.

The major nuclei in the ascending auditory pathway are shown in Fig. 1.7. The three major subdivisions of the cochlear nucleus are the anteroventral cochlear nucleus (AVCN), the posteroventral cochlear nucleus (PVCN), and the dorsal cochlear nucleus (DCN). The auditory nerve bifurcates soon after reaching the brain stem sending an ascending branch to the AVCN and a descending branch to the PVCN and DCN. The terminations of afferent fibers within each subdivision recreates the orderly tonotopic organization of the organ of Corti. The principal neurons within each subdivision can be classified according to their characteristic morphology and response patterns.

Cell types in the cochlear nucleus with different response properties suggest a variety of functional roles. For example, DCN neurons show strong inhibitory interactions that allow them to encode sharp spectral features. Such features are introduced by the directionally dependent filtering effects of the head and outer ear, and it is likely that the DCN plays an important role in sound localization. However, PVCN neurons respond strongly to the onset of acoustic stimuli, and it has been hypothesized that this fast conduction pathway contributes to acoustic startle reflexes. The encoding of speech has been studied most extensively in the AVCN, and this section examines the structure and function of neurons found there.

The two basic synaptic configurations of auditory nerve inputs to the AVCN are shown in Fig. 1.8. Bushy cells, so named because of the bush-like appearance of their stunted dendritic arborization, are located in the anterior portion of the nucleus. The cell bodies of these second-order neurons are practically engulfed by enormous synaptic contacts with auditory nerve fibers. These synaptic specializations (*i.e.*, endbulbs of Held) ensure a strong link between action potentials of a small number of auditory nerve fibers and the cochlear nucleus neuron. In light of this synaptic morphology, it is not surprising that bushy cells show patterns of responses that are nearly identical to those of their auditory nerve inputs. Because auditory nerve fibers are the primary afferents of the auditory system, the response patterns of bushy cells are called primarylike. It has been hypothesized that primarylike neurons in the cochlear nucleus maintain the precise timing of discharge rates in the peripheral auditory system. In support of this interpretation, anatomic studies have traced the pro-

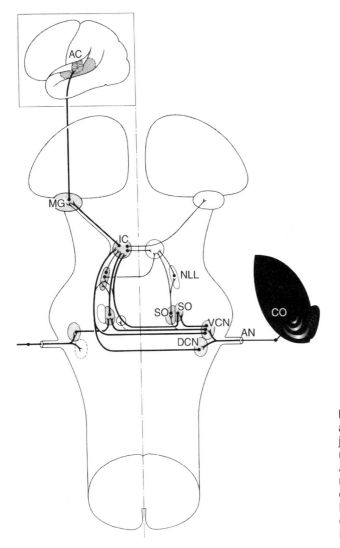

FIG. 1.7. The diagram of the central auditory system summarizes the major ascending projections from the right ear to the left auditory cortex. AC, auditory cortex; AN, auditory nerve; CO, cochlea; DCN, dorsal cochlea nucleus; IC, inferior collicolus; MG, medial geniculate; NLL, nucleus of lateral lemniscus; SO, superior olive; VCN, ventral cochlear nucleus.

jections of AVCN bushy cells to the superior olive, which is believed to be an important site of binaural temporal processing in the central auditory system (for stimuli that are perceived by both ears). Binaural temporal cues are essential for the accurate localization of low-frequency sounds and the perception of pitch.

Stellate cells can be found throughout the more posterior regions of the AVCN. These multipolar cells have elaborate dendritic fields compared with bushy cells and receive extensive auditory nerve inputs on dendrites and cell bodies through conventional bouton synapses. When recording from stellate cells, electrophysiologists have noticed their regular discharge patterns, which have been called chopper responses. The weak inputs from a single auditory nerve fiber are not likely to drive a chopper unit into a state of activity; rather, these neurons require the convergence of many inputs. Temporal information is lost by this process of neural integration, but there can be a substantial

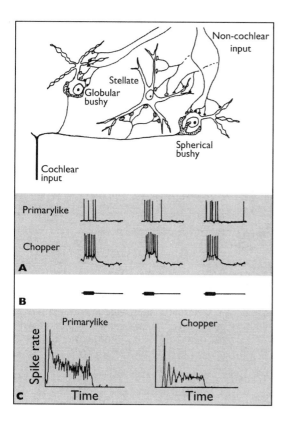

FIG. 1.8. Neural response types in the anteroventral cochlear nucleus. Bushy cells and stellate cells receive different patterns of cochlear input *(top)*. **A:** Sparse auditory nerve projections to bushy cells create irregular trains of actions potentials that are similar to those seen in the auditory nerve (primarylike responses), and the highly convergent cochlear inputs to stellate cells produce regularly timed activity (chopper responses). **B:** Peristimulus time histograms (PSTHs) display average spike rates during the stimulus presentation. Notice the multimodal "chopping" PSTH that is associated with stellate cells. (Adapted from Sachs and Blackburn, 1991, with permission.)

increase in the resolution of stimulus levels that are encoded by the neuron's discharge rates.

It has been suggested that chopper units expand their dynamic range limits by "selective listening" to the inputs of the low-threshold, high–spontaneous rate auditory nerve fibers at low stimulus levels and to the high-threshold, low–spontaneous rate fibers at high stimulus levels. The major dynamic range differences between AVCN primarylike and chopper units are evident in the effects of stimulus level on the quality of their vowel representations.

Representative rate profiles for the two unit types are shown in Fig. 1.9. To produce this figure, the vowel-driven responses for a population of primarylike neurons have been segregated according to spontaneous rate and averaged. The resulting rate profiles show the same dynamic range limitations as auditory nerve fibers. Primarylike neurons with high spontaneous rates encode the formant structure of the vowel at low levels, but saturation effects degrade such representation at high levels. Primarylike neurons with low spontaneous rates fail to respond to low levels of stimulation, but excellent peak-to-trough rate differences are observed at high vowel levels. The best representation of the vowel is provided by chopper units. These neurons show good sensitivity, high rates of firing before saturation, and strong suppression effects; as a result, an excellent representation of the vowel's formant peaks is observed across a wide range of stimulus levels.

ASCENDING AUDITORY PATHWAY

Projection neurons exit the cochlear nucleus by distinct pathways and terminate in different target structures. The axons of pyramidal cells in the dorsal cochlear nucleus enter the dorsal acoustic stria and project to the con-

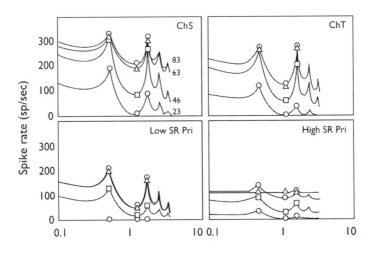

FIG. 1.9. Effects of level on the vowel representations of cochlear nucleus neurons. Stellate cells in the anteroventral cochlear nucleus can be classified as sustained choppers (ChS) or transient choppers (ChT) based on their temporal properties. Bushy cells can be separated into low and high spontaneous rate (SR) categories. Across most stimulus levels and in the presence of background noise, the best vowel representations in the cochlear nucleus are provided by chopper neurons and the poorest representations by primarylike (Pri) units with high rates of spontaneous activity. (Adapted from May *et al.*, 1998, with permission.)

tralateral inferior colliculus (IC). Octopus cells in the posteroventral cochlear nucleus ascend to the contralateral nucleus of the lateral lemniscus by way of the intermediate acoustic stria. Bushy cells in the anteroventral cochlear nucleus send axons to the superior olivary complex on both sides of the brain stem. Stellate cells project to the contralateral IC. The anatomy and physiology of the central auditory pathway beyond the cochlear nucleus is intricate and complex. This section summarizes some major projections and their presumed functional roles.

Bipolar neurons in the medial superior olive (MSO) receive bilateral excitatory inputs from spherical bushy cells in the AVCN. The tight synaptic coupling in this pathway suggests that MSO neurons are specialized for the processing of binaural time differences. These temporal cues for sound localization are created by the relative time of arrival of a sound pressure wave at the two ears. If a sound emanates from a source outside the

median plane that bisects the head, it arrives at one ear before the other. Neurons in the MSO are exquisitely sensitive to binaural time differences and presumably enhance the localization of low-frequency tones or complex sounds with low-frequency temporal features. These contributions to directional hearing are suggested in the tonotopic organization of the nucleus, which shows a strong bias toward low frequencies. The MSO may be entirely absent in species such as the hedgehog and some bats that are unable to process binaural temporal disparities.

Neurons in the lateral superior olive (LSO) receive excitatory inputs from spherical bushy cells in the ipsilateral AVCN and inhibitory inputs from principal cells of the ipsilateral medial nucleus of the trapezoid body (MNTB). The major ascending projection to the MNTB is an excitatory input from globular bushy cells in the contralateral AVCN; the large calyceal synaptic coupling in this projection is reminiscent of the end bulbs of Held that connect spiral ganglion cells to bushy cells. The combination of direct excitatory and indirect inhibitory projections from the cochlear nuclei establish a sensitivity to differences in level between ears among LSO neurons. If a sound is louder in one ear than the other, the response of LSO neurons on that side of the brain are dominated by their ipsilateral excitatory inputs. LSO neurons in the contralateral brain stem are inhibited.

The binaural analysis performed by the LSO is critical for localization at high frequencies, which are strongly attenuated by the sound shadow of the head when sound sources are located outside the median plane. In contrast to the MSO, the tonotopic organization of the LSO is biased toward high frequencies.

Most of the primary nuclei of the central auditory system exhibit a central core structure that is composed of ascending afferent projections that input information and a surrounding belt of descending efferent projections that provide outgoing relays. The periolivary belt around the MSO and LSO is the source of the olivocochlear bundle, which is an efferent projection linking the auditory brain stem to the cochlea. Within the cochlea, these efferent neurons terminate on the peripheral processes of spiral ganglion cells and the outer hair cells. The principal neurotransmitter of the olivocochlear bundle is acetylcholine, and outer hair cell potentials can be altered by the effects of acetylcholine on membrane conductances. Presumably, by changing the potassium conductances of the outer hair cells, olivocochlear efferents can regulate the active mechanical properties of the basilar membrane. These processes are necessary to maintain the sharp frequency tuning and sensitivity of the inner hair cells. When the olivocochlear bundle is destroyed by surgical manipulation, the discrimination of speech sounds is compromised in the presence of background noise. It also has been shown that olivocochlear feedback can play an organizing role in the developing auditory system and protect the cochlea from acoustic injury.

The IC receives convergent inputs from virtually all of the ascending and descending auditory pathways. The central nucleus at the core of the IC receives afferent projections from stellate and pyramidal cells in the contralateral cochlear nucleus, bilateral projections from neurons in the MSO and LSO, and inputs from the nuclei of the lateral lemniscus. Synaptic domains can be identified within the central nucleus, where these diverse sources of input are segregated or mixed in different combinations.

Little is known about how the IC integrates its multiple sources of input. The basic response properties of neurons in the central nucleus are similar to those of cell types found in other nuclei of the auditory brain stem and appear to reflect direct monosynaptic inputs from the cochlear nucleus, MSO, and LSO. Pharmacologic agents do not alter these fundamental properties, but overall levels of neural activity can change dramatically when neurotransmitters are manipulated in the IC. These results suggest that the nucleus may serve as a mechanism for gating levels of input to higher auditory centers.

The medial geniculate body (MGB) of the thalamus is an obligatory synaptic relay for all afferent inputs to the auditory cortex. The most dense ascending projection to the MGB originates in the the central nucleus of the ipsilateral IC. Although the cellular organization of the MGB is complex and has been the subject of several classification systems, it is well established that the ventral division of the MGB serves as the major thalamocortical relay carrying information from IC to primary auditory cortex. The systematic physiologic characterization of the MGB is limited in comparison to other auditory structures because of its particular sensitivity to the effects of anesthesia.

Some of the most detailed electrophysiologic studies have been performed on unanesthetized bats, and it has been shown that neurons in the belt areas of the MGB respond selectively to the spectral temporal combinations of bat sonar signals. Similar response patterns may contribute to the auditory processing of communication signals, such as human speech.

The major auditory cortical fields are located on the temporal lobe of the cerebral cortex (Fig. 1.10). In most primate species, including humans, auditory cortex is buried deep within the sylvian fissure. Primary audi-

tory cortex, or area A1, forms the central core of the auditory field. Physiologic responses in area A1 show a mapping of high to low frequencies as the site of recording moves from posterior to anterior locations. The tonotopic organization of A1 is presumed to arise from the mechanical tuning of the cochlea; however, the essentially one-dimensional cochlear frequency map is transformed into a two-dimensional cortical field.

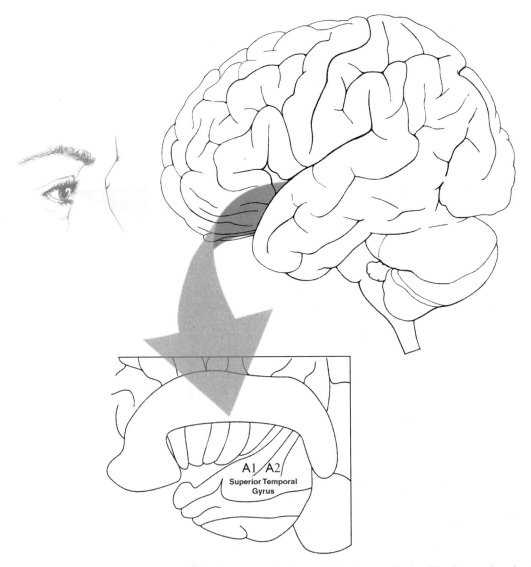

FIG. 1.10. Auditory fields on the superior temporal gyrus of the human brain. The lower view is obtained by retracting the temporal lobe and looking down on the brain from above. A1, primary auditory cortex; A2, secondary auditory cortex. (Adapted from Webster, 1992, with permission.)

The more complex topography of auditory cortex has led to the speculation that other stimulus dimensions may be mapped at right angles to the frequency axis. For example, the laterality of the dominant excitatory ear, sharpness of frequency tuning, and a selective sensitivity to spectral shapes that emphasize high or low frequencies have all been found to change in an organized manner along the orthogonal axis. This topographic organization suggests that neurons in different cortical regions may serve as feature extractors for specific combinations of the acoustic elements that form biologically significant sounds.

Systematic parametric analyses have not supported this interpretation; instead, it appears that cortical neurons play a more generalized role in the auditory processing of sounds with spectral and temporal complexity. Acoustic patterns of this nature are important in vocal communication, but effective stimuli are not necessarily limited to biologic signals.

Pioneering neurosurgeons such as Broca, Wernicke, and Penfield were the first to identify regions for language comprehension and speech production in the secondary cortical fields surrounding area A1. These early clinical investigators inferred functional localization by relating perceptual deficits, or aphasias, to the sites of cortical injury or electrical stimulation during brain surgery. Modern noninvasive research methods such as otoacoustic emissions, positron emission tomography (PET scans), and evoked auditory potentials allow scientists to map auditory function from cochlea to cortex in humans.

With each technologic advancement in our ability to image the functioning brain, our understanding of the centers that contribute to human language becomes increasing complex. For example, when physiologic and psychophysical measures of speech discrimination are performed simultaneously in human listeners, cortical areas that are usually linked to cognitive functions such as attention and emotion show stronger correlations with behavioral performances than tradi-

tional language centers. For this reason, most contemporary models of speech perception have been shaped by psychophysical phenomena and not by direct physiologic evidence.

SENSORINEURAL HEARING LOSS

The most common form of sensorineural deafness involves the loss of cochlear hair cells in the auditory periphery. Because the central auditory system remains functional, there is the potential to restore some percept of hearing by providing the brain with alternative forms of input. Assistive devices attempt to achieve this goal by transforming sounds into the range of residual hearing or, in the case of profound hearing loss, by direct stimulation of the auditory nerve with electrical currents.

A better understanding of the advantages and disadvantages of both clinical interventions can be gained by examination of the physiologic consequences of SNHL in animal models. Experimental studies of SNHL typically use loud sounds or ototoxic drugs to destroy hair cells. Outer hair cells and basal regions of the cochlea show a greater susceptibility to these insults creating a gradient of pathology along the cochlear partition. Regions with normal anatomic features make the transition to regions with partial deficits involving outer or inner hair cells, which give way to regions where the cochlea is devoid of hair cells. Although it is intuitively obvious that this topographically organized pattern of hair cell trauma can be used to infer the functional implications of structural changes in th damaged cochlea, early attempts to link structural changes with functional deficits found poor correlations between patterns of hair cell survival and hearing sensitivity. The stereocilia of surviving hair cells can exhibit a variety of morphologic changes that have profound implications on signal transduction.

The classic laboratory study of the ultrastructural basis of SNHL was published by Liberman and Dodds in 1984. These investigators combined electron micrographic analysis of hair cell stereocilia with electrophysiologic recording in the auditory nerve to identify four states of stereocilia damage and their effects on auditory processing. Conceptual models of their observations are depicted by the tuning curves shown in Fig. 1.11. Loss or disarray of inner hair cell stereocilia results in an elevation of the tips and tails of auditory nerve fiber tuning curves (left panels), but damage to the stereocilia of outer hair cells leads to decreased sensitivity at the tip of the tuning curve and a hypersensitive tail (right panels). All of the hypothetical examples in Fig. 1.11 are presumed to have a preexposure BF near 25 kHz; nevertheless, fibers that originate in cochlear regions with outer hair cell damage show maximum sensitivity to much lower frequencies after acoustic trauma. Changes in frequency

tuning disrupts the normal tonotopic organization of the auditory nerve representation for complex sounds.

Effects of acoustic trauma on the auditory nerve representation of a steady-state vowel are shown in Fig. 1.12. Different symbols identify the spontaneous discharge rates of individual fibers, but the average rate profile is computed across all fibers with similar BFs, regardless of spontaneous rate. This abeyance of the classification system is necessary because loud sound exposure changes spontaneous rates in the auditory nerve.

In contrast to Fig. 1.5, the rate profiles obtained from sound-exposed animals fail to show clearly defined peaks at the vowel's formant frequencies. Simple amplification strategies can compensate for this loss of sensitivity but do nothing to restore cochlear frequency selectivity. Notice how the poor

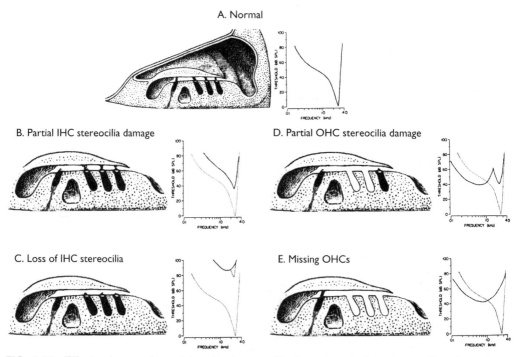

FIG. 1.11. Effects of sensorineural hearing loss on the frequency tuning curves of auditory nerve fibers. **A:** The normal complement of hair cells is shown in cross section with a representative frequency tuning curve. **B,C:** Loss of the inner hair cell (IHC) stereocilia leads to a loss of the sensitive tip of the tuning curve. **D,E:** Outer hair cell (OHC) losses create a broadly tuned response with increased low-frequency sensitivity. (Adapted from Liberman and Dodds, 1984, with permission.)

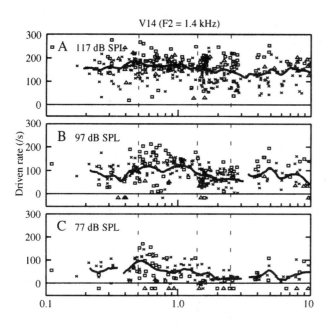

FIG. 1.12. Effects of sensorineural hearing loss on vowel representations of auditory nerve fibers. Average rate profiles *(lines)* fail to encode the formant structure of the vowel /ɛ/ even at very high levels of amplification (*e.g.*, 117 dB SPL). Plotting conventions are described in Fig. 1.5. (Adapted from Miller *et al.*, 1999; with permission.)

quality of the representation shows no improvement when the vowel is presented at highly amplified sound pressure levels.

Psychoacousticians have described the task of listening in real world environments as auditory scene analysis. Even quiet situations are likely to present a soundscape that is complex and pervasive: multiple conversations in a restaurant, the whirl of an overhead fan, and the clatter of plates all compete for the attention of a diner. Loud ambient noise levels and reverberant environments offer further impediments to effective communication. Perceptual studies have shown that listeners with normal auditory function segregate these competing sounds into meaningful streams of information by attending to the unique acoustic properties that identify the multiple sound sources. For example, speech sounds produced by a conversational partner may have a distinctive pitch and harmonic relation. Frequency and amplitude changes within the speech stream are correlated in time. They arrive from a specific direction. If the listener can observe movements of the speaker's mouth and lips, acoustic cues can be supplemented with visual

information. Specialized processing mechanisms at virtually all levels of the auditory system contribute to auditory scene analysis by enhancing the spectral, temporal, and spatial resolution of hearing.

Adaptive systems require functional inputs from the cochlea and can be disrupted by SNHL in the auditory periphery. As a result, communication in a noisy environment represents a serious challenge for the hearing impaired even when assistive devices operate satisfactorily under ideal listening conditions.

Advances in microprocessor technology have led to the development of hearing aids and cochlear implants that have the capacity to perform heretofore impossible feats of signal processing before sounds are delivered to the auditory system. Modern digital aids and multichannel implants can filter a complex sound into its multiband components and adaptively adjust the amplification in individual bands of the filter array. These processing algorithms have major implications for lessening loudness recruitment and sharpening the spectral features of speech sounds for better communication. Calling on designs that exist in the normal system, the deleterious effects of background noise can be reduced with directional binaural microphones and by processing strategies that use spectrotemporal correlations to separate signal from noise. Notwithstanding these remarkable achievements, the human brain remains the essential computational device for finding perceptual organization in auditory sensation; consequently, the designers of the next generation of hearing aids will continue to look to the normal physiologic function of the cochlea for processing strategies that use the full potential of human cognition.

SUGGESTED READINGS

Bregman AS. *Auditory scene analysis: the perceptual organization of sound.* Cambridge, MA: MIT Press, 1994.

Brugge JF. An overview of central auditory processing. In: Popper AN, Fay RR, eds. *The mammalian auditory pathway: neurophysiology.* New York: Springer-Verlag, 1992:1–33.

Liberman MC, Dodds LW. Single-neuron labeling and chronic cochlear pathology. III. Stereocilia damage and alterations of threshold tuning curves. *Hear Res* 1984;16:55–74.

Miller RL, Schilling JR, Franck KR, Young ED. Effects of acoustic trauma on the representation of the vowel ε in cat auditory nerve fibers. *J Acoust Soc Am* 1997; 101:3602–3616.

Moore BCJ. *An introduction to the psychology of hearing.* San Diego, CA: Academic Press, 1997.

Pickles JO. *An introduction to the physiology of hearing.* San Diego, CA: Academic Press, 1988.

Rosen S, Fourcin A. Frequency selectivity and the perception of speech. In: Moore BCJ, ed. *Frequency selectivity in hearing.* San Diego, CA: Academic Press, 1986.

Sachs MB. Neural coding of complex sounds: speech. *Annu Rev Physiol* 1984;46:261–273.

Suga N. Auditory neuroethology and speech processing: complex-sound processing by combination-sensitive neurons. In: Edelman GM, Gall WE, Cowan WM, eds. *Auditory function, neurobiological bases of hearing.* New York: Wiley, 1988:679–720.

Webster DB. An overview of mammalian auditory pathways with an emphasis on humans. In: Webster DB, Popper AN, Fay RR, eds. *The mammalian auditory pathway: neuroanatomy.* New York: Springer-Verlag, 1992:1–22.

Appendix 1A

Correlates Sensorineural Hearing Loss and Their Effect on Hearing Aid Use:
The Problem of Recruitment

Ginger D. Grant

Although the number of cochlear implants has grown significantly during the past decades, this number represents only a tiny fraction of devices used to assist those with sensorineural hearing loss (SNHL). Hearing aids continue to be the principal management tool to improve auditory access. Tech-

G. D. Grant: Department of Otolaryngology—Head and Neck Surgery, The Johns Hopkins Medical Institutes, Baltimore, Maryland 21205-1809.

nologic improvements in circuitry have led to advanced signal processing in smaller hearing aids. However, the impaired auditory system presents certain boundaries that limit use of even the most advanced hearing aids.

While SNHL usually manifests with reduced sensitivity, a common source of frustration relates to constrained dynamic ranges (Boothroyd, 1998). SNHL often affects perceived changes in intensity. A healthy auditory system normally provides a wide dynamic range for sound intensities. The normal range from detecting soft sounds to withstanding loud sounds is more than 100 dB. Within this dynamic range of hearing lies a narrower dynamic range for speech. Vocalizations span an intensity range from low-intensity, high-frequency consonant sounds to high-intensity, low-frequency vowel sounds. This range, approximating 30 dB, is easily represented in a healthy cochlea to provide access to the softest and loudest speech sounds.

SNHL imposes a reduced dynamic range by raising the threshold of audibility and by lowering the ceiling of tolerance to high-intensity sounds (Boothroyd, 1988). Boothroyd (1998) offers the following formula for predicting dynamic range based on the amount of hearing loss:

For losses below 60 dB:
$$\text{dynamic range} = (100 - \text{the loss})$$

For losses below 60 dB:
$$\text{dynamic range} = (70 - \text{half the loss})$$

Consider the following examples in calculating dynamic range for a moderate (50 dB) hearing loss and a severe (90 dB) hearing loss:

$$\text{Dynamic range} = (100 - 50)$$
$$= 50 \text{ dB dynamic range}$$
$$\text{Dynamic range} = (70 - 45)$$
$$= 25 \text{ dB dynamic range}$$

A more severe SNHL constrains the dynamic range. The result is an inadequate representation of soft and loud sounds and a phenomenon known as recruitment.

Recruitment is defined as an abnormal growth in loudness (Moore, 1991). It is perhaps one of the great ironies of SNHL. Although low-intensity sounds are inaudible, slight increases in intensity, even to threshold level, may cause sounds to become a source of physical discomfort. Re-

cruitment is typically more severe for those frequencies of hearing most impaired. Most often it is observed in the high frequencies, which carry critical information for speech understanding. For example, high-frequency consonant sounds such as *f*, *s*, *th*, and *p* are of low intensity. Providing adequate amplification to make these sounds audible can also make them uncomfortably loud and distorted. At average speaking levels, an individual with recruitment may ask a talker to speak more loudly, but with even a slight increase in vocal intensity the speech becomes uncomfortably loud.

The mechanism underlying recruitment is a change in patterns of response in auditory nerve fibers (Pickles, 1988). When a hearing loss occurs as a consequence of hair cell loss, the sharpness of the nerve fiber tuning curves is diminished (Fig. 1A.1). At the threshold level, only the tips are activated. As the intensity of the stimulus is raised the tails are reached quickly, and the number of nerve fibers that respond surges (Evans, 1975).

Hearing aids were once considered the only option for addressing the functional communication problems imposed by the loss of hearing sensitivity from SNHL. However, despite improved circuitry in modern hearing aid design, recruitment continues to challenge aural rehabilitation (Moore, 1991). Even the most advanced hearing aids cannot replicate the complex, nonlinear system of a healthy cochlea, much less compensate for the abnormal frequency and temporal resolution associated with a SNHL.

Amplification may provide sufficient power to compensate for the loss of sensitivity. Compression circuitry may limit the amount of amplification for loud sounds and increase the amount of amplification for soft sounds. However, loudness compression has a price in that important elements in the speech signal may be distorted by compression (Moore, 1990; Boothroyd, 1988). When a recruiting ear makes speech at conversational levels intolerable, a hear-

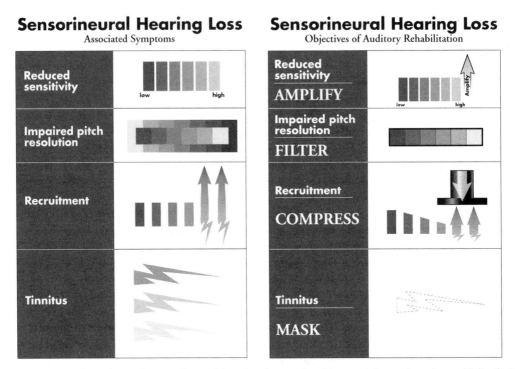

FIG. A1. Manifestations of sensorineural hearing loss extend beyond the reduced sensitivity that results from hair cell damage. Although simple amplification can address reduced sensitivity to sound, other symptoms can hamper effective rehabilitation. For example, impaired pitch resolution results in sound distortion because of impairment of hair cell responsiveness and efferent control of hair cell activity. Recruitment results from the abnormally rapid growth in the amount of activity of auditory fibers. Tinnitus is a phantom perception, often thought to be the result of the loss of supply of auditory inputs to the brain. Contemporary hearing aids amplify, filter sounds, and compress, the goal of which is to provide more amplification for low-level signals and to decrease the amplitude of high-level signals to compensate for recruitment. They mask tinnitus by supplying improved perception of environmental and speech sounds and promoting tinnitus adaptation. Hearing aids developed in the past decade use expanded frequency response characteristics to suppress high-level distortion and achieve faster and more effective means of compression.

ing aid is rendered useless for important speech sounds.

A cochlear implant directly activates the auditory nerve fibers in a manner that is limited by gain controls and avoids surges of neural activation and loudness recruitment characteristic of the impaired cochlea. Electrical hearing does not recruit. A primary consideration in the cochlear implant candidacy process is the measurement of benefit from hearing aids for speech understanding. Recruitment must be considered when evaluating this benefit. Although reproducible, measurement of benefit in a controlled environment, such as a sound-proof testing suite, provides little information about a patient's functional communication abilities. For patients who are unable to regularly wear hearing aids because of discomfort from loudness recruitment, cochlear implantation may provide greater receptive benefit.

REFERENCES

Boothroyd A, Springer N, Smith L, Schulman J. Amplitude compression and profound hearing loss. *J Speech Hear Res* 1998;31:362–376.

Evans EF. The sharpening of cochlear frequency selectivity in the normal and abnormal cochlea. *Audiology* 1975;14:419–442.

Moore B. Characterization and simulation of impaired hearing: Implications for hearing aid design. *Ear Hear* 1991;2:6[Suppl l]:154S–161S.

Moore B. How much do we gain by gain control in hearing aids? *Acta Otolaryngol Suppl* 1990;469: 250–156.

Pickles J. *An introduction to the physiology of hearing.* London: Academic Press, 1988.

Cochlear Implants: Principles & Practices, edited by John K. Niparko, Karen Iler Kirk, Nancy K. Mellon,
Amy McConkey Robbins, Debara L. Tucci, and Blake S. Wilson. Lippincott Williams & Wilkins, Philadelphia © 2000.

2

Brain Plasticity

The Impact of the Environment on the Brain as It Relates to Hearing and Deafness

David K. Ryugo, Charles J. Limb, and Elizabeth E. Redd

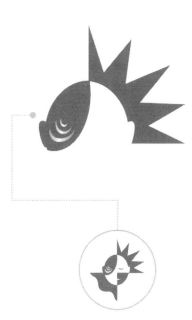

The brain is the organ of behavior. Perhaps the most important aspect of behavior is learning, defined as any change in behavior as a result of experience. Behavior is shaped by interactions between genetics and environment, and the relative influence of nature and nurture vary in ways yet to be determined. The environment can modify even the most stereotyped behavior, and all behavior is bound by genetic factors. Different behaviors depend on separate classes of nerve cells having specialized functions with highly organized and specific interconnections between them. The brain forms the physical substrate for our ability to hear, which is involved in the acquisition of language and social communication, the localization of sounds in space, and the appreciation of music. Changes in brain function

mediate changes in behavior, and vice versa. In this chapter, we discuss the malleability or plasticity of these mutually dependent functions, focusing on factors that underlie the brain mechanisms of hearing.

The brain is constantly changing throughout our lives. The adult brain is composed of approximately 100 billion nerve cells, with characteristic gyri and sulci where certain functions can be attributed to certain locations.

- How do neural cells acquire their specific identities, and how do they form their patterns of neural connections?

These daunting questions are frequently asked because mammals, with all their complexity, arise embryologically from the merging of only two germ cells. The brain develops in an orderly progression of steps, with a precise temporal sequence that is characteristic for each neural entity and system. Moreover, individual neurons connect with only a selected subset of potential target neurons, and these connections are made only at specific regions along the surface of the target cell.

The total genetic information available to an animal, roughly 100,000 genes in mammals, is insufficient to specify on a one-to-one

D. K. Ryugo: Center for Hearing and Balance Sciences, Department of Otolaryngology—Head & Neck Surgery, The Johns Hopkins University, Baltimore, Maryland 21205.

C. J. Limb: Department of Otolaryngology—Head & Neck Surgery, The Johns Hopkins University, Baltimore, Maryland 21205.

E. E. Redd: Department of Otolaryngology—Head & Neck Surgery, The Johns Hopkins University, Baltimore, Maryland 21205.

basis the total number of neural connections that are made in the brain, estimated to be about 10^{15}. To accommodate this mismatch, the nervous system relies on environmental triggers to activate different subsets of genes at specific times during development. The orchestration of these environmental signals with the normal time course of brain development controls neural differentiation. The external environment provides nutritive factors, sensory and social experiences, and learning. These internal and external signals impinge on the developing cell in the form of diffusible factors and surface molecules. In this way, a complex array of specific factors is timed to induce the proper differentiation of individual neurons. It is thought that brain cells continue to be produced until shortly after birth. In humans, after 2 to 3 years of age, new neurons are no longer generated, and all of the basic neural connections are thought to be completed by the late teenage years. The consequence is that most of the changes in brain function occur through modification of the wiring at the level of cells and molecules. Proper development and proper maintenance of the brain depend on an interactive balance between genetic makeup and environmental influences.

CRITICAL PERIODS
OF DEVELOPMENT

More than 100 years ago, it was reported that newly hatched chickens, as soon as they were able to walk, would follow any moving object (Spalding, 1873). This sight-guided behavior endowed the chick with no more disposition to follow a hen than to follow a duck or a human. When hatchlings were blinded by placing an opaque hood over their head, this indiscriminate following of the first object they saw endured for the first 3 to 3.5 days. At 4 days and later, however, the chicks exhibited the opposite response on unhooding and fled from the first object they encountered. The normal attachment of newborn chicks to their parents was called imprinting (Heinroth, 1911). The brief period during

which imprinting could occur was called the *critical period* in the life of the organism (Fig. 2.1).

The concept of a critical period has been applied to explain other phenomena that occur or are affected most severely during restricted time windows of development. These critical periods reinforce the notion that there are clearly defined times when the physiologic readiness of the organism must coincide with the occurrence of specific externally derived experiences. To understand the human brain, neuroscientists often study the brains of other mammals, such as rats or monkeys. With animal models, it is possible to examine experimentally the cellular mechanisms of sensory processing such as vision, touch, or hearing and motor functions such as spinal reflexes, paralysis, or recovery of function. Language, however, is a largely human characteristic, and the study of rats and monkeys provides little insight into its development or neural substrate. However, birds have a natural song, and although clearly different from human language, it is nevertheless a highly complex production derived from auditory-motor interactions and serves critical communication functions. Investigations of bird song have provided highly instructive examples of how genetic factors interact with the environment.

The song of the white crowned sparrow has a distinctive and elaborate acoustical pattern when learned in a natural environment. A male sparrow raised in social isolation develops an abnormal song. Birds deafened at birth produce an even more distorted song (Konishi, 1985). To mitigate the effects of social isolation on song development, the experimenter can play recorded songs to the isolated male. After 3 weeks of listening to 60 songs per day, the male develops a normal song. This result suggests that an auditory template of the natural song resides in the brain against which the bird's song is compared and that birds need to be able to hear themselves sing to perfect their song. A template must exist because, even when the bird is deafened, the resulting abnormal song is

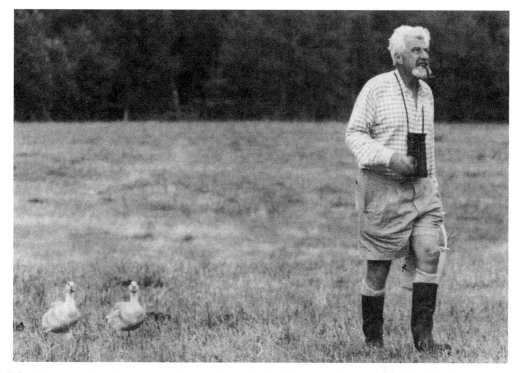

FIG. 2.1. Imprinting is a curious form of learning that is quick to develop and difficult to reverse. The best known and most illuminating example of imprinting comes from the pioneering experiment performed by ethologist Konrad Lorenz in Austria in 1935. He first divided a clutch of eggs laid by a single graylag goose into two groups. One group of hatched goslings was permitted to associate with their mother goose. A test group of goslings were hatched in an incubator, and the first living creature they saw was Lorenz. In the first few days of their lives, they were allowed to follow Lorenz as if he were their parent. Later, the goslings were marked according to their early post-hatching experience and placed together under a box. When released, the two groups separated from each other and sought their respective, adopted parent. (H. Karcher)

not random but has some crude resemblance to the normal song. Variations in the song that a young bird hears results in corresponding variations in the song produced. These variations are called dialects, such that groups of birds living only a few miles apart sing with distinctly different song patterns (Marler and Tamura, 1962). Heredity limits the effects that the environment can have and facilitates experienced-based learning.

The importance of auditory experience is crucial for vocal learning in songbirds. Young songbirds innately recognize and prefer to learn the songs of their own species. In fledgling white-crowned sparrows lacking song experience, it was revealed that songs composed of parts of the total song or songs played in reverse elicited behavioral responses as strongly as did normal song (Whaling *et al.*, 1997). In all cases, these responses surpassed those to other species songs. The discrimination by baby birds of songs of their species seems to parallel a process observed in human infants, who recognize individual phonemes common to their language before they learn words, phrases, and sentences (Kuhl, 1991; Goodsitt *et al.*, 1993). These studies lie at the heart of how the environment interacts with neural substrate and provide insight into aspects of brain function that support language learning in humans.

There have been reports on the lack of language development in humans reared in apparent social isolation or under adverse conditions. Perhaps the most noteworthy example concerns *Le Sauvage de l'Aveyron* (*The Wild Boy of Aveyron*), a report of a boy, 12 or 13 years old, captured by hunters in the southern part of France in the central Pyrenees Mountain range near Lourdes (Lane, 1976; Shattuck, 1980) (Fig. 2.2). This boy, later named Victor, seemed to be feral, living in the wild without clothes, social companions, or spoken language. He was initially thought to be deaf but was later shown to have highly developed sensory and motor skills but no aptitude for spoken language or other social skills.

Victor's story is important because of reports from his tutor of 5 years, Dr. J. M. G. Itard. Itard used his experience as an educa-tor of the handicapped to attempt to provide Victor with communication skills. Itard had developed novel strategies for teaching language to deaf and retarded individuals, and he advocated the use of sign language. Despite the success and international acclaim that Itard enjoyed as an educator for the hearing and mentally impaired, he was unable to help Victor develop language. The general inference from this and other similar cases is that spoken language cannot develop in a vacuum, whether from social isolation or deafness. Instances of social isolation are understandably infrequent, and considerably more data are available addressing language development in the deaf population. The main conclusion is that congenitally deaf individuals rarely acquire normal spoken language. Those who retain a certain measure of hearing and even those who lose hearing

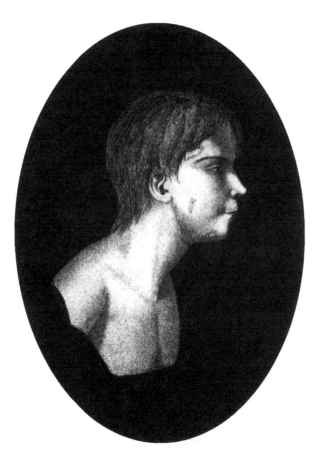

FIG. 2.2. Le Sauvage de l'Aveyron. This portrait shows the only surviving depiction of the savage of Aveyron, a boy approximately 12 to 13 years old who was found living alone in the wilderness of southern France. Although his exact origins remained a mystery, the boy, later named Victor, was believed to have spent his entire young life in isolation from civilization. Victor was unable to acquire any language skills despite exhaustive attempts to teach him how to speak. (Courtesy of Bibliothéque Nationale.)

shortly after birth often acquire functional levels of spoken language. Exposure to speech early in life, however brief, seems to be a necessary requirement for the acquisition of spoken language, and the longer the exposure, the better the outcome (Shattuck, 1980).

BRAIN PLASTICITY UNDERLIES BEHAVIORAL PLASTICITY

Behaviors, whether they are imprinting or language development, have their bases in modifications of brain function. Concepts of critical periods reflect brain processes. As we consider features of auditory plasticity that operate through critical periods, we naturally turn to the brain to understand the relevant mechanisms. Much of what we understand about brain plasticity is derived from experiments in nonauditory systems such as the visual and somatosensory systems. One example of the detrimental effects on the brain has been illustrated in the visual system, in which uncorrected amblyopia, myopia, or crossed-eyedness results in functional blindness in one eye.

In normal conditions, the two eyes function together so that the world appears as a single, unified whole even though it is seen with two separate eyes that project slightly different images on the two retinas. We perceive a single perspective because proper alignment of the eyes causes convergence of the separate images on corresponding loci of the retinas. The result of this convergence is called fusion. Even with normal convergence, fusion is not perfect for images that lie outside the focal plane of fixation. This small amount of noncorrespondence is called binocular disparity and is used by the visual system to perceive depth. The projection of the visual pathway from each eye through the lateral geniculate nucleus and up to layer IVc of visual cortex remains segregated and monocular. In the cortex, projections are organized into distinct but parallel stripes, where alternating stripes represent the inputs from each eye (Wiesel *et al.*, 1974).

These stripes are called ocular dominance columns (Fig. 2.3). Connections within and across these columns are thought to form the substrate for visual perception. Blocking input to the cortex from one eye during the first 6 months of age renders this deprived eye functionally blind. The result of the deprivation is that the projections from the deprived eye are atrophic (the ocular dominance stripes are abnormally thin) compared with the robust projections from the intact eye (their projections have characteristically expanded). The deprived eye loses its ability to activate cortical neurons, and visual perception from that eye is lost. If left uncorrected, this loss is permanent and irreversible.

These experimental conditions in animal models resemble monocular amblyopia, cross-eyedness, or monocular myopia in newborn infants. In such cases, it is hypothesized that the inability of the system to fuse the separate visual fields leads to a crisis in the cortex (Raviola and Wiesel, 1985). Both eyes are functioning, and both have robust projections into the cortex. Because the images are disparate, however, the brain selects the inputs from one eye and suppresses the inputs from the other so that a single image is achieved. Over time, the suppressed eye behaves as if it were blind. Visual stimuli to that eye can no longer activate cortical neurons (the eye loses its ocular dominance stripes), and no visual stimuli are perceived through that eye. Consistent with other developmental processes that involve a critical period, a similar visual deprivation in an adult has no effect on cortical responses to visual stimulation and no effect on visual perception (reviewed by LeVay *et al.*, 1981). These are the kinds of data that have guided the decision to correct surgically some forms of amblyopia as soon as it is detected in infants.

The blindness produced in the deprived eye is of central rather than peripheral origin. Consequently, even though the peripheral sensory structures may be intact, normal vision is impossible. These findings emphasize

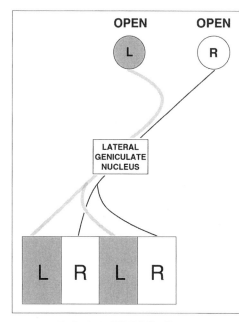
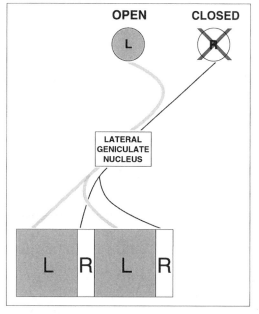

BOTH EYES OPEN   **RIGHT EYE CLOSED**

FIG. 2.3. Diagram of the effects of monocular deprivation on visual cortex development. **A:** Schematic representation of the visual pathway from the eye to the visual cortex illustrates the normal development of ocular dominance columns, as occurs when both eyes are left open during development. The gray circle represents the left (L) eye, and the open circle represents the right (R) eye. The gray and black lines represent afferent nerve fibers from the eyes that pass through the lateral geniculate nucleus of the thalamus and travel to the ocular dominance columns in primary visual cortex. As shown in the rectangles, the ocular dominance columns representing left and right eyes alternate with one another. Because both eyes are open in this case, the ocular dominance columns are equal in size. **B:** Schematic representation of the visual pathway in the case of a monkey raised under conditions of monocular deprivation. The X over the right eye represents forced eye closure during development. As a result of monocular deprivation, the ocular dominance columns from the closed eye fail to form properly, and they are abnormally thin. In contrast, the ocular dominance columns representing the left eye have expanded into the regions formerly activated by the right eye. These schemes illustrate the importance of sensory input for proper development of the brain.

the point that even a perfect sensory prosthesis can be inadequate if the central nervous system is not amenable to receiving and processing the specific sensory inputs. Moreover, the results of these studies highlight the crucial importance of environmental stimuli during periods of development. Further experiments by Wiesel and Hubel (1974) showed that the monkey was most vulnerable to monocular deprivation during the first 6 weeks of life. Because this early period represented the greatest susceptibility of the visual system to experimental manipulations, they applied the term *critical period* to de-

scribe this aspect of visual development. The effects of monocular deprivation were less severe if deprivation took place after the critical period, presumably because the brain and environment had already interacted sufficiently to establish the basic organization of the system. Such periods are often referred to as sensitive periods by other investigators to denote the time during which a system is most vulnerable to deprivation.

Central changes produced by sensory deprivation are not limited to the visual system. Unlike humans, rodents have whisking facial hairs called vibrissae through which a great deal of tactile information is received. Vibrissae differ from whiskers by virtue of the presence of striated muscle at the base of the vibrissa follicle that enables movement. Each vibrissa acts as an independent sensory structure, and a spatial map of the vibrissa pad is topologically represented in the somatosensory cortex by distinct cytoarchitectonic units known as barrels (Welker and Woolsey, 1974). The barrels are composed of organized accumulations of cells in layer IV that receive a correspondingly organized projection from the thalamus (Killackey, 1973). The barrel region of the somatosensory cortex undergoes an age-related differentiation from birth to maturity under normal conditions (Rice and Van der Loos, 1977). If, however, an individual vibrissa is selectively injured at birth, the barrel, which corresponds to that damaged vibrissa, fails to develop (Van der Loos and Woolsey, 1973) (Fig. 2.4). This effect has a relatively narrow time window, such that by 5 days after birth, vibrissae damage does not disrupt cortical organization (Weller and Johnson, 1975). Damage to vibrissae after the critical period produces no loss of cortical barrels. This disruption of cortical organization by vibrissae damage seems to be mediated at least in part by the thalamus because neonatal vibrissae removal results in a failure of thalamocortical barrel projections to form (Killackey *et al.*, 1976).

Because there are no identifiable barrels at birth in normal animals, these studies suggest that deprivation of vibrissae input at birth interrupts the process of morphogenesis. Resembling vision in monkeys, the developing cortical structures that process vibrissae input depend on proper functioning of the peripheral end organ during growth. If peripheral structures are damaged during the critical period, the brain fails to form normally, and subsequent modifications in peripheral structures cannot ameliorate the changes in the central nervous system. In the case of barrel cortex, the organizational loss is obvious, and the impact on cortical processing is expected

to be profound. The very matrix by which individual vibrissae maintain segregated information channels is lost.

COMPETITION AND THE PLURIPOTENT CORTEX

The studies described previously were seminal works that opened new lines of scientific investigation. The notion of neuronal competition was introduced and suggested that the function of a given region of the brain was not necessarily established at birth. Rather, neurons themselves were integral in determining what function they would eventually serve by virtue of the signals they carried. The idea of the pluripotent neuron, a cell whose function was unassigned and therefore plastic, raised fascinating possibilities regarding the brain.

Anatomic and physiologic methods were employed to extend the basic findings of ocular dominance. Using a monocular deprivation paradigm, the visual cortex of cats was studied by making injections of radioactive label into the eyes of visually deprived cats (Shatz and Stryker, 1978). These researchers saw a decrease in the number of geniculocortical afferents from the deprived eye and an increase in the number of such afferents from the nondeprived eye.

In addition to anatomic changes in the afferents serving the eyes, single unit microelectrode recordings from cortical neurons revealed that the nondeprived eye exclusively drove most of the cells in primary visual cortex. This finding is consistent with their anatomic data and suggests that early monocular deprivation of vision produces a visual cortex in which very few neurons represent the visual field of the deprived eye. The investigators postulated a physical reorganization of thalamocortical neurons to account for their observations. These studies provided experimental data to support the notion that regions of the cortex that would normally serve a particular function (*e.g.*, left eye vision) could be recruited for other uses if necessary. This work helped to refine the

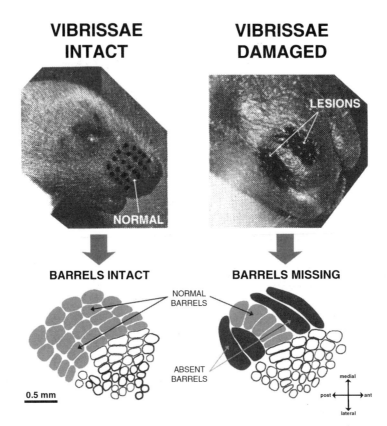

FIG. 2.4. The effects of damage to vibrissae (whiskers) on the development of barrels, the cortical structures that receive input from each mouse pup vibrissa; ink is placed on each vibrissa to help visualization. Below is a schematic diagram showing the somatosensory cortex with individual barrels (*gray ovals*) corresponding to the main mustacial vibrissae and other minor facial vibrissae (*open ovals*). There is a one-to-one relationship between vibrissae and barrels, and the cortical barrels are discrete and normally developed. The photograph shows a close-up of a mouse pup with lesions of selected vibrissae. The lesions are arranged in two parallel stripes, flanking a row of normal vibrissae. The cortical barrels corresponding to the damaged vibrissae fail to develop and appear to have merged together. These data emphasize the importance of the intact peripheral sensory structure on the normal development of cortical organization. (Adapted from ref. 16, with permission.)

idea of neuronal pluripotential, by showing specific, quantifiable alterations in brain anatomy and physiology in response to environmental manipulation.

These studies of visual deprivation suggest that competition and pluripotency are closely related phenomena, but the full extent of the brain's malleability still remains to be determined. Deafferentation experiments helped to define exactly how cortical areas evolve to serve their designated functions (Roe *et al.*, 1990). In neonatal ferrets, the investigators ablated the normal target of retinal neurons by surgical lesions of the superior colliculus (with subsequent degeneration of the lateral geniculate nucleus, a visual synaptic station) and blocked the normal input to primary auditory cortex by selective transections of ascending auditory fibers to the medial geniculate nucleus (a higher auditory synaptic station). These lesions removed auditory fibers as a source of competition for retinal fibers in the medial geniculate nucleus while also eliminating the normal recipient of retinal information. As a result of these lesions, retinal axons successfully invaded the medial geniculate nucleus, and the medial geniculate nucleus projected to auditory cortex representing a two-dimensional map of visual space, not the expected acoustic representation of frequency (Roe *et al.*, 1990).

This dramatic change in cortical topography, such that auditory cortex begins to function as visual cortex, reveals that a single, immature cortical area is capable of supporting different types of sensory maps. The final fate of any cortical region may be mediated in part by the type and nature of its inputs. Although the space map in the auditory cortex exhibited some variability in receptive field location, the two-dimensional visual map was fairly accurate, showing that the responsiveness of the auditory neurons to visual stimuli was not random or useless but instead produced a functional visual cortex. The cortex may be modular in design, with its function depending on the particular inputs it receives.

GENETIC FACTORS: PREPROGRAMMED DEVELOPMENT

Interaction between genomic and environmental factors is responsible for normal development, and the studies described have illustrated dramatic effects from selective loss of environmental stimuli. Although the conditions under which an animal is raised have pervasive effects, these effects are constrained by genetic determinants. For example, a terrestrial mammal raised under avian conditions is unlikely to learn to fly as a result. In experiments of binocular deprivation, cats were raised under two contrasting conditions with both eyes open or closed. The cortical maps for orientation and ocular dominance developed normally for the first 3 weeks of life regardless of the conditions (Crair *et al.*, 1998). In fact, early pattern vision had no effect on the formation of cortical maps during this period, a finding that suggests the existence of a strong and definite

program that dictates initial development. These experiments also showed that central changes from sensory deprivation took place only after this initial period of development. The critical period of ocular dominance development may therefore begin after a brief initial period of environmental insensitivity.

EFFECTS OF EARLY EXPERIENCES ON ADULT BEHAVIOR AND ADAPTATION

Although sensory deprivation is a useful paradigm for the study of plasticity, such conditions are somewhat extreme. A more subtle but equally relevant issue focuses on the effects that juvenile experience has on mature behavior.

- Do different methods of upbringing affect the ability to adapt to new situations in adulthood?

The barn owl provides an animal model in which sound localization ability is extraordinarily sophisticated. Barn owls can locate a mouse in complete darkness using sound cues alone (Payne, 1971). The remarkable localization ability of the barn owl has provided the basis for an interesting series of experiments (Knudsen, 1998). Prisms were placed over the eyes of young barn owls, such that vision was offset by a fixed number of degrees in a given direction. As a consequence of prism placement, a discrepancy was created between the auditory and visual cues received by the owl. The prisms remained on the eyes of young owls until the animals had learned to adjust for the auditory-visual discrepancy. After removal of prisms, these owls were in time able to adjust and correctly localize sounds. If, however, prisms were placed over the eyes of adult owls, only those owls with juvenile prism experience were able to adapt. Owls without prior experience were unable to adjust their auditory map to the new changes in visual input and could not accurately localize sounds.

The conclusion from these studies is that

juvenile experience has a significant effect on adult plasticity and that the information learned as a young animal can be selectively applied as an adult when required. An adult that has had experiences while young appears to be able to use the early functional connections with relative ease. An adult without prior experience finds adaptation largely beyond the capacity of his or her brain.

ANIMAL MODELS OF DEAFNESS

We have learned from animal studies of the visual system that peripheral lesions produce central nervous system changes. Similar changes occur in the central auditory system under conditions of deafness. Several animal models have been examined in studies aimed at characterizing the anatomic changes found in deafness and the molecular mechanisms that underlie these changes. There are many studies of peripheral deafening induced by experimental manipulation, including cochlear ablation, acoustic trauma, and application of ototoxic agents. Other studies of deafness have examined naturally occurring models of deafness, such as the congenitally deaf white cat and various strains of deaf mice.

The cochlea contains the sensory epithelium that transduces acoustic information and sends it to the brain in the form of electrical signals through the auditory nerve. Studies have shown a close relationship between peripheral sensory structures and the central nervous structures that receive inputs from them. The cochlear nucleus provides the first interface between peripheral and central auditory system and is the initial site of central processing of auditory signals within the brain. Deafferentation of the auditory system produces significant changes in the structure and function of the central auditory pathways. After unilateral cochlear aspiration in 6-day-old mice, 39 days later there was a 46% overall reduction in size of the cochlear nucleus and a 34% decrease in overall number of neurons (Trune, 1982). Co-

chlear ablation in gerbils also shows an age-dependent response, emphasizing vulnerability to peripheral cochlear ablation (measured by changes in neuron number and size in the anteroventral cochlear nucleus). The effect on the cochlear nucleus was most pronounced in the first week of life, even before the onset of hearing or cochlear functionality (Hashisaki and Rubel, 1989). Ablations in older animals resulted in less drastic effects (Powell and Erulkar, 1962). The main conclusions from these kinds of data is that the developing brain is significantly more vulnerable to sensory deprivation compared with the mature brain and that, regardless of age, the longer the duration of sensory deprivation, the greater was the degree of degenerative changes.

Similar kinds of results were obtained by ablating the basilar papilla of newborn chickens, illustrating the much more severe effects of neonatal manipulations compared with those in adults (Born and Rubel, 1985). Deafferentation before 6 weeks of age caused a 25% to 30% decrease in neuron number and 10% to 20% decrease in ipsilateral cell size. Deafferentation at 66 weeks of age, however, produced a less than 10% decrease in neuron number and no change in cell size. These studies addressed the idea of a critical period in the auditory system and suggested that early sensory ablation produced marked central changes in the auditory brain stem that were minimized if ablation occurred at a later age.

Cochlear removal has age-dependent functional consequences (Moore et al., 1993). The investigators studied the response of neurons in the inferior colliculus and superior colliculus of the ferret to unilateral cochlear removal. They showed that the age at which cochlear ablation occurred (postnatal day 5 versus postnatal day 40) affected the responses seen, with earlier deafferentation producing lower thresholds and broader dynamic responsivity. Superior colliculus neurons showed a volume-dependent response to acoustic stimuli presented to the intact ear, with loud sounds producing broader spatial tuning in animals subjected to early deafferentation. These results support the notion that physiologic properties of auditory neurons in the brain stem are also susceptible to cochlear ablation, and the age-graded nature of the influences implicates a critical period of heightened vulnerability.

These studies employed cochlear ablation as the method of inducing sensory deprivation, but the results must be interpreted with caution. Cochlear ablation produces other changes in the developing organism, including disruption of the blood supply, direct damage to spiral ganglion neurons, and traction on auditory nerve axons. It is therefore difficult to isolate the specific cause for the changes observed in the cochlear nucleus. One study addressed the issue of whether activity in particular was responsible for the central changes seen in cochlear ablation (Sie and Rubel, 1992). These researchers applied tetrodotoxin, a sodium channel blocker, to the perilymph of developing gerbils and compared their findings to cochlear ablation. Analysis of protein synthesis (measured by change in incorporation of tritiated leucine) and cell size revealed that similar transneuronal changes occurred in both experimental groups, although the time course of the changes differed somewhat. These data suggest that the blockade of activity alone is sufficient to produce the central changes seen in cochlear ablation and support the idea that neural activity is a crucial variable for proper development of the auditory system.

Animal models of congenital deafness provide an alternative means of addressing issues pertaining to the effects of deafness on development. An advantage of studying animals with congenital cochlear defects is that cochlear ablation or traumatic insults are not necessary to produce deafness. It may be concluded that the pathologic changes seen in the central nervous system are produced by the peripheral deafness. The deaf white cat represents a congenital model of deafness and mimics the Scheibe deformity seen in humans (Bosher and Hallpike, 1965; Mair, 1973). Studies of this cat revealed a 50% reduction of cochlear nuclei volume compared with that of normal cats and a 30% to 40% decrease in cochlear nucleus cell size (West and Harrison, 1973; Saada et al., 1996). Although these studies do not directly address critical periods, they are relevant to development because the changes seen are the result of lifelong acoustic deprivation. Other studies of the deaf white cat have focused on endbulb synapses (Ryugo et al., 1997) and their correlation to single unit activity in the auditory nerve and cochlear structure (Ryugo et al., 1998). The endbulb of Held is a large axosomatic (auditory nerve fiber to cell body) synapse located in the anteroventral cochlear nucleus and has a distinctive, treelike shape (Fig. 2.5). This synapse is thought to be involved in the preservation of timing information, an important cue for the comprehension of speech and localization of sound. The endbulbs of deaf white cats were atrophic, with decreased complexity compared with normal hearing cats. Ultrastructural examinations using electron microscopy confirm the degenerate nature of endbulbs in deafness, showing near depletion of synaptic vesicles together with a hypertrophy of the neurotransmitter receptor sites.

These structural changes suggest that the endbulb of Held may not faithfully transmit afferent activity. A fundamental question regarding natural animal models of deafness pertains to causality:

- Does the state of deafness induce changes seen, or are deafness-associated changes the result of direct effects of the genetic abnormality on the central nervous system?

This question can best be addressed by the study of naturally deaf animal models throughout development. It has been found that the endbulbs of Held of a deaf young cat (6 months old) exhibit morphologic abnormalities resembling those of a 6-year-old deaf adult cat (Ryugo et al., 1997). This observation reveals that synaptic abnormalities are fully apparent by 6 months of age and

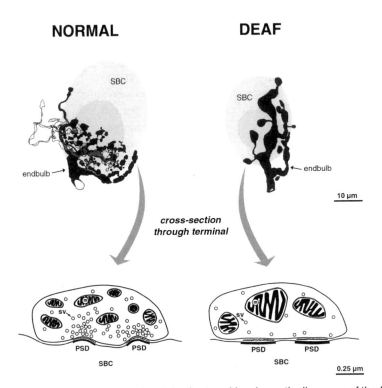

FIG. 2.5. Endbulb synapses from normal and deaf cats, with schematic diagrams of the fine structure of each ending. **A:** A typical, normal endbulb terminal (*black*) is shown as it synapses onto a spherical bushy cell (SBC) (*gray silhouette*). The slightly darker circle within the cell represents the cell nucleus. The endbulb terminal is a highly arborized and complex structure, with numerous branches and points of apposition between it and the recipient cell. A cross section through the terminal (*lower left*) depicts the normal ultrastructure of the ending. Synaptic vesicles (sv) are clustered around the postsynaptic density (PSD), indicating the site of neurotransmitter release and reception. The postsynaptic densities are characteristically curved toward the presynaptic ending. **B:** This endbulb (*black*) is typical of a congenitally deaf white cat. The postsynaptic bushy cell body (*gray*) is characteristically smaller than normal. The endbulb is atrophied, with a loss of complexity and tertiary branching. The number of appositional points between the ending and the postsynaptic cell is decreased. Ultrastructural analysis reveals deafness-induced changes, including the relative absence of synaptic vesicles and hypertrophied postsynaptic densities. m, mitochondria.

that there is no progressive deterioration with age. The implication is that a critical period for the developing auditory system has already passed by 6 months of age. During this time, a lack of organized neural activity caused synaptic remodeling in the form of hypertrophy and loss of synaptic vesicles in the auditory nerve fibers that terminate in the cochlear nucleus. We need to know how these neural changes affect the efficacy of cochlear implants. Because the cochlear nucleus initiates the ascending auditory

pathways, any corruption of information processing would necessarily be transmitted throughout the system.

NEURAL COMPENSATION: A FORM OF PLASTICITY IN HUMANS

It is natural to question the applicability of so much animal research to human pathology. Studies of the developing brain as it relates to human behavior have been less frequent compared with animal studies. However, some evidence illustrates cross-modal, developmental plasticity in humans afflicted with some forms of sensory loss. Functional imaging studies with blind humans reveal striking differences in cortical activation between those blinded at an early age and normal, sighted individuals (Sadato *et al.*, 1996). Subjects who were blind from an early age use their visual cortex when reading Braille, a task normally requiring primarily somatosensory activity. In contrast, sighted individuals do not exhibit visual cortical activity when presented with somatosensory stimulation (Uhl *et al.*, 1991). Disruption of the visual cortex using transcranial magnetic stimulation did not interfere with tactile discrimination in normal subjects but did distort tactile perceptions of blind subjects. Transient stimulation of the visual cortex had no effect on tactile performance in normal sighted subjects, although similar stimulation is known to disrupt their visual performance. The results demonstrate that visual cortex is recruited during early blindness to have a role in somatosensory processing (Cohen *et al.*, 1997). It appears that the developing brain, if deprived of a specific input, undergoes compensatory changes in other modalities so that deprived regions do not go unused (Kujala *et al.*, 1995).

Anecdotal notions hold that individuals with certain deficits compensate by having extraordinary refinements of their other senses. For example, blind subjects are often considered to have hearing that is better than normal. Scientific validation of such notions, however, is only preliminary. In a study of human subjects, people with and without vision were tested for their ability to identify sound sources in space (Lessard *et al.*, 1998). The investigators found that early-blind people were better at monaural localization of sound sources than normal sighted subjects. The ability to localize sounds in space with one ear relies on spectral cues created by interference patterns created by the external ear canal and the folds of the pinna. A person must learn to use these pinna spectral cues to locate sounds with one ear. When binaural

timing cues are not available, such as when the sound originates directly overhead or behind the head, pinna spectral cues are also useful for localization. The enhanced performance by blind subjects is consistent with the idea that selective sensory deprivation induces the remaining intact sensory systems to sharpen as a form of compensation.

ADULT PLASTICITY

Although we have discussed plasticity as it relates to the immature, developing brain, we have not yet addressed the mature adult nervous system. Adult animals and humans are able to learn new skills and modify their behavior throughout life, but there does appear to be a clear distinction between the respective abilities of the young and old in processing new information and acquiring new skills.

• Is such learning in adults associated with structural or functional brain alterations?

Although neurobiologists have made significant progress over the past 20 years in defining and characterizing the nature of adult plasticity, it is unclear to what degree these plastic changes are related to behavioral changes. Even less clear is the feasibility of manipulating plasticity to improve how the brain functions or how it responds to pathology, such as that introduced by deafness.

To approach some of these issues, we must begin by defining the nature of adult plasticity. Fortunately, many of the principles that govern one region of the brain apply to others. Certain common themes of plasticity are helpful to auditory researchers because some techniques used to study the auditory system have significant limitations. For example, methods of auditory deprivation involve manipulations of the inner ear, a structure buried deep within the extremely dense and hard temporal bone. In contrast, experiments of the visual system involve manipulations of the eyes, which are readily accessible. Broadly speaking, sensory systems are characterized by many shared features. One example is that sensory cortex exhibits topographic representations of the peripheral receptors. For instance, adjacent regions of the skin are represented by adjacent areas of somatosensory cortex. Similarly, auditory cortex is organized as a tonotopic map that mimics the frequency organization of the basilar membrane, and visual cortex exhibits a spatial representation of the visual field known as a retinotopic map.

Evidence suggests that the adult sensory cortex is not necessarily static. Under experimental conditions, sensory exposure can be limited or eliminated altogether. In response, the topography of the brain undergoes organizational changes such that the new sensory maps reflect conditions of the periphery. Lesion studies in many different animals have demonstrated that the somatosensory, visual, and auditory cortices of adult brains have some degree of plasticity. Some general mechanism might be in effect by virtue of these plastic changes occurring in each of these sensory systems.

Somatosensory cortical plasticity in the adult has been demonstrated in numerous experiments. In one particular series of experiments in the monkey, cortical representations of the hand were examined before and after the amputation of one or two digits (Merzenich et al., 1984). By 2 to 8 months after amputation, the sensory region that had responded to the skin of the amputated digits had reorganized and exhibited novel responses to tactile stimulation from adjacent digits or the subjacent palm. There was no significant increase, however, in the representation of nonadjacent digits. Other examples of similar reorganization in the adult somatosensory cortex have been reported in response to denervation or amputation in many different mammals, including the cat (Kalaska and Pomeranz, 1979), the raccoon (Rasmusson, 1982), the rat (Wall and Cusick, 1984), and the flying fox (Calford and Tweedale, 1988). Several studies in humans have also indicated large-scale remodeling in the somatosensory and motor cortical areas in the weeks and months after limb amputation (Fuhr et al., 1992; Kew et al., 1994; Yang et al., 1994; Knecht et al., 1995).

Deprivation studies of the visual system in the adult demonstrate robust cortical plasticity. The experimental removal of normal retinal input to a portion of the primary visual cortex (V1) in the cat results in the reorganization of the retinotopic map. In one study, a 5- to 10-degree area of one retina was lesioned, and the other retina was removed entirely. Several weeks later, the cortical field previously responsive to the area of the lesioned retina acquired new receptive fields corresponding to areas surrounding the retinal lesion (Kaas et al., 1990). Further studies showed that focal lesions in one eye produce an altered retinotopic map in response to the lesioned eye while simultaneously retaining a normal retinotopic map for the normal eye (Schmid et al., 1996). The denervated region of cortex adopts the properties of neurons contained in the adjacent, intact cortical region.

Of special interest to auditory sciences, the adult auditory cortex has shown similar capacities for reorganization. Unilateral lesions to the cochlea of adult guinea pigs produced a rearrangement of the tonotopic map of the ipsilateral cortex (Roberston and Irvine, 1989). Immediately after the lesion, that part of cortex that normally responded to the frequencies contained in the damaged portion of the cochlea was silent (Fig. 2.6). By 1 month after the lesion, however, neurons in the deprived cortex responded to tone frequencies that corresponded to intact cochlear regions adjacent to the lesion site.

In addition, the intensity thresholds of neurons in the reorganized zone were similar to those recorded in normal cortex (Roberston and Irvine, 1989). These types of changes in tonotopicity as a response to cochlear lesions have also been reported in cats (Rajan et al., 1993) and monkeys (Schwaber et al., 1993).

The previously discussed studies focus on remodeling at the cortical level. Although

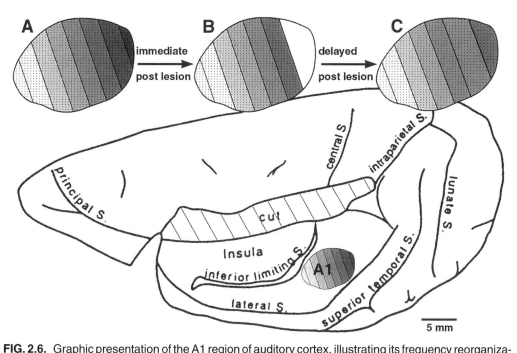

FIG. 2.6. Graphic presentation of the A1 region of auditory cortex, illustrating its frequency reorganization after high-frequency cochlear damage. The superior temporal gyrus of a monkey brain is viewed from a dorsolateral perspective after removal of the overlying parietal cortex (*cross-hatching*). The gray areas are shaded from light to dark, representing the tonotopic progression of low to high frequencies. The normal A1 **(A)** before and immediately after cochlear ablation **(B)** shows loss of high-frequency responsiveness (*white area*). Some time later, the intact, adjacent frequencies take over the denervated cortical region **(C)**. (Adapted from ref. 54, with permission.)

such studies are important and revealing, they do not necessarily describe what happens at lower levels of the central nervous system.

• In what other areas of the brain may plasticity occur?

If plastic changes originate in the midbrain or medulla, changes at the cortical level may primarily reflect the passive expression of plasticity at lower levels. It is important to determine the nature and the site of plasticity.

Different mechanisms may underlie plastic changes evident in deprived areas of sensory cortex. One study investigated the distributions of thalamic and cortical connections in macaque monkeys with long-standing, accidental trauma to their peripheral forelimb. Injections of dyes into the neocortex revealed a normal thalamocortical projection but significant sprouting of horizontal cortical connections by the normal areas into adjacent deprived areas (Florence *et al.*, 1998). A parallel study used macaque monkeys that had long-term denervation of an upper limb caused by severing the sensory nerve root as it entered the spinal cord. This manipulation led to degeneration of the primary sensory neurons, which consequentially produced the degeneration of axons in the dorsal columns and the transneuronal degeneration of topographically related sectors of the brain stem and thalamic nuclei. The thalamic nuclei were reorganized such that the representations of the face and body were directly adjacent to the body trunk, a pattern that was mirrored by a new arrangement of thalamocortical projections. The cortex reflected this remodeled somatosensory map (Jones and Pons, 1998).

The most interesting result to emerge from these studies is that electrophysiologic mapping of the cortex produced maps in which responses of normal, adjacent regions appeared in the deprived regions. The mechanisms providing this remodeling, however, were quite different depending on whether the primary neurons degenerated. In the case where there was no primary neuron degeneration (Florence et al., 1998), cortical sprouting of new horizontal connections from the adjacent, intact areas provided the remodeling. When there was primary neuron degeneration, remodeling occurred around transneuronal degeneration, and the new cortical map was produced by remodeled thalamocortical projections (Jones and Pons, 1998). These studies indicate the many faces of plasticity and that the nature of a lesion can determine the mechanism of subsequent remodeling.

These examples of cortical reorganization have all been produced by sensory deprivation of the cortex through peripheral loss. This situation has direct relevance to individuals who have suffered extreme loss of function because of trauma or disease, but perhaps the most common form of plasticity is the frequent occurrence of learning new material and developing new abilities. The acquisition of new skills in response to specific tasks or situations is called the *training effect* and is of particular relevance to helping adult cochlear implant users reestablish hearing and language skills.

Changes in the auditory cortical map have been seen after training monkeys on a frequency discrimination task. After several weeks of behavioral training, a monkey's ability to discriminate between different frequencies improved significantly. Detailed mapping of the tonotopic representation of the primary auditory cortex (A1) revealed that the representation of the conditioned frequency band was several times larger in trained monkeys than in controls. A substantial correlation was found between the suc-

cessful behavioral performance of the monkeys and the size of the cortical area representing the trained frequencies (Recanzone et al., 1993).

Classic conditioning involves the systematic pairing of a neutral signal (e.g., sound of a bell) to a reward (e.g., food) or punishment (e.g., shock), thereby giving significance to previously neutral signal (Pavlov, 1927). Frequency-specific receptive-field plasticity in the auditory system has been demonstrated using just such a protocol (Weinberger et al., 1993). The researchers paired a tone of a given frequency with an aversive electrical shock. Tuning curves recorded from the auditory cortex before and after conditioning revealed a shift in the best frequency responses toward the frequency of the conditioned stimulus (Fig. 2.7). This result suggests that conditioning caused the recruitment of extra neurons to be sensitive to the important stimulus.

Given the evidence for adult plasticity, the question of an age-related effect still remains:

• Why should a younger brain have greater plasticity than an older brain?

It is almost as if the mechanisms of plasticity, present at birth, become progressively restrained with age. Examination of some of the components of brain tissue suggest possible mechanisms that underlie plasticity.

Myelin is a cellular substance that surrounds the axons of neurons throughout the nervous system. Myelin is essential for the timely propagation of electrical signals along the course of an axon. Evidence supports the notion that myelination, a process that takes place throughout early life, may be partially responsible for the gradual restriction of plasticity over time. Myelin-associated neurite growth inhibitory proteins (MNGIPs) prevent regeneration of nerve fibers. Although such proteins may seem maladaptive, closer consideration reveals that there must be stable components of the brain whose neural connections, once formed, remain

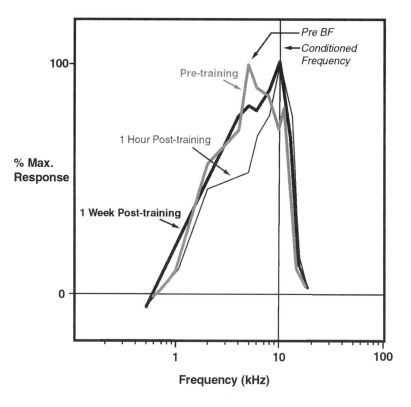

FIG. 2.7. Short-term (1 hour) and long-term (1-week) changes in neuronal tuning after training. These plots show that a neuron originally tuned to a best frequency (BF) of 5 kHz changes its optimal responsiveness after training to a 10-kHz conditioned stimulus. The light gray line indicates the pretraining BF of 5 kHz. (Adapted from ref. 59, with permission.)

permanent. One group of researchers used a monoclonal antibody to neutralize the MNGIP in adult rats in conjunction with a unilateral lesion of the corticospinal tract. This lesion caused a motor paralysis of the right forelimb in the rat. Rats treated with antibody-secreting cells at the site of damage produced new sprouts, or collateral fibers, into the damaged area from the remaining intact fibers (Fig. 2.8). Rats without antibody treatment showed no such collateral growth (Schwab *et al.*, 1998).

The most intriguing aspect of this study is the effect of antibody treatment on the animal's motor skills, even in the presence of a lesion in the corticospinal tract. On various tests designed to isolate right forelimb motor skills, rats treated with antibodies to MNGIP showed performance that was equal to that of normal, unlesioned rats. In other words, the inhibition of MNGIP in adult rats produced a state of heightened plasticity within

the damaged spinal cord, the result of which was the full recovery of gross motor abilities (Schwab *et al.*, 1998).

PLASTICITY AND THE TREATMENT OF HEARING DISORDERS

Remedies for the treatment of hearing loss have evolved from the early use of the ear trumpet, a funnel placed in the external auditory canal, to the modern multichannel cochlear implant. Although skeptics may question the crudity of such a device for a process as complex as audition, it is widely accepted that properly selected recipients of cochlear implants can benefit tremendously from this intervention.

• Why should a cochlear implant work at all?

It seems that the tight temporal coupling of environmental sounds to neural events represents a key element for the proper de-

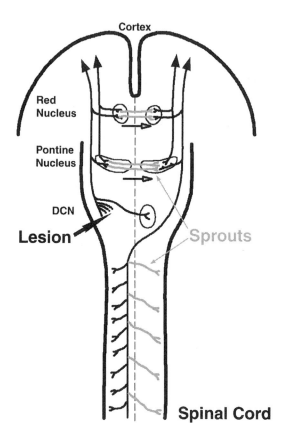

FIG. 2.8. A lesion of the corticospinal tract on the left side (*arrow*) denervates the right side of the spinal cord. After treatment with monoclonal antibody IN-1, newly sprouted fibers cross the midline of the spinal cord to innervate the denervated hemicord. Sprouts also crossed into the contralateral red nucleus, pontine nuclei, and dorsal column nucleus (DCN). (Adapted from ref. 60, with permission.)

velopment of auditory function and validation of the auditory pathways. We speculate that the cognitive appreciation of this timing is learned, that it begins early in postnatal life, and that congenital deafness impairs auditory system development by removing these timing cues. During development, the plasticity of the brain is at its maximum. The brain is primed to receive input. In a sense, the brain acts as a sponge during early life and absorbs any useful information it receives from the environment. It is likely that the most important factor for proper development of the brain, especially the auditory system, is stimulation.

For the auditory system, stimulation normally occurs in the form of sounds. However, the malleability of the brain at a young age is extraordinary, and the brain can use areas of cortex deprived of input for other purposes. The brain is remarkably capable of extracting useful information from seemingly sparse input. It follows that the stimulation received by the auditory system need not be acoustic in nature. Electrical stimulation, as provided by cochlear implants, is triggered by external cues. This stimulation has a firm basis in and a relationship to the real world, and a developing child can learn to associate visual, somatosensory, and other environmental cues with those provided by a cochlear implant. Cochlear implants therefore prevent a state of sensory deprivation, even though they do not replace the normal mechanism of the ear. We have discussed the importance of environmental input for proper brain development. Cochlear implants can provide this crucial information. Whereas the exact requirements for proper development of the auditory system have not been defined, evidence suggests that the single most important variable may be the presence or absence of activity, rather than its type, nature, or cause.

IMPLANT PERFORMANCE AND PLASTICITY

- What accounts for the success of a cochlear implant in some individuals and not in others?

These findings are far from arbitrary. The success of auditory rehabilitation methods such as the cochlear implant lies in their ability to present sound as a physiologically useful code to the auditory pathway. The ability to comprehend speech with a cochlear implant requires that the central auditory pathways encode, process, and organize the patterns of electrical stimulation into an auditory percept. Moreover, this processing must occur effectively in quiet and noisy conditions. Results of cochlear implantation in children (Quittner and Steck, 1991; Fryauf-Bertschy *et al.*, 1992) and in adults (Waltzman *et al.*, 1993; Gantz *et al.*, 1994; Tyler and Summerfield, 1996) suggest that young children represent the best candidates for a cochlear implant. Delayed implantation after the early onset of deafness predicts lower levels of speech reception. The available evidence further suggests that children with even minimal hearing abilities tend to perform better than congenitally deaf children (Waltzman *et al.*, 1994, 1997; Waltzman and Cohen, 1998).

This effect of timing of cochlear implantation is even more striking in cases of long-term deprivation. Clinical trials have confirmed that profoundly deaf adult recipients who have benefited most from the implants are those who developed linguistic skills before becoming deaf (Waltzman *et al.*, 1991; Zwolan *et al.*, 1997). The 1988 and 1995 National Institutes of Health Consensus Development Conferences on Cochlear Implants recognized that congenitally deaf adult recipients often demonstrate few or no objective gains in speech recognition from preoperative to postoperative conditions. Although

speech-reading assessments reveal a trend toward improved lip reading in this population, there is little indication that pure auditory speech discrimination is achieved.

These findings suggest that stimulus coding in this subpopulation of subjects often fails to provide adequate combinations of temporal and spectral cues to support comprehension.

- Can we exploit our understanding of critical periods and the phenomenon of plasticity in adults to increase the benefits of cochlear implants?

Efforts to treat congenital deafness need to address deafness onset and the progressive degeneration that appears within the auditory pathway as a result of plasticity. A growing body of animal and human data suggests that cognitive and perceptual disorders may be based on an inability to perform temporal segmentation and spectral (frequency) discrimination despite normal auditory thresholds. One of the fundamental tasks in designing strategies for hearing rehabilitation is to understand how to compensate for the reduced temporal precision and frequency specificity of deafness. Frequency discrimination is critical for the proper perception of vowel sounds. Cortical plasticity in response to partial damage to the cochlea might impair frequency specificity because adjacent intact areas spread into the deprived areas. Such reactive plasticity might serve to diminish frequency separation. The faithful representation of timing information conveyed in speech is also essential to language understanding, and high-fidelity timing cues may be lost by plastic remodeling of synapses in the cochlear nucleus.

Auditory reception in children with impaired language-learning capabilities is associated with the regular occurrence of certain perceptual effects. Among the more consistent patterns are limitations in identifying phonetic elements that are relatively brief in their presentation. Performance is often poor in sequencing short-duration acoustic signals presented with short interstimulus intervals (Tallal *et al.*, 1996; Merzen-ich *et al.*, 1996). Language learning–impaired children show improvements in identifying and distinguishing brief phonetic elements and in properly sequencing stimuli when stimulus presentation occurs at a slower speed. Intensive practice with stimuli pre-sented at progressively shorter intervals ap-pears to result in significant improvements in temporal processing. This result indicates that the recognition of rapid speech elements can be improved with properly configured, incremental training paradigms.

The ability to treat hearing loss is often thwarted by an inability to restore speech comprehension, a sensory task that requires effective transfer of encoded speech infor-mation from the auditory nerve throughout the appropriate central pathways. Although total deafness does not appear to alter the basic tonotopicity of the auditory system, chronic electrical stimulation of deafened cats does produce profound alterations of spatial frequency representation in the audi-tory midbrain (Snyder *et al.*, 1990; Leake *et al.*, 1995). There may be other complications in temporal and spectral processing induced by reactive changes in primary synapses as a consequence of ear dysfunction (Gerken, 1979; Moore *et al.*, 1994, 1997; Ryugo *et al.*, 1997, 1998).

Observations from the studies discussed in this chapter may have direct relevance to neural mechanisms that underlie limitations in speech processing capabilities on sensory restoration. Difficulties in pitch perception and frequency discrimination among im-planted patients have been well documented in psychophysical studies (Simmons *et al.*, 1965; Townsend *et al.*, 1987). These studies emphasize that frequency encoding involves place and temporal information (Eddington, 1983; Hartmann *et al.*, 1984; Niparko *et al.*, 1993). Basic science and clinical studies sug-gest some degree of variability in the preci-sion with which temporal cues are encoded by electrical stimulation (Shannon, 1989; Waltzman *et al.*, 1990; Snyder *et al.*, 1991), but temporal discrimination capabilities are

important in predicting speech comprehen-sion in implant users (Hochmair-Desoyer *et al.*, 1985). The synaptic interface between endbulbs of Held and spherical bushy cells is one key site where temporal cues intro-duced in the periphery are relayed to as-cending auditory pathways (Pfeiffer, 1966). Pathologic atrophy at this site, as shown in the studies of deaf white cats (Ryugo *et al.*, 1997), probably would compromise the abil-ity of synapses to transmit information accu-rately, thereby reducing the temporal fidelity with which auditory cues are processed.

Synaptic changes in deafness may repre-sent a fundamental obstacle to sensorineural rehabilitation. It has been tempting to pre-sume that restored input by itself is capable of reconstituting auditory connections, but the task remains a complicated problem of knowing the processing capabilities of the neural network and the optimal time and form of prosthetic intervention. Much re-search has tried to define structural corre-lates of abolished activity of the auditory re-ceptors and primary afferent fibers. Such studies provide insight into fundamental mechanisms by which activity influences neu-ronal form and lead us to consider exactly how and when intervention may ameliorate or reverse central auditory pathway degener-ation induced by the loss of peripheral audi-tory activity.

Adult cochlear implant users provide clini-cal examples of the decline of neural plastic-ity with age. Prelingually deafened adults have passed their period of maximum plastic-ity by the time they reach adulthood. They also have been unable to form the necessary neural structures required to process lan-guage. For these reasons, truly satisfying re-sults in prelingually deafened adults have not been achieved with the current technology. Successful implantation of this group in the future may depend wholly on our ability to manipulate the plasticity of the brain. Al-though the reasons why plasticity is greatest at early ages remain unclear, there must be an underlying principle that is responsible for such features of the brain. The example of MNGIP neutralization with resultant sprouting of neurons suggests that recovery of plasticity in the adult human may eventually become possible. With further research, the mature brain may some day be sufficiently understood such that language skills can be acquired by prelingually deafened adults as easily as they are by normal children.

THE PARADOX OF PLASTICITY

The process of learning inherently depends on brain plasticity. The more pliable our brains are, the better they are at processing new information, forming neural connections, and modifying neuronal response properties as a result of this information.

• How well would a brain function if it were entirely plastic?

A brain in which all connections are malleable and none are permanent could never learn from prior experiences. It could not place discrete pieces of new information into an overall concept of the external world gained through experience. Memory stabilizes the world by providing permanence. With all that we learn on a regular basis coupled with fluid adjustments of brain structure and activity, it is a wonder that we wake up each morning the same person as the previous day. These ideas, although somewhat absurd, direct us toward more relevant questions.

• How much plasticity is too much?
• If our brains are truly plastic, how do our external and internal worlds stay largely constant in the mind's eye?

The data we need to address such questions are being collected at a rapid pace. Whereas these types of questions previously constituted little more than intellectual exercises, evolving technology and insights into the brain have pushed these abstract considerations of plasticity into the sphere of reality. Cochlear implants validate many questions regarding plasticity that are raised by intel-

lectual discourse. In addition to providing a major opportunity for us to help the deaf, cochlear implantation also helps enable us to learn how plasticity of the human brain works. The success of cochlear implants places emphasis on the importance of increasing our understanding of plasticity its nature, mechanisms, extent, and applicability so that the full implications of our therapeutic modalities may be appreciated.

CONCLUSIONS

We have described the extraordinary degree of plasticity in the developing organism, a feature of life that appears present in some form throughout all species and that seems to be an integral component of early development. This plasticity is required for normal development to occur, and the period of greatest plasticity, the critical period, is primarily responsible for the proper formation of those brain regions needed for sensory processing. We also discussed evidence to support the notion that even adult brains exhibit plasticity. Although all critical periods of development have passed, the adult brain still maintains a large degree of plasticity that enables adaptation to new experiences. To what extent electrical stimulation of the auditory nerve prevents brain stem or cortical degeneration has not been established, nor is it known what particular components of the auditory pathway are most negatively affected by deafness or positively affected by cochlear implants. The outcome of cochlear implantation largely depends on the natural course of plasticity that exists in the brain. As our understanding of plasticity evolves, our ability to provide useful hearing through implant technology should evolve in kind.

ACKNOWLEDGMENTS

The authors were supported by National Institutes of Health grants RO1 DC00232 (DKR) and T32 DC00027 (CJL, EER) while preparing this manuscript.

REFERENCES

Born DE, Rubel EW. Afferent influences on brain stem auditory nuclei of the chicken: neuron number and size following cochlea removal. *J Comp Neurol* 1985;231:435–445.

Bosher S, Hallpike C. Observations on the histological features, development and pathogenesis of the inner ear degeneration of the deaf white cat. *Proc R Soc B* 1965;162:147–170.

Calford MD, Tweedale R. Immediate and chronic changes in responses of somatosensory cortex in adult flying-fox after digit amputation. *Nature* 1988;332:446–448.

Cohen LGP, Celnik P, Pascual-Leone A, *et al.* Functional relevance of cross-modal plasticity in blind humans. *Nature* 1997;389:180–183.

Crair MC, Gillespie DC, Stryker MP. The role of visual experience in the development of columns in cat visual cortex. *Science* 1998;279:566–570.

Eddington DK. Speech recognition in deaf subjects with multichannel intracochlear electrodes. *Ann NY Acad Sci* 1983;405:241–258.

Florence SL, Taub HB, Kaas JH. Large-scale sprouting of cortical connections after peripheral injury in adult macaque monkeys. *Science* 1988;282:1117–1121.

Fryauf-Bertschy H, Tyler RS, Kelsay DM, *et al.* Performance over time of congenitally deaf and postlingually deafened children using a multichannel cochlear implant. *J Speech Hear Res* 1992;35:913–920.

Fuhr P, Cohen LG, Dang N, *et al.* Physiological analysis of motor reorganization following lower limb amputation. *Electroencephalogr Clin Neurophysiol* 1992;85:53–60.

Gantz BJ, Ryler RS, Woodworth GG, *et al.* Results of multichannel cochlear implants in congenital and acquired prelingual deafness in children: five-year follow-up. *Am J Otol* 1994;2[Suppl 1]:1–7.

Gerken GM. Temporal summation of pulsate brain stimulation in normal and deafened cats. *J Acoust Soc Am* 1979;66:728–734.

Goodsitt JV, Morgan JL, Kuhl PK. Perceptual strategies in prelingual speech segmentation. *J Child Lang* 1993;20:229–252.

Hartmann R, Topp G, Klinke R. Discharge patterns of cat primary auditory fibers with electrical stimulation of the cochlea. *Hear Res* 1984;13:47–62.

Hashisaki GT, Rubel EW. Effects of unilateral cochlea removal on anteroventral cochlear nucleus neurons in developing gerbils. *J Comp Neurol* 1989;283:465–473.

Heinroth O. *Beiträge zur Biologie, nahmentlich Ethologie und Psychologie der Anatiden,* Verh. 5 int. orn. Kongr. Berlin: Deutsche ornithologische gesellschaft, 1910:589–702.

Hochmair-Desoyer E, Hochmair-Desoyer I, Stiglbrunner H. Psychoacoustic temporal processing and speech understanding in cochlear implant patients. In: Schindler RA, Merzenich MM, eds. *Cochlear implants.* New York: Raven Press, 1985:291–304.

Jones EG, Pons TP. Thalamic and brainstem contributions to large-scale plasticity of primate somatosensory cortex. *Science* 1998;282:1121–1125.

Kaas JH. Krubitzer LA, Chino YM, *et al.* Reorganiza-

tion of retinotopic cortical maps in adult mammals after lesions of the retina. *Science* 1990;248:229–231.

Kalaska J, Pomeranz B. Chronic paw denervation causes an age-dependent appearance of novel responses from forearm in paw cortex of kittens and adult cats. *J Neurophysiol* 1979;42:618–633.

Kew JJ, Ridding MC, Rothwell JC, *et al.* Reorganization of cortical blood flow and transcranial magnetic stimulation maps in human subjects after upper limb amputation. *J Neurophysiol* 1994;72:2517–2524.

Killackey HP, Belford G, Ryugo R, *et al.* Anomalous organization of thalamocortical projections consequent to vibrissae removal in the newborn rat and mouse. *Brain Res* 1976;104:309–315.

Killackey HP. Anatomical evidence for cortical subdivisions based on vertically discrete thalamic projections from the ventral posterior nucleus to cortical barrels in the rat. *Brain Res* 1973;51:326–331.

Knecht S, Henningsen H, Elbert T, *et al.* Cortical reorganization in human amputees and mislocalization of painful stimuli to the phantom limb. *Neurosci Lett* 1995;201:262–264.

Knudsen EI. Capacity for plasticity in the adult owl auditory system expanded by juvenile experience. *Science* 1998;279:1531–1533.

Konishi M. Birdsong: from behavior to neuron. *Annu Rev Neurosci* 1985;8:125–170.

Kuhl PK. Human adults and human infants show a perceptual magnet effect for the prototypes of speech categories; monkeys do not. *Percept Psychophys* 1991;50:93–107.

Kujala T, Alho K, Kekoni J, *et al.* Auditory and somatosensory event-related brain potentials in early blind humans. *Exp Brain Res* 1995;104:519–526.

Lane H. *The wild boy of Aveyron.* Cambridge, MA: Harvard University Press, 1976.

Leake PA, Snyder RL, Hradek GT, *et al.* Consequences of chronic extracochlear electrical stimulation in neonatally deafened cats. *Hear Res* 1995;82:65–80.

Lessard N, Par JM, Lepore F, *et al.* Early-blind human subjects localize sound sources better than sighted subjects. *Nature* 1998;395:278–280.

LeVay S, Wiesel TN, Hubel DH. The postnatal development and plasticity of ocular-dominance columns in the monkey. In: Schmitt FO, Worden FG, Adelman G, Dennis SG, eds. *The organization of cerebral cortex: proceedings of a neuroscience research program colloquium.* Cambridge, MA: MIT Press, 1981;29–45.

Mair IW. Hereditary deafness in the white cat. *Acta Otolaryngol* 1973;31:41–48.

Marler P, Tamura M. Song variation in three populations of white-crowned sparrow. *Condor* 1962;64:368–377.

Merzenich MM, Nelson RJ, Stryker MP, *et al.* Somatosensory map changes following digit amputation in adult monkeys. *J Comp Neurol* 1984;224:591–605.

Merzenich, MM, Jenkins WM, Johnston P, *et al.* Temporal processing deficits of language-learning impaired children ameliorated by training. *Science* 1996;271:77–81.

Moore DR, King AJ, McAlpine D, *et al.* Functional consequences of neonatal unilateral cochlear removal. *Prog Brain Res* 1993;97:127–133.

Moore JK, Niparko JK, Miller MR, *et al.* Effect of profound hearing loss on a central auditory nucleus. *Am J Otol* 1994;15:588–595.

Niparko JK, Pfingst B, Johansson C, *et al*. Extracochlear stimulation with a lateral cochlear-wall titanium implants. *Ann Otol Rhinol Laryngol* 1993;102:447–454.

Pavlov IP. *Conditioned reflexes*. New York: Dover, 1927.

Payne RS. Acoustic location of prey by barn owls (*Tyto alba*). *J Exp Biol* 1971;54:535–573.

Pfeiffer RR. Classification of response patterns of spike discharges for units in the cochlear nucleus: tone burst stimulation. *Exp Brain Res* 1966;1:220–235.

Powell TPS, Erulkar SD. Transneuronal cell degeneration in the auditory relay nuclei of the cat. *J Anat* 1962;96:219–268.

Quittner AL, Steck JT. Predictors of cochlear implant use in children. *Am J Otol* 1991;12[Suppl 1]:89–94.

Rajan R, Irvine DRF, Wise LZ, *et al*. Effect of unilateral partial cochlear lesions in adult cats on the representation for lesioned and unlesioned cochleas in primary auditory cortex. *J Comp Neurol* 1993;338:17–49.

Rasmusson DD. Reorganization of raccoon somatosensory cortex following removal of the fifth digit. *J Comp Neurol* 1982;205:313–326.

Raviola E, Wiesel TN. An animal model of myopia. *N Engl J Med* 1985;312:1609–1615.

Recanzone GH, Schreiner CE, Merzenich MM. Plasticity in the frequency representation of primary auditory cortex following discrimination training in adult owl monkeys. *J Neurosci* 1993;13:87–104.

Rice FL, Van der Loos H. Development of the barrels and barrel field in the somatosensory cortex of the mouse. *J Comp Neurol* 1977;171:545–560.

Robertson D, Irvine DRF. Plasticity of frequency organization in auditory cortex of guinea pigs with partial unilateral deafness. *J Comp Neurol* 1989;282:456–471.

Roe AW, Pallas SL, Hahm JO, *et al*. A map of visual space induced in primary auditory cortex. *Science* 1990;250:818–820.

Ryugo DK, Pongstaporn T, Huchton, DM, *et al*. Ultrastructural analysis of primary endings in deaf white cats: morphologic alterations in endbulbs of Held. *J Comp Neurol* 1997;385:230–244.

Ryugo DK, Rosenbaum BT, Kim PJ, *et al*. Single unit recordings in the auditory nerve of congenitally deaf white cats: morphological correlates in the cochlea and cochlear nucleus. *J Comp Neurol* 1998;397:532–548.

Saada AA, Niparko JK, Ryugo DK. Morphological changes in the cochlear nucleus of congenitally deaf white cats. *Brain Res* 1996;736:315–328.

Sadato N, Pascual-Leone A, Grafman J, *et al*. Activation of the primary visual cortex by Braille reading in blind subjects. *Nature* 1996;380:526–528.

Schmid LM, Rosa MGP, Calford MD, *et al*. Visuotopic reorganization in the primary cortex of adult cats following monocular and binocular retinal lesions. *Cereb Cortex* 1996;6:388–405.

Schwab ME, Thallmair M, Metz GAS, *et al*. Neurite growth inhibitors restrict plasticity and functional recovery following corticospinal tract lesions. *Nat Neurosci* 1998;1:124–131.

Schwaber MK, Garraghty PE, Kaas JH. Neuroplasticity of the adult primate auditory cortex following cochlear hearing loss. *Am J Otol* 1993;14:252–258.

Shannon RV. Detection of gaps in sinusoids and pulse trains by patients with cochlear implants. *J Acoust Soc Am* 1989;85:2587–2592.

Shattuck R. *The forbidden experiment*. New York: Farrar Straus Giroux, 1980.

Shatz CJ, Stryker MP. Ocular dominance in layer IV of the cat's visual cortex and the effects of monocular deprivation. *J Physiol* 1978;281:267–283.

Sie KCY, Rubel EW. Rapid changes in protein synthesis and cell size in the cochlear nucleus following eighth nerve activity blockade or cochlea ablation. *J Comp Neurol* 1992;320:501–508.

Simmons FB. Auditory nerve: electrical stimulation in man. *Science* 1965;148:104–106.

Snyder RL, Rebscher SJ, Cao K, *et al*. Chronic intracochlear electrical stimulation in the neonatally deafened cat. I: Expansion of central representation. *Hear Res* 1990;50:7–33.

Snyder RL, Rebscher SJ, Leake PA, *et al*. Chronic intracochlear electrical stimulation in the neonatally deafened cat. II. Temporal properties of neurons in the inferior colliculus. *Hear Res* 1991;56:246–264.

Spalding DA. Instinct, with original observations on young animals. *Macmillan's Magazine* 1873;27:282–293. [Reprinted in *Br J Anim Behav* 1954;2:2–11.]

Tallal P, Miller SL, Bedi G, *et al*. Language comprehension in language-learning impaired children improved with acoustically modified speech. *Science* 1996;271:81–84.

Townshend B, Cotter N, Van Compernolle D, *et al*. Pitch perception by cochlear implant subjects. *J Acoust Soc Am* 1987;82:106–115.

Trune DR. Influence of neonatal cochlear removal on the development of mouse cochlear nucleus: I. Number, size, and density of its neurons. *J Comp Neurol* 1982;209:409–424.

Tyler RS, Summerfield AQ. Cochlear implantation: relationships with research on auditory deprivation and acclimatization. *Ear Hear* 1996;17[Suppl 3]:38S–50S.

Uhl F, Franzen P, Lindinger G, *et al*. On the functionality of the visual deprived occipital cortex in early blind persons. *Neurosci Lett* 1991;124:256–259.

Van der Loos H, Woolsey TA. Somatosensory cortex: structural alterations following early injury to sense organs. *Science* 1973;179:395–398.

Wall JT, Cusick CG. Cutaneous responsiveness in primary somatosensory (S-I) hindpaw cortex before and after partial hindpaw deafferentation in adult rats. *J Neurosci* 1984;4:1499–1515.

Waltzman S, Cohen NL, Gomolin RH, *et al*. Open-set speech perception in congenitally deaf children using cochlear implants. *Am J Otol* 1997;18:342–349.

Waltzman S, Cohen NL, Shapiro WH, *et al*. The prognostic value of round window electrical stimulation in cochlear implant patients. *Otolaryngol Head Neck Surg* 1990;103:102–106.

Waltzman S, Cohen NL. Cochlear implantation in children younger than 2 years old. *Am J Otol* 1998;19:158–162.

Waltzman S, Fisher S, Niparko JK, *et al*. Predictors of postoperative performance with cochlear implants. *Ann Otol Rhinol Laryngol* 1994;165:15–18.

Weinberger NM, Javid R, Lepan B. Long-term retention of learning-induced receptive field plasticity in the auditory cortex. *Proc Natl Acad Sci USA* 1993; 90:2394–2398.

Welker C, Woolsey TA. Structure of layer IV in the somatosensory neocortex of the rat: description and comparison with the mouse. *J Comp Neurol* 1974; 158:437–454.

Weller WL, Johnson JI. Barrels in cerebral cortex altered by receptor disruption in newborn, but not in five-day-old mice (*Cricetinae* and *Muridae*). *Brain Res* 1975;83:504–508.

West CD, Harrison JM. Transneuronal cell atrophy in the deaf white cat. *J Comp Neurol* 1973;151:377–398.

Whaling CS, Solis MM, Doupe AJ, *et al.* Acoustic and neural bases for innate recognition of song. *Proc Natl Acad Sci USA* 1997;94:12694–12698.

Wiesel TN, Hubel DH, Lam D. Autoradiographic demonstration of ocular dominance columns in the monkey striate cortex by means of transsynaptic transport. *Brain Res* 1974;79:273–279.

Yang TT, Galleon CC, Cobb, *et al.* Noninvasive detection of cerebral plasticity in adult human somatosensory cortex. *Neuroreport* 1994;5:701–704.

Zwolan TA, Collings LM, Wakefield GH. Electrode discrimination and speech recognition in postlingually deafened adult cochlear implant subjects. *J Acoust Soc Am* 1997;102:3673–3685.

SUGGESTED READINGS

Kajula T, Alho K, Kekoni J, *et al.* Auditory and somatosensory even-related brain potentials in early blind humans. *Exp Brain Res* 1995;104:519–526.

Lorenz K. Der Kumpan in der Umwelt des Vogels; die Artgenosse als auslòsendes Moment sozialer Verhaltungsweisen. *J Ornithol* 1935;83:137–213. [Also in English translation: Companionship in bird life; fellow members of the species as releasers of social behavior. In: Schiller CH, ed. *Instinctive behavior.* New York: International University Press, 1957.]

Moore JK, Niparko JK, Perazzo LM, *et al.* Effect of adult-onset deafness on the human central auditory system. *Ann Otol Rhinol Laryngol* 1997;106:385–390.

Wiesel TN. Postnatal development of the visual cortex and the influence of environment. *Nature* 1982;299: 583–592.

Cochlear Implants: Principles & Practices, edited by John K. Niparko, Karen Iler Kirk, Nancy K. Mellon, Amy McConkey Robbins, Debara L. Tucci, and Blake S. Wilson. Lippincott Williams & Wilkins, Philadelphia © 2000.

3

Inner Ear Pathology in Severe to Profound Sensorineural Hearing Loss

Matthew Ng, John K. Niparko, and George T. Nager

This chapter describes the forms of sensorineural deafness that are likely to be found in persons who may become candidates for cochlear implants. We discuss the clinical presentation and treatment of each form of deafness and the known or postulated mechanisms of sensorineural impairment. We summarize current views on the pathologic changes in the inner ear, auditory nerve, and central auditory pathway that may affect cochlear implant candidacy and performance.

SURVIVAL OF AUDITORY NEURAL ELEMENTS

Severe to profound deafness is associated with a range of pathologies of sensory structures within the cochlea and their associated nerve fibers. The degree of nerve survivabil-

M. Ng: Department of Otolaryngology—Head and Neck Surgery, The Johns Hopkins University, Baltimore, Maryland 21205-1809.

J. K. Niparko: Department of Otolaryngology—Head and Neck Surgery, The Listening Center at Johns Hopkins, The Johns Hopkins University, Baltimore, Maryland 21205-1809.

G. T. Nager: Department of Otolaryngology—Head and Neck Surgery, The Johns Hopkins University, Baltimore, Maryland 21205-1809.

ity reported for these cases has been broad, from less than 10% to more than 70% of normal. Although greater populations would seem to predict improved performance, hard experimental evidence is lacking. The degree and pattern of nerve loss that accompanies severe to profound hearing loss varies with several factors. The normal number of auditory nerve fibers within the auditory nerve trunk for individuals under the age of 20 is slightly more than 35,000 (Otte *et al.*, 1978). More than 95% of these fibers are responsible for reporting information from inner hair cells of the cochlea to the brain (Fig. 3.1).

Injury to cochlear structures is associated with degeneration of auditory nerve fibers to the extent that support cells within the inner ear are lost (Suzuka and Schuknecht, 1988; Johnsson, 1974). That is, there is a direct correlation between the degree of damage to the supporting cells (*i.e.*, pillar cells and inner phalangeal cells) of the organ of Corti and the number of neuronal fibers lost. The process of nerve degeneration within the cochlea reveals unique features. It is not unusual for dendritic extensions of the auditory fiber to be lost despite a preserved neuronal cell body, and axonal extension of this indicates that the cell body portion of the neuron can survive independent of its den-

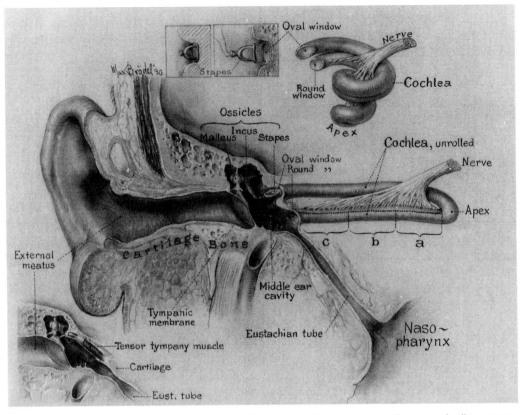

FIG. 3.1. The human cochlea has been unrolled to illustrate frequency-specific areas. Auditory nerve fibers serve low, middle, and high frequencies in segments a, b, and c, respectively.

dritic extension into the cochlea. This pattern of partial nerve survival is unusual and unlike the process of retrograde degeneration commonly associated with nerve injury. Preserved neuronal cell bodies provide an alternative to the dendritic extension of the nerve fiber for prosthetic stimulation and may be all that is necessary for adequate stimulation by a cochlear implant.

Normally, auditory neuronal loss occurs at a rate of 2,000 cells per decade because of aging effects alone. Most temporal bone studies of cases of profound sensorineural hearing loss reveal substantial survival of populations of spiral ganglion cells (Fig. 3.2). Although neuronal survival varies somewhat with cause (Table 3.1), microscopic studies have revealed surviving spiral ganglion counts of 10% to 70% of the normal complement of 35,000 to 40,000 cells.

In general, retained neural elements are widely distributed through most regions of the cochlea except for the region of basal turn corresponding to severe high-frequency hearing loss (Hinojosa and Marion, 1983; Nadol, 1984). For example, neuronal survival is greatest in deafness induced by ototoxicity and least in cases of deafness from bacterial infections of the inner ear. In profound deafness, advanced age and longer duration of deafness are associated with smaller populations of retained nerve fibers (Nadol *et al.*, 1989).

The importance of the size of the spiral ganglion population is uncertain insofar as there is no clear relationship between the cause of deafness and success in speech recognition with a cochlear implant (Gantz *et al.*, 1988). Light microscopic evidence of spiral ganglion cell presence or spiral

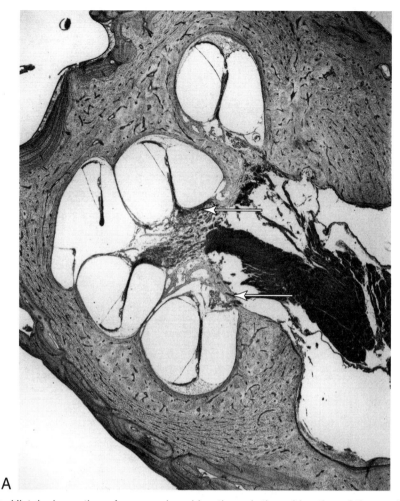

A

FIG. 3.2. A: Histologic section of a normal cochlea through the midportion of the modiolus (*i.e.*, mid-modiolar section) (hematoxylin and eosin stain, ×10).

ganglion nerve counts provide only limited assessment of auditory nerve functionality. Other attributes of the neuron, including the state of the peripheral processes, degree of myelinization, and the condition of the terminal axon, are not addressed by basic light microscopic evaluation of the temporal bone. Moreover, temporal bone microscopic evaluation provides no information regarding the integrity of the central auditory circuits.

The requisite number of residual, responsive neurons to effectively encode speech has been estimated in studies that correlate per-

formance on speech tests with neuronal reserves found on postmortem examination. Correlative studies indicate that approximately one-third to one-sixth of the neuronal population is necessary for socially useful speech recognition (Ylikoski and Savolainen, 1984). Kerr and Schuknecht (1968) suggested that neurons in the region of the upper basal and second turn (15 to 22 mm from the round window membrane) appear to provide the most support in enabling speech recognition. Otte *et al.* (1978) concluded that at least 10,000 spiral ganglion cells, with 3,000 or more in the apical 10 mm

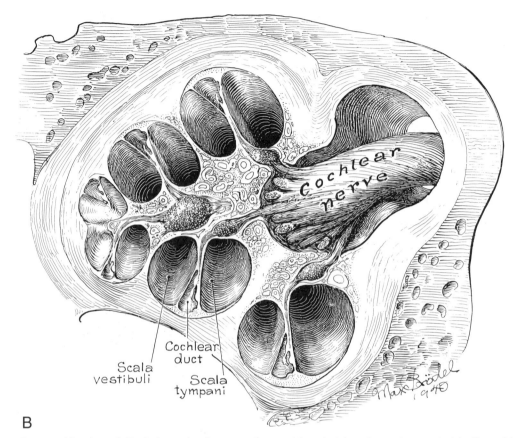

B

FIG. 3.2. *(Continued)* **B:** Schematic diagram of a cochlea that has been transected in the mid-modiolar plane, similar to the histologic section seen in **A**. Nerve cell bodies occupy Rosenthal's canal *(arrow)*, which lies between the cochlear nerve and the organ of Corti. (Courtesy of Max Brödel Archives, Johns Hopkins School of Medicine, Baltimore, MD.)

of the cochlea, were required for discrimination of speech to be preserved in cases of severe sensorineural hearing loss (with residual hair cell populations).

The minimal number of auditory neurons needed to facilitate speech recognition with a cochlear implant is less certain. However, the number probably is small, given observations of speech understanding in cases with only a modest number of residual neurons (*e.g.*, less than 10% of the normal complement of auditory neurons) from histologic studies of temporal bones after cochlear implants (Linthicum *et al.*, 1991; Fayad *et al.*, 1991).

Determining what stimulable neural elements most likely exist with each pathologic process is useful to know before cochlear implantation, and morphologic studies over a wider range of pathologies are needed to elucidate this issue more clearly. Much is unknown about the postimplant effects on the inner ear neural elements. The potential for further loss of neuronal elements within the cochlea after placement of the cochlear implant electrode exists. Placement of the cochlear implant electrode conventionally begins within the scala tympani through cochleostomy adjacent to the round window. During the course of advancing the electrode, the electrode takes the pathway of least resistance and lies against the most-lateral, outer bony cochlear wall within the scala tympani. In postmortem examination

TABLE 3.1. *Spiral ganglion cell counts in various pathologies*

Diagnosis	Ganglion cell counts	No. of temporal bones	Study
Labyrinthitis ossificans			
Meningogenic	6,310–28,977 (mean = 14,903)	7	Hinojosa *et al.*, 1992
	1,530–21,303 (mean = 12,906)	6	Nadol and Hsu, 1991
	21,700	1	Pollak and Felix, 1985
Tympanogenic	21,846–24,681 (mean = 22,859)	3	Hinojosa *et al.*, 1992
Otosclerosis	10,127–22,525 (mean = 15,400)	3	Hinojosa *et al.*, 1992
Wegener's	14,564–25,369 (mean = 19,967)	2	Hinojosa *et al.*, 1992
Infectious			
Bacterial labyrinthitis	11,968 ± 4,367	15	Nadol *et al.*, 1989
	0	1	Hinojosa and Marion, 1983
	22,125	1	Hinojosa and Marion, 1983
Postviral labyrinthitis	7,880 ± 5,760	13	Nadol *et al.*, 1989
	7,305	1	Hinojosa and Marion, 1983
	19,826	1	Hinojosa and Marion, 1983
Congenital rubella syndrome	13,127 ± 261	3	Nadol *et al.*, 1989
Congenital syphilis	5,733 ± 2,915	3	Nadol *et al.*, 1989
Sudden idiopathic deafness	21,844 ± 11,637	6	Nadol *et al.*, 1989
Meniere's disease	12,726 ± 3,080	2	Nadol *et al.*, 1989
	24,885	6	Otte *et al.*, 1978
Otosclerosis, presbycusis, or both	18,885 ± 4,612	5	Nadol *et al.*, 1989
Otosclerosis	25,695	18	Otte *et al.*, 1978
	10,127 and 13,139	2	Hinojosa and Marion, 1983
Presbycusis			
Neural	13,086	8	Otte *et al.*, 1978
Strial	26,667	18	Otte *et al.*, 1978
Unspecified	18,621	12	Otte *et al.*, 1978
	25,783	1	Hinojosa and Marion, 1983
Aminoglycoside toxicity			
Unspecified	21,628 ± 5,113	13	Nadol *et al.*, 1989
Neomycin	23,700	1	Pollak and Felix, 1985
Streptomycin	19,608	1	Hinojosa and Marion, 1983
Congenital or genetic forms			
Unspecified	11,197 ± 6,823	15	Nadol *et al.*, 1989
	9,738	1	Schmidt 1985
Mondini	9,200	1	Pollak and Felix, 1985
	16,055	1	Hinojosa and Marion, 1983
	7,677–16,110 (mean = 11,216)	5	Schmidt 1985
Scheibe	9,471 and 23,912	2	Hinojosa and Marion, 1983
Kearns-Sayre	10,849	1	Hinojosa and Marion, 1983
Alport's	18,687	1	Hinojosa and Marion, 1983
	22,914 and 22,347	2	Schmidt 1985
Usher's	18,171 and 21,870	2	Schmidt 1985
Rubella (congenital)	13,311	1	Schmidt 1985
DiGeorge's	19,035, 19,800, 30,753	3	Schmidt 1985
DiGeorge with Mondini	13,734	1	Schmidt 1985
Trisomy 22 with Mondini	13,572	1	Schmidt 1985
Down's syndrome	9,612	1	Schmidt 1985
Klippel-Feil	29,025	1	Schmidt 1985
Klippel-Feil with Mondini	27,414	1	Schmidt 1985
Other forms			
Temporal bone fracture			
Transverse	~28,000 and ~25,000	2	Marsh *et al.*, 1992
Unspecified	11,468 ± 9,152	4	Nadol *et al.*, 1989
Head trauma	13,110	1	Hinojosa and Marion, 1983
Temporal bone tumor or cerebellopontine angle tumor	17,620 ± 8,385	10	Nadol *et al.*, 1989
Paget's disease	18,117	1	Hinojosa and Marion, 1983
Normal values			
Adult	28,620	16	Otte *et al.*, 1978
Adult	29,802–39,520 (mean = 33,915)	12	Hinojosa and Marion, 1983
Adult—normal audiograms	29,802–38,352 (mean = 33,623)	16	Hinojosa *et al.*, 1985
Young	35,028	3	Otte *et al.*, 1978

of implanted temporal bones, the electrode has been found in this particular area, often disrupting the spiral ligament and basilar membrane by the shearing action of the electrode tip during electrode advancement (Kennedy, 1987; Welling *et al.*, 1993) (Fig. 3.3). The effect could further disrupt the organ of Corti and the dendritic processes emanating from the osseous spiral lamina, but the effect on the spiral ganglion is unknown. Deep cochlear implant electrode insertion, beyond 30 mm, has been attempted, resulting in injury no greater than that from the standard 20-mm insertions (Gstoettner *et al.*, 1997). However, when attempts have been made to pass the electrode farther than the first point where resistance is met, severe injury, such as osseous spiral lamina disruption, has occurred. This may influence the

survivability of the spiral ganglion cells located within the modiolus.

In a case report of an individual deafened by gentamicin therapy and implanted for a total of 10 weeks before dying of an unrelated cause, the spiral ganglion counts between the implanted and nonimplanted side did not differ significantly (Nadol *et al.*, 1994). Although this report may indicate that there are no acute postimplantation effects on the spiral ganglion counts, the long-term effects are unknown. In another case report involving histologic examination of a temporal bone implanted for 10 months, spiral ganglion counts were found to be the lowest in the basal turn compared with the nonimplanted side (Zappia *et al.*, 1991). The organ of Corti in the corresponding basal turn region was also the lowest. These low counts

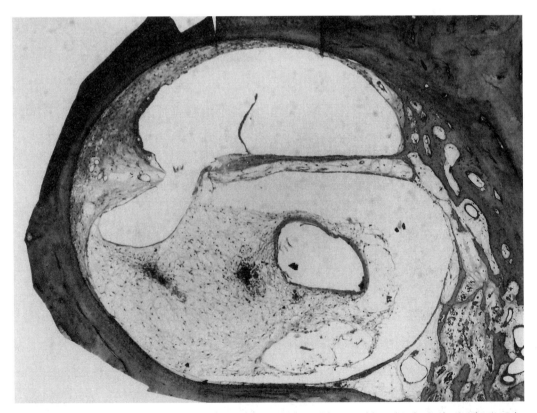

FIG. 3.3. Photomicrograph of the basal turn of a cochlea with a cochlear implant electrode tract in the scala tympani. Notice the disrupted basilar membrane (hematoxylin and eosin stain, ×75).

might have resulted from electrode insertion damage or an underlying pathology that led to deafness.

GENETIC HEARING LOSS

Hereditary hearing loss encompasses a wide diversity of hearing losses induced by genetic alterations or interactions of genetics and environment. There are many ways to view and classify hereditary hearing loss. Genetic hearing loss may be present at birth (congenital) or may manifest later in life (delayed). It can be progressive or nonprogressive, unilateral or bilateral. Syndromic forms of hearing loss refer to those in which other organ systems exhibit an abnormality of form or function in a recognizable pattern across generations. Heritable hearing loss may be classified by the pattern of inheritance. Autosomal dominant disorders are passed to one-half of the offspring in each generation at various levels of expression. Autosomal recessive disorders occur only when both parents carry a genetic abnormality that is not expressed until the gene pair is matched in an offspring. Sex-linked transmission yields a disorder as a result of genetic abnormality within a gender-determining chromosome (typically the X chromosome). A comprehensive discussion of the forms of hereditary hearing loss is beyond the scope of this text.

Approximately two-thirds of cases of hereditary hearing loss are nonsyndromic. A similar proportion of cases assume an autosomal recessive inheritance pattern (Grundfast and Josephson, 1997). Determining whether heredity plays a causative role in the hearing impairment relies on a detailed history (*e.g.*, onset and pattern of hearing loss, birth history, family history, related medical conditions) and accurate physical examination (*i.e.*, search for syndromic features). Syndromic features may range from the obvious to the very subtle to the casual examiner evaluating hearing loss. The key is to look for particular and common features. The options for aural rehabilitation for each patient depend on the severity of the disease and the surviving neural elements.

Autosomal dominant disorders typically reflect structural abnormalities that affect several organ systems. The more common types of hereditary sensorineural hearing loss associated with the autosomal dominant inheritance pattern include Waardenburg's syndrome, brachial-otorenal syndrome, Stickler's syndrome, Alport's disease, neurofibromatosis, and nonsyndromic, autosomal dominant, delayed-onset hereditary hearing impairment.

Waardenburg's syndrome includes characteristic physical features of white forelock, dystopia canthorum, heterochromia iridis, premature graying of the hair, vitiligo, and broad nasal root. Approximately 20% of individuals with Waardenburg's syndrome possess bilateral symmetric sensorineural hearing loss reflective of cochlear involvement. A person with type I Waardenburg syndrome possesses the classic physical features previously described, and this form is more common. Hearing loss occurs in about 58% of affected persons; it can be unilateral or bilateral, is usually nonprogressive, and can vary from mild to profound levels (Smith *et al.*, 1998). The less common type II form does not include dystopia canthorum. There is a greater incidence of hearing loss (51% to 77%) in this latter group of patients, who typically have progressive, bilateral, moderate to severe sensorineural hearing loss (Liu and Newton, 1995; Hildesheimer, 1989). Temporal bone studies from patients with Waardenburg's syndrome demonstrate variable degrees of atrophy of the organ of Corti, stria vascularis, and cochlear nerve (Fisch, 1959; Rarey and Davis, 1984; Ahmad *et al.*, 1991).

The brachial-otorenal syndrome, also known as the Melnick-Fraser syndrome, manifests with ear pits or tags, cervical fistulas, and varying degrees of renal dysplasia. Seventy-five percent of patients have significant hearing loss: sensorineural (20%), conductive (30%), or mixed (50%). The Mondini deformity has been reported to occur with this particular syndrome.

Stickler's syndrome (*i.e.*, Marshall-Stickler

syndrome or hereditary arthro-ophthalmopathy) includes micrognathia, myopia or detached retina, Robin sequence, hypermobile and enlarged joints, and a predisposition to develop arthritis. Sensorineural (high-frequency loss) or mixed hearing loss occurs in 15% of these patients. Genes responsible for this syndrome have been identified as the collagen genes *COL2A1* on chromosome 12 and *COL11A2* on chromosome 6 (Ahmad *et al.*, 1991; Brunner *et al.*, 1994).

Persons with types I, V, and VI of Alport's disease have the autosomal dominant inheritance pattern, and those with types II, III, and IV have the X-linked inheritance pattern. Patients with Alport's disease usually have some degree of renal impairment from nephritis. The gene for the X-linked type of Alport's disease has been linked to the *COL4A5* collagen gene. Hearing loss is typically progressive and sensorineural. Schmidt described preservation of the organ of Corti with spiral ganglion neuronal counts of approximating 20,000 in both ears in a patient with Alport's disease and mild to moderate symmetric sensorineural hearing loss (Schmidt, 1985). Other temporal bone studies have reported degeneration in the organ of Corti and cochlear neurons, with unidentified basophilic deposits in the stria vascularis (Fujita and Hayden, 1969; Mayers and Tyler, 1972; Johnsson and Arenberg, 1981).

The sensorineural hearing loss of neurofibromatosis originates from a central nervous system lesion, rather than a cochlear abnormality. Neurofibromatosis type I, also known as von Recklinghausen's disease, occurs at a frequency of 1 case per 3,000 members of the population. Patients usually demonstrate the characteristic features of café-au-lait spots and multiple fibroma tumors (*i.e.*, cutaneous, central or peripheral nervous system, or visceral). Acoustic neurofibromas occur in about 5%. Neurofibromatosis type II is a genetically distinct entity, with 95% of patients having bilateral acoustic neuromas. Attempts at aural rehabilitation for this latter form have mostly concentrated on the auditory brain stem

implant (Brackmann *et al.*, 1993) (see Chapter 10.)

Autosomal dominant, delayed-onset hearing loss usually progresses to severe or profound sensorineural hearing loss. This form is nonsyndromic and manifests at variable ages with variable patterns of progression. Different types of this entity have been described based on the type of hearing loss and audiometric configuration (Konigsmark and Gorlin, 1976). There is no common audiometric pattern or type of hearing loss. In temporal bone studies, degeneration of the peripheral auditory elements (*i.e.*, dendrites) have been described (Khetarpal *et al.*, 1991).

The spectrum of autosomal dominant structural malformations of the inner ear includes Mondini's and Michel's aplasia. These contrast with Scheibe's dysplasia (*i.e.*, cochleosaccular dysplasia), which is typically inherited in an autosomal recessive pattern but was reported in one case with autosomal dominant inheritance to have near-normal spiral ganglion populations, although with a degenerated organ of Corti (Nadol and Burgess, 1982). Michel's aplasia is the most severe, and it represents complete agenesis of the petrous temporal bone. The presence of this condition is a contraindication for cochlear implantation. Deformities in Mondini's aplasia include absent interscalar septum in the upper cochlear coils while maintaining a developed basal coil (Fig. 3.4). This deformity may be unilateral or bilateral and may coexist with Pendred's, Waardenburg's, Treacher Collins, and Wildervaank's syndromes.

The number of surviving neural elements in Mondini's aplasia depend on the severity of the deformity (Fig. 3.5). In Schmidt's report (1985) examining spiral ganglion counts in eight temporal bones with the Mondini's deformity, the number of neurons was smallest in cases that appeared most severe. Nevertheless, satisfactory experience with implantation of intracochlear prosthesis in patients with the Mondini's deformity is reported (Suzuki *et al.*, 1998; Turrini *et al.*, 1997; Silverstein *et al.*, 1988). The potential for a

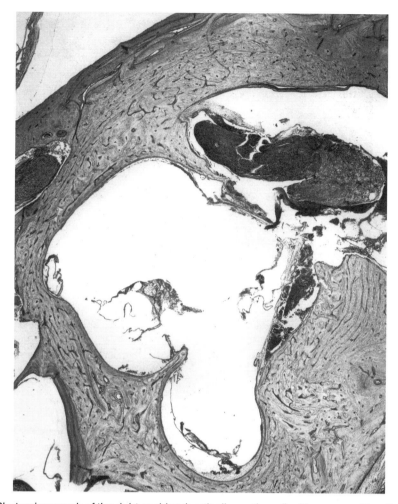

FIG. 3.4. Photomicrograph of the right cochlea (vertically sectioned) with a severe Mondini deformity. The largest space is the common cochlear cavity without any interscalar septa. The auditory nerve root appears in the superior aspect of the cavity (hematoxylin and eosin stain, ×20).

perilymphatic gusher resulting from a widely patent cochlear aqueduct has been raised during cochlear implantation, which may present a problem with persistent cerebrospinal fluid leak (Nadol, 1984).

A condition related to the Mondini's deformity is the large vestibular aqueduct syndrome (LVAS), first clinically described by Valvassori and Clemis (1978) purely as a radiologic finding (see Chapter 9). In this report, the condition was found with other anomalies of the labyrinth, and LVAS was initially believed to be part of the spectrum

of inner ear dysplasias. Its occurrence as an isolated finding with its separate constituency of clinical symptoms led to the recognition as its own syndrome (Levenson et al., 1989). A genetic pattern for its inheritance (autosomal recessive or X-linked) has been suggested (Griffith et al., 1996). The clinical features include progressive, bilateral sensorineural hearing loss with various levels of severity. The anomaly is found bilaterally twice as often as unilaterally. In one study of 17 patients with LVAS, Jackler and De La Cruz (1989) reported normal hearing was

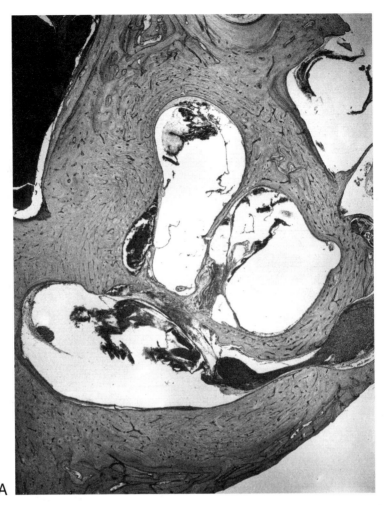

A

FIG. 3.5. A: Photomicrograph of a right cochlea with a Mondini deformity, demonstrating $1\frac{1}{4}$ basal turn of the cochlea (hematoxylin and eosin stain, ×20). **B:** Photomicrograph of the residual neural elements within the primitive Rosenthal canal, demonstrating scant spiral ganglion cells. In this high-power view of the temporal bone seen in **A**, the arrow demarcates myelinated axonal fibers (hematoxylin and eosin stain, ×150).

found in 4% and profound hearing loss in 39%, with progression of hearing loss in 65% of the patients over a follow-up period of 7.3 years. The most common audiometric configuration was a downsloping shape. In another study, 46% of the patients demonstrated progression of the hearing loss (Arcand *et al.*, 1991). Experience with cochlear implantation in two patients with LVAS brought attention to the common finding of a slight perilymphatic gusher that did not present a problem during electrode insertion (Aschendorff *et al.*, 1997).

Relatively commonly encountered autosomal recessive types of hereditary sensorineural hearing loss include Pendred's syndrome, Jervell and Lange-Nielsen syndrome, and Usher's syndrome. Less common types responsible for sensorineural hearing loss include Hurler's disease, Hunter's syndrome, Klippel-Feil syndrome, and Refsum's disease.

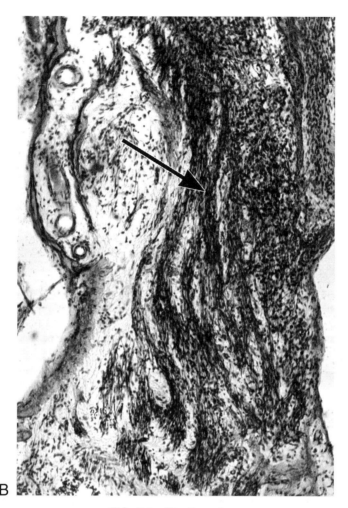

B

FIG. 3.5. *(Continued)*

Pendred's syndrome occurs at a frequency of about 1 case per 50,000 persons. It is characterized by a defect in iodine metabolism. The hearing loss typically lies in the high frequencies and is usually severe to profound in more than 50% of cases. The hearing loss may be progressive in 15% to 20% of affected persons. The Mondini malformation was identified in six temporal bones from five patients with Pendred's syndrome (Hvedberg-Hansen and Jorgensen, 1968).

Jervell and Lange-Nielsen syndrome features cardiac conduction defect and severe congenital sensorineural hearing loss. Histopathologic studies reveal atrophy of the organ of Corti and spiral ganglion and demonstrate periodic acid–Schiff–staining deposits in the stria vascularis region (Briedmann *et al.*, 1966).

Usher's syndrome occurs at a prevalence of approximately 3 cases per 100,000 persons. It may be associated with retinitis pigmentosa. Of the patients with retinitis pigmentosa, 10% develop sensorineural hearing loss. Hearing loss is typically bilateral, congenital, and sensorineural. Type I is characterized by congenital bilateral profound hearing loss with absent vestibular function, and type II (less common) is characterized by moderate to severe hearing loss and normal vestibular function. There occasionally may be bilateral, progressive sensorineural hearing loss associated with type II. As with the Mondini deformity, attempts at cochlear implantation have been made, demonstrating overall benefit (Young *et al.*, 1995; Hinderlink *et al.*, 1994).

An autosomally recessive, nonsyndromic cause of hearing loss has been linked to mutations in the connexin-26 gene *DFNB1* locus on chromosome 13q12, which encodes for the gap-junction protein (Kelsell *et al.*, 1997; Liu *et al.*, 1997; Estivill *et al.*, 1998). This one type of inheritance pattern represents the largest constituency of genetic hearing loss and is probably the least understood. In this one group, it is often difficult to identify the specific causes of hearing loss and which family members may be carriers for the affected gene, if that particular gene is known. Patients possessing a mutation in the connexin-26 gene have an abnormal gap junction protein, which has been localized in the murine inner ear stria vascularis, basement membrane, limbus, and spiral prominence (Kelsell *et al.*, 1997). Because gap junctions are responsible for ion exchange, defective gap junctions can disrupt the strictly maintained ionic environment in the cochlea, leading to hearing loss. The hearing loss in patients who possess this defect is profound or predominantly high-frequency hearing loss (Kelsell *et al.*, 1997; Liu *et al.*, 1997).

The more common causes of heredity sensorineural hearing loss with a sex-linked inheritance pattern include Norrie's syndrome and Wildervaank's syndrome. The hearing loss in Norrie's syndrome is progressive, with onset in the second to third decade of life. A mixed or sensorineural hearing loss may be found in Wildervaank's syndrome. The Mondini deformity can coexist with Wildervaank's syndrome.

AGING

Presbycusis comprises the summed effects of the aging process on the ear and hearing and may involve the tissues of the inner ear and auditory nerve and the the central auditory pathway. Most often, the organ of Corti and the stria vascularis show the greatest changes. The hearing loss is typically sensorineural and slow to evolve. Schuknecht (1964, 1974) postulated four basic types of presbycusis:

1. *Sensory*, in which the hair cells of the organ of Corti degenerate first
2. Neural, in which the cochlear neurons degenerate first
3. Strial or *metabolic*, with associated with atrophy of the stria vascularis
4. Inner ear conductive or *mechanical*, with thickening of the basilar membrane

From our own observations and those of others (Johnsson and Hawkins, 1972; Johnsson, 1974), it is clear that individual types of presbycusis are seldom seen in isolation. Most ears have mild to complete degeneration of the organ of Corti in the lower basal turn and mild degeneration of some auditory nerve fibers in the osseous spiral lamina. There is considerable individual variation, but in general, advancing age is associated with more extensive loss of sensory cells and supporting structures. As Schuknecht pointed out, strial degeneration is more often present in the upper turns and unaccompanied by hair cell loss in the basal turn. The inner ear conductive type of pathology is rare. Nomura (1970) described lipidosis of the basilar membrane in aging cochleas, and Nadol (1979) reported that the basilar membrane can be thickened at its basal end, but there was also loss of Corti's organ in the same region, so that the case for isolated forms of the inner ear conductive type of loss is not strong.

The material examined by Bredberg (1968) is exemplary. Material from donors older than 60 years of age revealed various degrees of presbycusis, often exaggerated when there was a history of noise exposure. The inner ears of one 73-year-old man with no history of noise exposure showed an almost complete degeneration of organ of Corti and nerve fiber loss in the lower half of the basal turn. He had a low-frequency loss of 35 dB at 500 Hz and a virtually complete loss of hearing above 3 kHz.

In the temporal bones of 17 patients with the spontaneous and gradually progressive bilateral hearing loss that is characteristic of presbycusis, Suga and Lindsay (1976) found evidence of variable degeneration of the spiral ganglion cells of the auditory nerve. Despite neural degeneration and a diffuse loss of sensory cells, the general form of the organ of Corti as seen in their celloidin sections was well preserved. The loss of spiral ganglion cells, although never complete, extended throughout the cochlea in several cases. These findings appear to be exceptional and differ significantly from those of Bredberg (1968) and of Johnsson and Hawkins (1972).

Well-coordinated studies of temporal bone pathology and auditory brain stem pathology are needed to close the gaps in our understanding of human presbycusis, because aging appears to be associated with subtle but measurable changes in the central auditory pathway. Although candidacy for cochlear implantation may be questioned on the basis of extensive degeneration of the auditory nerve in neural presbycusis, evidence of an absence of neural responsiveness in individuals with extensive presbycusis is lacking. As a group, individuals older than 65 years demonstrated characteristics of cochlear implant use that were similar to those of younger adult populations and favorably rated their cochlear implant use as an improvement in their overall quality of life (Horn *et al.*, 1991).

NOISE

Noise, in a variety of modern forms, is generally regarded as the second most common cause of all levels of hearing impairment. Noise-induced hearing loss results from noise sustained over long periods and from a single exposure (*i.e.*, acoustic trauma). The duration and the intensity of the sound are important factors. Guidelines based on the duration of exposure and sound intensity have been established to help reduce the incidence of noise-induced hearing loss at the workplace as a result of the awareness of the consequences of noise.

Patients who are evaluated for hearing loss may or may not volunteer the information regarding previous noise exposure. It is important to include this in routine history taking. The degree of hearing impairment usually depends on the characteristics of noise intensity and duration. Rarely does noise-induced hearing loss alone produce the profound level of hearing loss. Contributions from other processes that lead to hearing loss, such as presbycusis, should be taken into account. The hearing loss is typically bilateral, reflecting equivalent exposure to both ears at the same time and in the same manner. Unilateral hearing loss occurs if there is an unusual reason for preferential exposure or protection of one ear over the other, such as the long-barreled firearm that offers the right-handed shooter preferential protection by the right shoulder to the right ear. The hearing loss is stable and nonprogressive after the sound stimulus is halted. The audiometric configuration is characteristic, with a 4-kHz notch in the air conduction thresholds.

Temporary threshold shifts (TTS) and permanent threshold shifts (PTS) occur in response to acoustic trauma. TTS and PTS differences typically reflect the duration of noise exposure. Shorter exposures correlate with shorter threshold shifts. TTS often occurs in subjects exposed to pure tone stimuli greater than 110 dB for even short periods, and they demonstrate transient high-frequency hearing loss (Davis *et al.*, 1950). However, noise level beyond moderate intensities probably exerts a more permanent effect.

The effects of acoustic trauma on the ear have been extensively studied in a wide range of experimental animals and in temporal bones from patients with known history of noise exposure. Lurie *et al.* (1944) showed that the initial effect of intense pure tones on the cochlea of the guinea pig was hair cell loss, which could be followed by secondary degeneration of auditory nerve fibers, suggesting a retrograde neuronal degeneration pattern. Bredberg (1965) and Johnsson and Hawkins (1976) examined specimens that came from noise-exposed patients and evaluated the condition of the spiral ganglion cells and that of the organ of Corti and auditory nerve fibers. Neuronal cell bodies were preserved throughout the cochlea, except in the lower basal turn, where the organ of Corti and nerve fibers were missing. Igarashi *et al.* (1964) examined the temporal bones from three patients with losses of hair cells in the 5- to 13-mm region of Corti's organ. Two of them had a history of occupational or military noise exposure, and the other had a head injury as the result of a fall. Their audiograms had the typical high-frequency loss, centered at about 4 kHz. In all three cases, the neuronal cell body counts were recorded as normal. Egami *et al.* demonstrated loss of the organ of Corti, in the basal and middle cochlear turns in an individual with bilateral profound hearing loss with the exception of an audible 90-dB threshold at 250 Hz on the right (Egami *et al.*, 1978). There was a corresponding decrease in the dendritic fibers but with remaining spiral ganglion cells in the apical area.

In one of the larger human temporal bone studies with audiometric information available, McGill and Schuknecht (1976) identified hair cell loss in the 9- to 13-mm region of the cochlear duct (*i.e.*, basal turn). There was good correlation between increased auditory thresholds at the permanent threshold shift and loss of hair cells at the corresponding spatial area of the tonotopically arranged cochlea. There was greater degree of outer hair cell loss than inner hair cell loss.

The histopathologic findings of noise-induced hearing loss seem to point to degenerative changes centered on the organ of Corti at the basal turn of the cochlea. These changes occur at the level of the hair cells with variable patterns of spiral ganglion survival with severe depletion of neurons only in the basal-most aspect of the cochlea in the area serving the very high frequencies.

OTOTOXICITY

Identification of the cause of hearing loss resulting from the ototoxic effects of medication requires astute observation, careful review of the medical history, and an awareness of the more common, potential inciting agents. Each class of ototoxic agent is unique in its chemical structure, with its own propensity to attack different areas within the cochlea. Sometimes, the mere systemic presence of the medication is not enough to cause harm, but other factors may play a role in creating an ototoxic picture, including the body's ability to metabolize and clear the medication effectively. Patient's with impaired renal and hepatic function may have higher serum drug levels than normal (*i.e.*, longer drug half-life), and the usual dosing may create dangerously high serum levels of the drug. Particular attention must be paid to periodically checking serum drug levels during the course of therapy. Another factor is the patient's preexisting hearing loss. There may be prior cochlear injury from an unrelated process (*e.g.*, presbycusis) that may leave a minimal susceptible neural population. Exposure to the potentially ototoxic drug may destroy the remaining neural elements at doses typically not ototoxic to the normal individual.

Attempts have been made to identify early-onset cochleotoxic effects using high-frequency audiometric testing (>8 kHz) so that the serious consequences may be circumvented (Fausti *et al.*, 1994, 1998). The high frequencies, corresponding to neural injury in the basal cochlear turn, are usually affected first. However, this type of monitoring is not widespread.

Aminoglycosides

The pathologic changes in the inner ear that can be brought about by aminoglycoside antibiotics and other ototoxic agents have been extensively examined in laboratory animals.

Moreover, a sufficient number of human temporal bones from patients with ototoxic hearing loss have been examined to indicate that these drugs induce essentially similar changes in man. Our knowledge about the pathology of ototoxic deafness is probably at least as firmly established as that for any form of hearing impairment. Animals deafened by ototoxic drugs have been used as experimental models for studying the effects of cochlear implantation and of electrical stimulation of the auditory nerve (Duckert and Miller, 1984; Leake-Jones and Vivion, 1979).

Striking changes in the tissues of the inner ear are produced by the ototoxic action of the aminoglycosides, especially in the organ of Corti and in the end organs of the vestibular system. Injury to hair cells of the inner ear often include degeneration and disappearance of sensory and supporting cells. The organ of Corti in the lower basal coil is first affected, and injury progresses toward the apical coil with continued administration of the antibiotic. Outer hair cells are first affected, with inner hair cells affected by larger and prolonged doses. In the guinea pig, vigorous and prolonged treatment with amikacin can destroy Corti's organ completely, as shown by Cazals *et al.* (1979). The ototoxic action of streptomycin is exerted largely on the vestibular neuroepithelia, whereas that of neomycin, kanamycin, or amikacin is generally confined to the cochlea. Gentamicin and tobramycin tend to injure the cochlear and the vestibular neuroepithelia.

It appears that ototoxic degeneration of the distal portion of the peripheral processes (*i.e.*, distal processes) of the cochlear neurons can occur without necessarily involving the cell bodies of auditory neurons. Cell bodies that can remain for long periods, as suggested by the observations of Ylikoski and Savolainen (1984) of human material. Koitchev *et al.* (1981) showed that massive treatment with amikacin destroys the organ of Corti and leads to a loss of 30% to 55% of the spiral ganglion cells within a month after

treatment and up to 85% within 1 year. The relatively rapid disappearance of so many of these cells suggests that massive levels of the antibiotic may be capable of exerting its ototoxic effect directly on the ganglion. This pattern of wholesale destruction is presumably unseen in clinical experience, because every effort is made to maintain blood levels of aminoglycosides at levels necessary for effective antimicrobial effects.

Among Nadol's case series, there was one 27-year-old woman with profound hearing loss as a result of kanamycin treatment. After her death 3 months later, a complete loss of hair cells was seen in one ear and a 90% loss in the other, but neuronal cell body counts appeared normal in both ears. The ears of a 53-year-old woman, who had developed a profound hearing loss after prolonged treatment with neomycin administered orally, showed loss of about one-half of the spiral ganglion cells from the basal and middle cochlear turns.

Lowry *et al.* (1973) examined the temporal bones of a 57 year-old woman who had become totally deaf and had died in renal failure on the 17th day after receiving a single dose of 8 g of neomycin intramuscularly. They found a marked loss of inner and outer hair cells, but they considered the count of neuronal cell bodies normal for the patient's age.

Otte *et al.* (1978) found excellent ganglia in both ears of a patient who had become profoundly deaf from kanamycin treatment. In the left ear of a 12 year-old boy who had been deafened by intraperitoneal neomycin, Bergstrom *et al.* (1973) observed hair cell loss, especially in the basal turn, but the auditory nerve fiber reserves appeared normal.

In a review of human cochlear pathology in hearing impairment caused by aminoglycosides, Huizing and deGroot (1987) recorded that the hair cells and the ganglion cells were affected in 8 of the 15 cases studied by serial sectioning of the temporal bone. In the other seven, hair cells were missing, but the ganglion cells appeared to be intact. The reason for this difference between the two groups is unknown. However, there appears to be good reason to expect that, in patients with aminoglycoside-induced deafness, cells of the spiral ganglion have survived and are available for stimulation by a cochlear implant. The same cannot be said for the peripheral processes in the osseous spiral lamina, which may be absent in most of the basal turn.

Loop Diuretics

The loop diuretics, of which furosemide is the typical example, have an acute but usually short-lived ototoxic action that can cause a short-term deafness as a result of their effect on the ion transport system of the stria vascularis (Hawkins, 1976). Occasionally, when large doses have been given as a bolus injection intravenously, the hearing impairment has been permanent (Quick and Hoppe, 1975), but the ears of such patients seem not to have been examined postmortem. When a patient receiving an aminoglycoside is also given a loop diuretic, the effects on the ear appear to be additive.

Cisplatin

The ototoxic action of the antineoplastic agent cisplatin has been studied in animal experiments by a number of investigators. Effects on the ear resemble those of the aminoglycosides, with hair cell loss beginning in the lower basal turn and changes observed in the stria vascularis (Nakai *et al.*, 1982; Schweitzer *et al.*, 1984). Hearing loss, especially for the high frequencies, is well recognized in cancer patients receiving cisplatin, and a few human temporal bones have been examined (Schaefer *et al.*, 1985; Wright and Schaefer, 1982; Strauss *et al.*, 1983). Strauss *et al.* (1983) assessed the temporal bones of a 9-year old boy who had developed a moderately severe sensorineural loss for frequencies above 700 Hz and had died 4 weeks after cisplatin therapy. Both ears showed extensive loss of cochlear hair cells, and but the loss of cells of the spiral ganglion was restricted to the basal turn. In clinical use, the severity of the ototoxic action of cisplatin correlates with the dose and duration of treatment and with concurrent use of aminoglycosides and diuretics. It appears, however, that these hearing losses are seldom severe enough to warrant a cochlear implant, even when the patient's long-term prognosis may otherwise be good.

INFECTIOUS DISEASES

Infectious diseases constitute an important cause of deafness in children, whether contracted *in utero*, prenatally, or postnatally. The deafness acquired *in utero* from *maternal rubella* is well known, and its underlying pathology has been studied by several investigators (Tondury, 1951; Nager, 1952; Lindsay *et al.*, 1953; Ward *et al.*, 1968; Bordley *et al.*, 1968; Hemenway *et al.*, 1969). The developing ear, like the eye and the heart, is most susceptible in the first trimester and especially during the eighth to ninth week of pregnancy. These effects usually manifest as congenital cataracts, deafness, and congenital heart defects, known as the rubella triad. The tissue primarily affected appears to be the stria vascularis (Fig. 3.6), with secondary effects throughout the cochlea. There is a reduced formation of endolymph, causing Reissner's membrane and the wall of the saccule to be partly collapsed. Most of the changes occur within the cochlea and saccular, a pattern resembling the changes occurring in Scheibe's cochleosaccular aplasia. Various degrees of hair cell loss are found, but there is little interference with the development of the peripheral neurons. There is general agreement that the spiral ganglion is normal or degenerates only in the lower basal turn. The histologic presentation of congenital rubella in the temporal bone is the same as for postnatal acquisition, differentiated only by the absence of the other developmental abnormalities seen in the prenatal form (Linthicum, 1978).

With *mumps*, the deafness is most likely to be unilateral and may go undetected without audiologic testing. The common presenta-

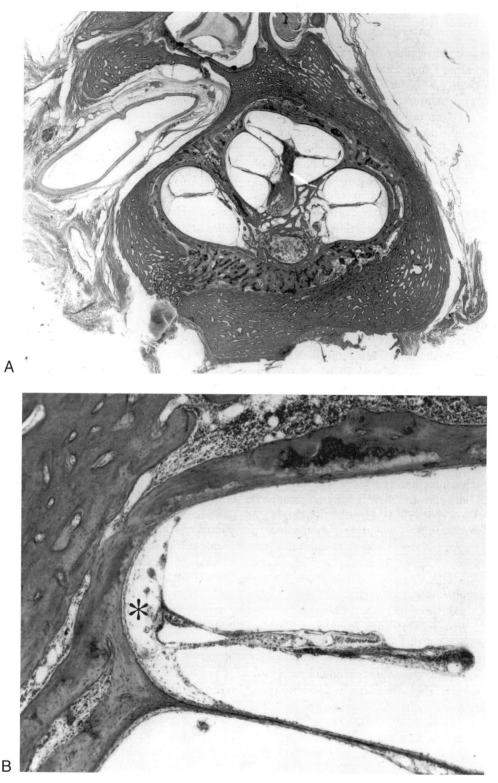

FIG. 3.6. A: Photomicrograph of a cochlea with congenital rubella infection. Notice the strial atrophy (hematoxylin and eosin, ×10). **B:** The photomicrograph demonstrates the characteristic strial atrophy of a cochlea affected with congenital rubella infection. The asterisk demarcates the area of strial atrophy representing vascular degeneration (hematoxylin and eosin stain, ×75).

tion is usually failure of a school audiogram, suggesting a unilateral hearing loss in a patient with past history of the mumps. Lindsay (1973) presented a case of bilateral mumps deafness in a boy 6 years old who had contracted the disease at 28 months. His temporal bone showed strial atrophy and hair cell loss in the basal and lower middle turns of the cochlea. The spiral ganglion and nerve fibers appeared normal in the upper turns but were fewer in the basal turn. Overall, the changes occur mainly in the cochlear duct with mild to moderate secondary degeneration of the cochlear neurons (Lindsay, 1973)

Measles is often associated with otitis media (Lindsay, 1973), but the virus can also affect the inner ear. It is a common cause of acquired profound hearing loss in children. Lindsay described its effects in a 3-month-old infant who died a few months later. The stria vascularis and organ of Corti were completely degenerated in the basal coil and in the lower half of the middle coil, although only partly so closer to the apex. The number of ganglion cells and nerve fibers was reduced in the basal coil but normal at higher levels. In the attempts to mimic an active measles infection, the virus was inoculated into hamsters and their inner ears examined (Fukuda *et al.*, 1994). Histologic changes included atrophy of the stria vascularis, loss of the organ of Corti, tectorial membranes that were rolled up, and presence of viral antigen identified by immunofluorescence in the endolymphatic compartment of the scala media (*i.e.*, endolymphatic labyrinthitis).

Hearing loss resulting from *bacterial meningitis* is a well-known complication. It affects 5% to 33% of the patients who are afflicted with this severe infection of the meninges. The source of the infection may take origin from various areas of the body, which disseminates and localizes in the central nervous system. The cause of hearing loss is purportedly spread of the bacterial infection to the inner ear through several routes: through the internal auditory canal, by hematogenous spread, or by means of the cochlear aqueduct (Bhatt *et al.*, 1991; Mer-

chant and Gopen, 1996; Dubs *et al.*, 1999). The result is labyrinthitis (Fig. 3.7), severe neural degeneration within the cochlea, and an inflammatory response leading to labyrinthitis ossificans (*i.e.*, new intracochlear bone formation). The common responsible microorganisms are *Haemophilus influenzae*, *Streptococcus pneumoniae,* and *Neisseria meningitidis*. The onset of the hearing loss after the acute bout of meningitis is unknown. However, in rabbit experiments with intrathecal inoculation of *Streptococcus,* hearing loss was detected as soon as 48 hours after infection (Bhatt *et al.*, 1991). Delayed progressive hearing loss or reversible hearing loss are uncommon. There is no predisposition for hearing loss in the high or low frequencies, but the level of hearing loss is usually severe and permanent, occurring in one or both ears (Berlow *et al.*, 1980).

Nerve injury in the setting of bacterial meningitis has historically been described as severe, with low spiral ganglion counts in temporal bone studies (Otte *et al.*, 1978; Nadol *et al.*, 1989; Kerr and Schuknecht, 1968). The appearance of new bone formation within the cochlea provides an additional factor that contributes to neural injury: *labyrinthine ossificans*. This process is not unique to meningitis. It may also be found in otosclerosis or in any situation of trauma to the cochlea. The common denominator is any stimulus for new bone growth within the cochlea (Kotzias and Linthicum, 1985). Studies have demonstrated that the amount of spiral ganglion cells in postmeningitic temporal bones correlates well with the severity of new bone formation in the inner ear (Nadol and Hsu, 1991; Lu and Schuknecht 1994; Nadol, 1997). Not all cases with bony occlusion have poor spiral ganglion counts; one study reported significant numbers present in the middle of severe bony occlusion in a minority of the cases (Nadol, 1997). In that same study looking at labyrinthine ossificans, there was never a total absence of spiral ganglion cells.

Hinojosa *et al.* (1991) noticed a correlation with the location of neo-ossification to loss of organ of Corti in the corresponding region

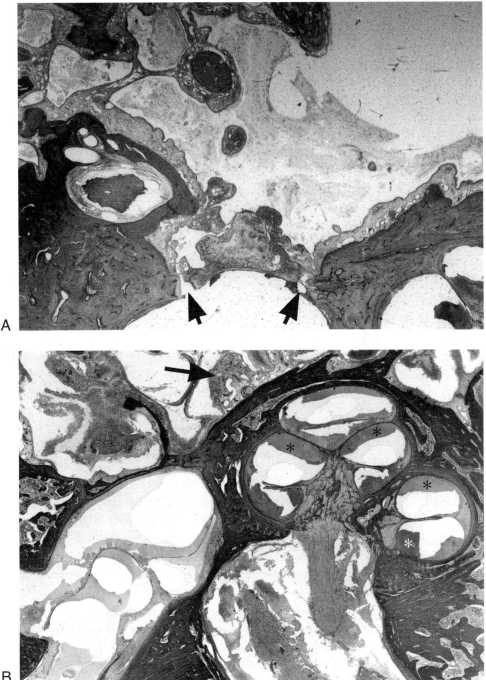

FIG. 3.7. A: Photomicrograph of otitis media that extended into the labyrinth through the oval window and subsequently developed into labyrinthitis. Notice the breach in the oval window annular ligament that creates an avenue for entry into the labyrinth *(arrows)* (hematoxylin and eosin stain, ×17). **B:** Photomicrograph of purulent inflammatory infiltrate within perilymphatic spaces of the cochlea. Extension of this infection led to meningitis. The arrow demarcates middle ear purulence, and the asterisk indicates otitis interna (hematoxylin and eosin stain, ×14).

but not with spiral ganglion loss. This finding may suggest that the ossification process is limited to the perilymphatic spaces but not Rosenthal's canal. Nevertheless, the process of labyrinthine ossificans appears to be most marked in the basal turn in the scala tympani.

Lindsay (1973) showed remarkable examples of bony cochlear changes that could potentially defeat the otologist's effort to implant an intracochlear prosthesis. There was a striking absence of ganglion cells in Rosenthal's canal in several of his specimens. If it would have been possible to insert an intracochlear prosthesis into the labyrinth, there would have been little or nothing to stimulate. This finding underlies the importance of the preoperative determination of cochlear anatomy and electrical responsivity in implant candidates with a history of meningitis. The implications of labyrinthine ossificans and cochlear implantation are further discussed in the Otosclerosis section.

Syphilis in its acquired or congenital form can cause hearing loss and deafness. In the acquired form, auditory symptoms may occur in the secondary or the tertiary stages. The temporal bones may show an extensive osteitis (Goodhill, 1939). In the first intracochlear prosthesis case to come to autopsy (Johnsson *et al.*, 1979), acquired syphilis was the cause of the patient's deafness, and the temporal bones showed extensive changes attributable in large part to the disease.

Although Schuknecht (1974) states that the pattern of cochlear involvement is not consistent from patient to patient, it is interesting that the one case he presented had the unusual combination of progressive degeneration of cochlear neurons beginning at the apex with apparently good preservation of the organ of Corti. In congenital syphilis, attacks resembling those characteristic of Meniere's disease are associated with endolymphatic hydrops; distension of the cochlear duct is obvious at autopsy. Atrophy of the spiral ligament and basilar membrane is accompanied by progressive degeneration of the organ of Corti and the cochlear neurons.

The extent to which *otitis media* can be held responsible for sensorineural hearing loss seems to be relatively slight, although Paparella *et al.* (1972) have made a strong case for some degree of association between the two. Subsequent studies have reported this phenomenon (Aviel and Ostefeld, 1982; Walby *et al.*, 1983; Paparella *et al.*, 1984). In children, bacterial toxins from an infection in the middle ear can cross the membrane of the round window and cause degeneration of hair cells in the lower portion of the basal turn. Histologic evidence of this was provided by Schachern *et al.* (1992). When streptococcal bacteria was placed in the guinea pig middle ear, the bacteria was found within the round window membrane and in the perilymphatic spaces. The resulting hearing loss is most likely to be restricted to the highest frequencies, and the patient may be unaware of it if the hearing loss is minimal.

Otitis interna in the form of suppurative labyrinthitis (Paparella and Sugiura, 1967) is one form of infectious disease of the ear in which degeneration of sensory structures within the cochlea may be extensive. Otitis interna may result from chronic otitis media and the entrance of bacteria into the inner ear through the round window or after erosion of the otic capsule by a cholesteatoma. Fortunately, with the widespread use of effective antibiotic treatment, this entity is rarely reported. Whether of tympanogenic or of meningogenic origin, suppurative labyrinthitis is an otologic emergency that can lead to destruction of the inner ear and replacement of fluid-filled spaces by newly formed bone (*i.e.*, labyrinthitis ossificans). These bony and neural changes can represent a significant challenge to successful cochlear implantation (Nadol, 1984) and require extended approaches to create a bony channel to accommodate the electrode carrier, as discussed previously.

OTOSCLEROSIS

Clinical otosclerosis manifests with gradually progressive hearing loss. The hearing loss is unilateral or bilateral and typically presents during the second decade of life. The diagnosis of otosclerosis is made almost twice as often in women than men. A family history of hearing loss may be elicited. On tuning fork examination or audiometry, a conductive hearing loss is revealed. The Carhart notch, which is an increase in bone conduction threshold most marked at 2 kHz, may be evident on the audiogram. Normal otoscopic findings are the rule, with the rare exception of Schwarze's sign, a reddish blush seen through the tympanic membrane in the area corresponding to an active otosclerotic focus of hypervascular bone on the promontory. If a component of sensorineural hearing loss is coincidentally found with the conductive loss, this may herald cochlear involvement by the otosclerosis.

Otosclerosis represents a bony disorder involving endochondral bone of the otic and labyrinthine capsule. In comparison, it is not found in bone that undergoes intramembranous sequence of development, such as long bones in the extremities. It is produced by a cycle of bony resorption and inflammation that is followed by a reparative response. It is unclear what initiates the bone resorption, but light microscopic features of this early stage typically include multinucleated osteoclasts and dilated vascular channels with increased perivascular spaces. New bone is then laid down in a disorganized manner by fibroblasts, imparting a woven bone appearance, which is the active otosclerotic lesion, sometimes known as otospongiosis. Replacement bone is abundant in gelatinous ground substance but lacks proper calcification. Ultimately, a more mature form of bone develops after remodeling occurs, and the end result of this cycle is bone that contains few osteocytes and small blood vessels and gives an appearance of a more compact lamellar bone (*i.e.*, inactive otosclerotic lesion).

Otosclerosis is most active in the area of the oval window at the annular ligament and footplate area, specifically at the fissula ante fenestram. This translates into fixation of the stapes, resulting in the characteristic conductive hearing loss. Bipolar fixation of the stapes may also occur with the additional involvement at the fossula post fenestram. More extensive involvement includes the entire footplate and may lead to "obliterative otosclerosis."

Treatment of otosclerosis is primarily surgical. Among the greatest triumphs of otologic surgery has been the restoration of useful hearing to patients with a severe conductive hearing loss as a result of otosclerotic fixation of the stapes. The first success came with Lempert's single-stage fenestration operation. An opening into the horizontal semicircular canal was created and covered with an external auditory canal skin flap so that the fluid wave, generated from sound stimulus, could be transmitted into the labyrinth through the fenestration site, bypassing the oval window with a fixed stapes. Rosen's stapes mobilization followed almost a decade later. Although this surgery showed much initial promise, refixation of the stapes led to the development of other techniques. These procedures represent various modifications of the stapedectomy, originally attempted by Blake and others late in the 19th century and then abandoned for more than 50 years, until revived by John Shea. Contemporary surgical treatment revolves around stapedotomy or stapedectomy, with placement of a stapes prosthesis to transmit sound energy to the underlying labyrinth.

Despite intense clinical interest and detailed scrutiny of temporal bone material for more than 100 years, the cause and nature of the otosclerotic process are still not fully understood, chiefly because no appropriate animal model has been discovered or devised. Otosclerosis may be of viral origin, though genetically modified, and occurs only in humans.

The existence of histologic otosclerosis (*i.e.*, otosclerotic foci within the otic capsule that have not affected the stapes or caused any elevation of auditory thresholds) has been known for more than 40 years (Guild, 1944). The spongiotic process can spread over and throughout the otic capsule (Fig.

3.8), and it can invade the inner ear, create new bone growth, and cause a severe sensorineural hearing loss. It is this population that eventually become candidates for cochlear implantation when they receive no benefit from surgery or amplification from conventional hearing aids. About one-fifth of the patients receiving cochlear implants before 1983 at one center had otosclerosis as the cause of their hearing loss (Fayad *et al.*, 1990). Some investigators have claimed that this endocochlear bony growth process can occur without stapes involvement, but the evidence for the existence of purely cochlear forms of otosclerosis is not convincing (Schuknecht, 1974).

Otosclerotic invasion can substantially alter the internal architecture of the cochlea (Johnsson *et al.*, 1978, 1982). When the anterior focus expands from the oval window toward the apex, it can affect the endosteal lining of the cochlea, particularly within the scala tympani of the middle cochlear turn. The focus can bulge into scala tympani, par-tially blocking it with spongy bone and perhaps hindering the insertion of a multiple channel cochlear implant. Occlusion or stenosis of the round window itself (*i.e.*, obliterative otosclerosis) can also occur, as illustrated in cases of capsular otosclerosis examined by Johnsson *et al.* (1978).

The cochlear ossification process is not exclusive to otosclerosis and may occur in the setting of infection such as labyrinthitis or trauma within the cochlea, including insertion of a cochlear implant electrode (Ibrahim and Linthicum, 1980). Nevertheless, successful cochlear implantation in the presence of labyrinthine ossification has been reported (Ibrahim and Linthicum, 1980; Gantz *et al.*, 1988; Balkany *et al.*, 1988; Balkany *et al.*, 1997). Techniques have included a drill-out procedure to achieve patency to the scala tympani. Several researchers have provided follow-up results indicating that labyrinthine ossificans does not preclude cochlear implant surgery. Particularly in cases with extension of the new bone to the proximal part of the

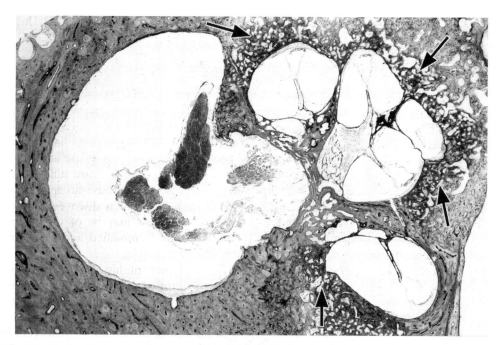

FIG. 3.8. Photomicrograph of capsular otosclerosis. Notice the foci of otosclerosis *(arrow)* on the periphery of the otic capsule surrounding the cochlea (hematoxylin and eosin stain, ×27).

scala tympani only, postimplant performance results compare favorably with those of patients without evidence of new bone formation (Fayad *et al.*, 1990).

Attempts at early medical treatment to halt the progression of the sensorineural component of the hearing loss in otosclerosis using fluoride was first reported by Shambaugh in 1964. The rationale for its use was inhibition of the resorptive enzymes, which are responsible for the otospongiotic process by conversion of active spongiotic bone to inactive sclerotic bone through deposition of the more dense fluorapatite compared with hydroxylapatite. Follow-up studies have emerged that report the reduction of progressive sensorineural hearing loss (Shambaugh and Causse, 1974; Forquer *et al.*, 1986; Bretlau *et al.*, 1985). However, there is a lack of evidence from temporal bone studies to confirm that progression of otosclerosis is arrested by fluoride (Kerr and Hoffman, 1989).

MENIERE'S DISEASE

Meniere's disease is a disorder characterized by attacks of vertigo, roaring tinnitus, fluctuating hearing loss, and sense of fullness within the ear. The patient with Meniere's disease may present with the entire spectrum of symptoms or may present atypically with one or several of the symptoms and with onset of the other symptoms much later. The condition usually begins in only one ear, but the other ear may be affected (Friberg *et al.*, 1984; Balkany *et al.*, 1980; Greven and Oosterveld, 1975; Palaskas *et al.*, 1988).

The hearing loss is sensorineural and primarily resides initially in the lower to middle frequencies, within the 250-Hz to 1-kHz range. Fluctuations in the hearing may be evident on serial audiograms, but progression of the disease usually results in a flat audiometric pattern. This so-called burned-out phase of Meniere's disease occurs when the hearing stabilizes at thresholds between 50 and 60 dB (Stahle, 1976). A few patients

with Meniere's disease (approximately 6% in one study [Shojaku *et al.*, 1995]) have profound hearing loss. Other auditory features of Meniere's disease include loudness recruitment, poor speech discrimination scores, and most notably, episodes of true vertigo that are usually far more disabling than the auditory symptoms.

In some patients, the symptoms can be controlled by medications (*e.g.*, diuretics, vestibular suppressants) or by a low-salt diet, but others have progressive exacerbation of the condition, and the loss of hearing may become complete with recurrent episodes of vertigo. In such cases, surgical options may be entertained. Options include endolymphatic sac decompression or shunt, vestibular nerve section, and unilateral surgical labyrinthectomy to bring relief from the vestibular symptoms. The latter procedure is usually chosen if the hearing loss is advanced or complete. In some patients, the use of ototoxic antibiotics by the intratympanic or parenteral route may effectively suppress function of the offending ear by virtue of the vestibulotoxic action of the aminoglycoside (Graham and Kemink, 1984).

The underlying pathology of Meniere's disease was unknown until 1938, when Hallpike and Cairns (1938) demonstrated the presence of hydropic swelling in the cochlear duct and the vestibular organs (*i.e.*, endolymphatic hydrops) (Fig. 3.9A). The scala media of the cochlea can appears distended, with balloon-like distortion of membranous boundaries (Fig. 3.9B). Theories on how the enlargement of the endolymphatic compartment may occur have focused on endolymph overproduction or underresorption. Another important advance was the demonstration by Kimura (1967) that endolymphatic hydrops could be produced in the guinea pig by surgical destruction of the endolymphatic sac. However, the condition observed in the animal temporal bone resembles Meniere's disease in some functional respects and not in others (Aran *et al.*, 1984).

The loss of sensory and neural elements of the cochlea does not appear to be an im-

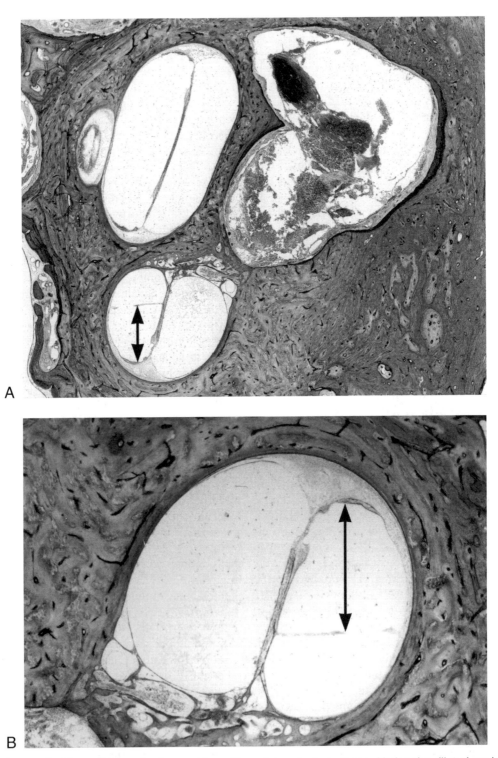

FIG. 3.9. A: Photomicrograph of a cochlea with endolymphatic hydrops. Notice the dilated scala media compartment *(arrows)* (hematoxylin and eosin stain, ×13). **B:** Higher-power photomicrograph of the dilated scala media compartment *(arrows)* from the same temporal bone (hematoxylin and eosin stain, ×35).

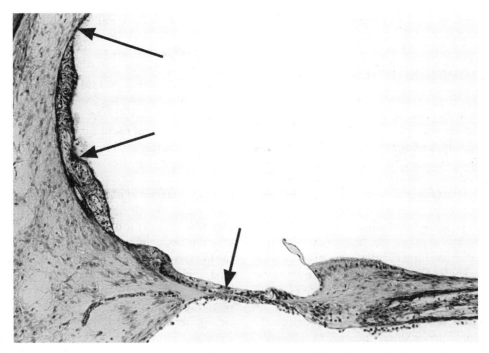

FIG. 3.10. High-power photomicrograph of a collapsed organ of Corti from a cochlea with endolymphatic hydrops *(lower arrow)*. The area of attachment of Reissner's membrane *(upper arrow)* and slight strial atrophy *(middle arrow)* are demonstrated. This represents end-stage Meniere's disease with associated hair cell loss (hematoxylin and eosin stain, ×150).

portant feature of Meniere's disease. Exceptions have been described in which there is severe hair cell loss (Fig. 3.10). Histologic examination of temporal bones from patients with Meniere's disease have surprisingly revealed minimal pathology in the cochlea for the degree of hearing loss actually observed. By light microscopic examination, the most notable features include loss of hair cells and spiral ganglion cells in the apical turn (Schuknecht 1975; Schuknecht, 1968; Schuknecht 1963). Electron microscopic evaluation of the neural elements show significantly reduced number of afferent endings for inner and outer hair cells (Nadol and Thornton, 1987) and reduced diameter of the axons and spiral ganglion nuclei compared with the non-Meniere's contralateral side (Nadol, 1990). However, in the latter study (Nadol, 1990), there was no difference in the spiral ganglion population between sides despite

better hearing (pure tone average: 15 dB versus 50 dB) and discrimination scores (speech discrimination score: 90% versus 34%) in the contralateral ear.

Patients with Meniere's disease who become candidates for cochlear implantation also possess poor speech discrimination. The above evidence seems to indicate that widespread spiral ganglion degeneration is not a feature in Meniere's disease and that cochlear implantation can stimulate the residual neural elements. Cochlear implantation may also occur in another setting with Meniere's disease.

In a patient who has undergone labyrinthectomy on one side and had a severe hearing loss on the other, an implant capable of stimulating the cochlear nucleus should be helpful. Studies (Kemink *et al.*, 1991, Zwolan *et al.*, 1993) indicate that auditory neural structures remain highly responsive to electrical stimulation after laby-rinthectomy.

AUTOIMMUNE INNER EAR DISEASE

Injury to the inner ear and its neural elements may occur as a result of inflammation in the absence of an identifiable infection. This entity has been characterized as an autoimmune process, reflecting the notion that the body itself initiates the inflammatory process, attacking native tissues as foreign or nonself as if to combat infection. Autoimmune processes that affect the ear may coexist with other, broader autoimmune disorders that can target virtually any tissue within the body. This process occurs in Cogan's syndrome with concurrent hearing loss (Cogan, 1945). Another example is rheumatoid arthritis, an autoimmune disorder of extremely high prevalence wherein tissues of the joints, most often those within the hands and knees, become inflamed, limiting mobility and producing pain and swelling (Heyworth and Liyanage, 1972; Kakani et al., 1990; Magaro et al., 1990; Kastanioudakis et al., 1995). Alternatively, the inflammatory process may be restricted to the inner ear.

Autoimmune sensorineural hearing loss has been suspected clinically for more than 20 years. The original description of this disorder is credited to Lenhardt in 1958, when he treated sudden bilateral hearing loss with steroids with improvement in some patients. McCabe (1979) of the University of Iowa presented a larger series of patients suspected to have autoimmune-associated hearing loss. He anecdotally described a patient who had undergone a mastoid procedure that had not healed despite repeated attempts to close the wound behind the ear. When the biopsy report indicated intense inflammation of the blood vessels within tissue surrounding the wound, steroid medications were administered. In addition to healing the wound, the medication improved the patient's sensorineural hearing loss. This bit of serendipity led to the description of a distinct, organ-specific autoimmune process that is now called autoimmune inner ear disease (AIED), and when restricted to the hearing portion of the inner ear, it is called autoimmune cochleopathy.

One of the most important lines of research of sensorineural hearing loss during the past decade has involved the mechanisms by which the inner ear may be damaged by autoimmunity. Harris and his research team identified mechanisms by which autoimmune-triggered inflammation may gain access to the inner ear (Harris et al., 1985). Previously, it was thought that the inner ear, like the brain, is separated from the blood circulation to preserve the biochemical environment needed to transduce sound waves into neurochemical signals. However, Harris has demonstrated that the inner ear environment is capable of triggering an inflammatory response that can damage sensory structures within the inner ear as an innocent bystander (Harris et al., 1985; Harris, 1984; Woolf and Harris, 1986). One such area within the inner ear that is immunologically active is the endolymphatic sac. Macrophages demonstrating active phagocytosis and local immunoglobulin production have been localized at this particular site (Rask-Andersen and Stahle, 1980; Tomiyama and Harris, 1987; Arnold et al., 1984; Altermatt et al., 1990).

Histopathologic examination of the intracochlear changes associated with certain types of autoimmune diseases have been reported with fairly common features in animals and humans. The features include loss of the organ of Corti, retrograde neural degeneration to the level of the spiral ganglion, endolymphatic hydrops, stria vascularis dystrophy, neofibro-osteogenesis in the basal turn of the cochlea, fibrosis of the endolymphatic sac, and lymphocytes in the labyrinthine membrane compartment (Hoistad et al., 1998; Schuknecht and Nadol, 1994; Harris, 1987; Trune et al. 1989, Orozco et al. 1990). Antibodies to type II collagen have been induced in laboratory animals with subsequent intracochlear injury to the nuclei of the spiral ganglion cells, vacuolization of the stria vascularis, and atrophy of the organ of Corti with immunofluorescent immune complex deposition of the inner ear blood vessels (Takeda *et al.*, 1996; Cruz *et al.*, 1990; Yoo *et al.*, 1983).

Although injury at the cochlear level has been observed, there is potential autoimmune injury to the cochlear nerve. Some of the established models of autoimmune injury that include neural damage are Guillain-Barré syndrome, multiple sclerosis, and some of the idiopathic demyelinating diseases. Immune-mediated injury in these forms may create direct nerve injury or, more often, injury to the supporting cells of the central (glial) or peripheral (Schwann) nerve fibers (Argall *et al.*, 1991; Ilyas *et al.* 1992; Banati *et al.* 1995). In the animal model with experimental allergic encephalomyelitis, an experimental model for multiple sclerosis, neural changes occurred at the spiral ganglion, cochlear nerve, cochlear nucleus, superior olive, lateral lemniscus, and inferior colliculus, with hearing loss documented by brain stem auditory evoked potentials (Watanabe *et al.*, 1996). Impressively, the hearing loss was prevented by administration of a specific antibody to the $V_\beta 8$ receptor on the T lymphocyte (Suzuki *et al.*, 1998), mitigating the degree of autoimmune injury.

The importance of recognizing an autoimmune disorder of the inner ear is that the disease may be treatable, particularly in its early stages. AIED typically presents in middle-aged individuals, more often women than men, and rapidly involves both ears (*i.e.*, sudden hearing loss) or develops in a progressive fashion. Different types of immune processes may be going on in these two latter types of hearing loss (Mayot *et al.*, 1993). There often is a history of an immune disease (*e.g.*, rheumatoid arthritis, lupus, polyarteritis) affecting the individual or another family member. Although this is the typical patient profile for AIED, atypical presentations do exist. The diagnosis is supported by information from blood tests that seek to identify the presence of alterations in immune function of humoral and cell-mediated types. These include high levels of nonspecific and specific antibodies (*i.e.*, inflammatory proteins) that are thought to be directed at cells within the inner ear (*e.g.*, antinuclear antibody, rheumatoid factor). Altered lymphocyte transformation and migration inhibition by *in vitro* testing may be found. A a possible inner ear antigen (MW 68,000) that the sensitized antibodies reacted to has been identified (Harris and Sharp, 1990).

The principal methods of treatment of AIED involve the use of potent anti-inflammatory medications. Steroids delivered intravenously or orally for 3 to 6 weeks are used most commonly. Nonsteroidal antiinflammatory agents may be used as well. For cases that require longer-term treatment, immunosuppressives such as the antimetabolite medication methotrexate or the alkylating agent cyclophosphamide have been used with some success (Sismanis *et al.*, 1994). However, these medications have significant side effects, and their use in maintaining hearing must be carefully monitored. When AIED fails to respond to antiinflammatory medications and useful hearing is lost, cochlear implantation is a viable alternative.

REFERENCES

Ahmad NN, Ala-Kokko L, Kowlton RG, *et al.* Stop codon in the procollagen II gene *(COL2A1)* in a family with the Stickler syndrome (artho-ophthalmopathy). *Proc Natl Acad Sci USA* 1991;88:6624–6627.

Altermatt HJ, Gebbers JO, Muller, *et al.* Human endolymphatic sac: evidence for a role in inner ear immune defense. *ORL J Otorhinolaryngol Relat Spec* 1990; 52:143–148.

Aran JM, Rarey KE, Hawkins JE Jr. Function and morphological changes in experimental endolymphatic hydrops. *Acta Otolaryngol (Stockh)* 1984;97:547–557.

Arcand P, Desrosiers M, Dube J, Abela A. The large vestibular aqueduct syndrome and sensorineural hearing loss in the pediatric population. *J Otolaryngol* 1991;20:247–250.

Argall KG, Armati PJ, King NJC, Douglas MW. The effects of West Nile virus on major histocompatibility complex class I and II molecule expression by Lewis rate Schwann cells *in vitro*. *J Neuroimmunol* 1991; 35:273–284.

Arnold W, Altermatt HJ, Gebbers JO, Laissue J. Secretory immunoglobulin A in the human endolymphatic sac. *ORL J Otorhinolaryngol Relat Spec* 1984;46:286–288.

Aschendorff A, Marangos N, Laszig R. Large vestibular aqueduct syndrome and its implication for cochlear implant surgery. *Am J Otol* 1997;18[Suppl 6]:S57.

Aviel A, Ostefeld E. Acquired irreversible sensorineural hearing loss in chronic otitis media and mastoiditis. *Am J Otolaryngol* 1982;3:217–222.

Balkany TJ, Gantz BJ, Nadol JB. Multi-channel cochlear implants in partially ossified cochleas. *Ann Otol Rhinol Laryngol* 1988;97[Suppl 135]:3–7.

Balkany TJ, Luntz M, Telischi FF, Hodges AV. Intact canal wall drill-out procedure for implantation of the totally ossified cochlea. *Am J Otol* 1997;18[Suppl];S58–S59.

Balkany TJ, Sires B, Arenberg IK. Bilateral aspects of Meniere's disease: an underestimated clinical entity. *Otoalryngol Clin North Am* 1980;13:603–609.

Banati RB, Gehrmann J, Lannes-Vieira J, Kreutzberg GW. Inflammatory reaction in experimental autoimmune encephalomyelitis (EAE) is accompanied by a microglial expression of the beta A 4-amyloid precursor protein (APP). *Glia* 1995;14:209–215.

Bergstrom L-V, Jenkins P, Sando I, English GM. Hearing loss in renal disease: clinical and pathological studies. *Ann Otol Rhinol Laryngol* 1973;82:555–576.

Berlow SJ, Caldarelli DD, Matz GJ, Meyer DH, Harsch GG. Bacterial meningitis and sensorineural hearing loss: a prospective investigation. *Laryngoscope* 1980;90:1445–1452.

Bhatt S, Hapin C, Hsu W, et al. Hearing loss and pneumococcal meningitis: an animal model. *Laryngoscope* 1991;101:1285–1292.

Bordley JE, Brookhouser PE, Hardy J, Hardy WG. Prenatal rubella. *Acta Otolaryngol (Stockh)* 1968;66:1–9.

Brackmann DE, Hitselberger WE, Nelson RA, et al. Auditory brainstem implant: I. Issues in surgical implantation. *Otolaryngol Head Neck Surg* 1993;108:624–633.

Bredberg G, Engstrom H, Ades HW. Cellular pattern and nerve supply of the human organ of Corti: a preliminary report. *Arch Otolaryngol* 1965;82:462–469.

Bredberg G. Cellular pattern and nerve supply of the human organ of Corti. *Acta Otolaryngol Suppl (Stockh)* 1968;236:1–135.

Bretlau P, Causse J, Causse J-B, Hansen HJ, Johnsen NJ, Salomon G. Otospongiosis and sodium fluoride. A blind experimental and clinical evaluation of the effect of sodium fluoride treatment in patients with otospongiosis. *Ann Otol Rhinol Laryngol* 1985;94:103–107.

Brunner HG, Van Beersum SE, Warman ML, Olsen BR, Ropers HH, Maruman EC. A Stickler syndrome gene is linked to chromosome 6 near the *COLIIA2* gene. *Hum Mol Genet* 1994;3:1561–1564.

Cazals Y, Aran JM, Erre JP, Guilhaume A, Hawkins JE Jr. Neural responses to acoustic stimulation after destruction of cochlear hair cells. *Arch Otol Rhinol Laryngol* 1979;224:61–70.

Cogan DG. Syndrome of nonsyphilitic interstitial keratitis and vestibuloauditory symptoms. *Arch Ophthalmol* 1945;33:144–149.

Cruz OLM, Miniti A, Cossermelli W, Oliveira RM. Autoimmune sensorineural hearing loss: a preliminary experimental study. *Am J Otol* 1990;11:342–346.

Davis H, Morgan CT, Hawkins JE Jr, Galambos R, Smith FW. Temporary deafness following exposure to loud tones and noise. *Acta Otolaryngol Suppl (Stockh)* 1950;88:1–57.

Dubs B, Niparko JK, Ng M, Nager GT. Mechanisms of meningitis-related hearing loss and effects on spiral ganglion cell populations. 1999 *(in preparation)*.

Duckert LG, Miller JM. Morphological changes following cochlear implantation in the animal model. *Acta Otolaryngol Suppl (Stockh)* 1984;411:28–37.

Egami T, Sando I, Sobel JH. Noise-induced hearing loss: a human temporal bone case report. *Ann Otol Rhinol Laryngol* 1978;87:868–874.

Estivill X, Fortina P, Surrey S, et al. Connexin-26 mutations in sporadic and inherited sensorineural deafness. *Lancet* 1998;351:394–398.

Fausti SA, Henry JA, Hayden D, Phillips DS, Frey RH. Intrasubject reliability of high-frequency (9–14 KHz) thresholds: tested separately vs. following conventional frequency testing. *J Am Acad Audiol* 1998;9:147–152.

Fausti SA, Larson VD, Noffsinger D, Wilson RH, Phillips DS, Fowler CG. High-frequency audiometric monitoring strategies for early detection of ototoxicity. *Ear Hear* 1994;15:232–239.

Fayad J, Linthicum FH, Otto SR, Galey FR, House WF. Cochlear implants: histopathologic findings related to performance in 16 human temporal bones. *Ann Otol Rhinol Laryngol* 1991;100:807–811.

Fayad J, Moloy P, Linthicum FH Jr. Cochlear otosclerosis: does bone formation affect cochlear implant surgery? *Am J Otol* 1990;11:196–200.

Fisch L. Deafness as part of an hereditary syndrome. *J Laryngol Otol* 1959;73:355–382.

Forquer BD, Linthicum FH Jr, Bennett C. Sodium fluoride: effectiveness of treatment for cochlear otosclerosis. *Am J Otol* 1986;7:121–125.

Friberg U, Stahle J, Svedberg A. The natural course of Meniere's disease. *Acta Otolaryngol Suppl (Stockh)* 1984;406:72–77.

Friedmann I, Fraser GR, Froggatt P. Pathology of the ear in the cardioauditory syndrome of Jervell and Lange-Nielsen (recessive deafness with electrocardiographic abnormalities). *J Laryngol Otol* 1966;80:451–470.

Fujita S, Hayden RC Jr. Alport's syndrome. Temporal bone report. *Arch Otolaryngol* 1969;90:453–466.

Fukuda S, Ishikawa K, Inuyama Y. Acute measles infection in the hamster cochlea. *Acta Otolaryngol (Stockh)* 1994;514[Suppl 514]:111–116.

Gantz BJ, McCabe BF, Tyler RS. Use of multichannel cochlear implants in obstructed and obliterated cochleas. *Otolaryngol Head Neck Surg* 1988;98:72–81.

Gantz BJ, Tyler RS, Knutson JF, et al. Evaluation of five different cochlear implant designs: audiologic assessment and predictors of performance. *Laryngoscope* 1988;98:1100–1106.

Goodhill V. Syphilis of the ear: histopathologic study. *Ann Otol Rhinol Laryngol* 1939;48:676–706.

Graham MD, Kemink JL. Titration streptomycin therapy for bilateral Meniere's disease: a progress report. *Am J Otol* 1984;5:534–535.

Greven AJ, Oosterveld WJ. The contralateral ear in Meniere's disease. *Arch Otolaryngol* 1975;101:608–612.

Griffith AJ, Arts HA, Downs C, et al. Familial large vestibular aqueduct syndrome. *Laryngoscope* 1996;106:960–965.

Grundfast KM, Josephson GD. Hereditary hearing loss.

In: Hughes GB, Pensak ML, eds. *Clinical otology,* 2nd ed. New York: Thieme Publishers, 1997.

Gstoettner W, Plenk H Jr, Franz P, *et al.* Cochlear implant deep electrode insertion: extent of insertional trauma. *Acta Otolaryngol (Stockh)* 1997;117:274–277.

Guild SR. Histologic otosclerosis. *Ann Otol Rhinol Laryngol* 1944;53:246–266.

Hallpike CS, Cairns H. Observations on the pathology of Meniere's syndrome. *J Laryngol Otol* 1938;53: 625–655.

Harris JP, Sharp PA. Inner ear autoantibodies in patients with rapidly progressive sensorineural hearing loss. *Laryngoscope* 1990;100:516–524.

Harris JP, Woolf NK, Ryan AF. Elaboration of systemic immunity following inner ear immunization. *Am J Otolaryngol* 1985;6:148–152.

Harris JP. Experimental autoimmune sensorineural hearing loss. *Laryngoscope* 1987;97:63–76.

Harris JP. Immunology of the inner ear: evidence of local antibody production. *Ann Otol Rhinol Laryngol* 1984;93:157–162.

Hawkins JE Jr. Drug ototoxicity. In: Keidel WD, Neff WD, eds. *Handbook of sensory physiology.* Vol V: *Auditory system.* Part 3: *Clinical and special topics.* Berlin: Springer-Verlag, 1976:707–748.

Hayworth T, Liyanage SP. A pilot survey of hearing loss in patients with rheumatoid arthritis. *Scand J Rheum* 1972;1:81–83.

Hemenway WG, Sando I, McChesney D. Temporal bone pathology following maternal rubella. *Arch Klin Exp Ohr Nas Kehlkheilk* 1969;193:287–300.

Hildesheimer M, Maayan Z, Muchnik C, Rubinstein M, Goodman RM. Auditory and vestibular findings in Waardenburg's type II syndrome. *J Laryngol Otol* 1989;103:1130.

Hinderlink JB, Brokx JP, Mens LH, vandenBroek P. Results from four cochlear implant patients with Usher's syndrome. *Ann Otol Rhinol Laryngol* 1994;103:288–293.

Hinojosa R, Green JD Jr, Marion MS. Ganglion cell populations in labyrinthitis ossificans. *Am J Otol* 1991;12[Suppl 12]:3–7.

Hinojosa R, Marion M. Histopathology of profound sensorineural deafness. *Ann NY Acad Sci* 1983;405: 459–484.

Hoistad DL, Schachern PA, Paparella MM. Autoimmune sensorineural hearing loss: a human temporal bone study. *Am J Otolaryngol* 1998;19:33–39.

Horn KL, McMahon NB, McMahon DC, Lewis JS, Barker M, Gherini S. Function use of the Nucleus 22-channel cochlear implant in the elderly. *Laryngoscope* 1991;101:284–288.

Huizing EH, deGroot JC. Human cochlear pathology in aminoglycoside ototoxicity—a review. *Acta Otolaryngol Suppl (Stockh)* 1987;436:117–125.

Hvedberg-Hansen J, Jorgensen MB. The inner ear in Pendred's syndrome. *Acta Otolaryngol (Stockh)* 1968;66:129–135.

Ibrahim RAA, Linthicum FH Jr. Labyrinthine ossificans and cochlear implants. *Arch Otolaryngol* 1980; 106:111–113.

Igarishi M, Schuknecht HF, Myers EN. Cochlear pathology in humans with stimulation deafness. *J Laryngol Otol* 1964;78:115–123.

Ilyas AA, Mithen FA, Dalakas MC, Chen Z-W, Cook SD. Antibodies to acidic glycolipids in Guillain-Barré syndrome and chronic inflammatory demyelinating polyneuropathy. *J Neurol Sci* 1992;107:111–121.

Jackler RK, De La Cruz A. The large vestibular aqueduct syndrome. *Laryngoscope* 1989;99:1238–1243.

Johnsson L-G, Arenberg IK. Cochlear abnormalities in Alport's syndrome. *Arch Otolaryngol* 1981;107: 340–349.

Johnsson L-G, Hawkins JE Jr, Linthicum FH Jr. Cochlear and otoconial abnormalities in capsular otosclerosis with hydrops. *Ann Otol Rhinol Laryngol Suppl* 1982;97:3–15.

Johnsson L-G, Hawkins JE Jr, Linthicum FH Jr. Cochlear and vestibular lesions in capsular otosclerosis as seen in microdissection. *Ann Otol Rhinol Laryngol Suppl* 1978;87:1–40.

Johnsson L-G, Hawkins JE Jr. Degeneration patterns in human ears exposed to noise. *Ann Otol Rhinol Laryngol* 1976;85:725–739.

Johnsson L-G, Hawkins JE Jr. Sensory and neural degeneration with aging, as seen in microdissections of the human inner ear. *Ann Otol Rhinol Laryngol* 1972;81:179–193.

Johnsson L-G, House WF, Linthicum FH. Bilateral cochlear implants: histological findings in a pair of temporal bones. *Laryngoscope* 1979;89:759–762.

Johnsson L-G. Sequence of degeneration of Corti's organ and its first-order neurons. *Ann Otol Rhinol Laryngol* 1974;83:294–303.

Kakani RS, Mehra YN, Deodhar SP, Manns B, Mehta S. Audiovestibular functions in rheumatoid arthritis. *J Otolaryngol* 1990;19:100–102.

Kastanioudakis I, Skevas A, Danielidis V, Tsiakou E, Drosos AA, Moustopoulos MH. Inner ear involvement in rheumatoid arthritis: a prospective clinical trial. *J Laryngol Otol* 1995;109:713–718.

Kelsell DP, Dunlop J, Stevens HP, *et al.* Connexin 26 mutations in hereditary non-syndromic sensorineural deafness. *Nature* 1997;387:80–83.

Kemink JL, Kileny PR, Niparko JK, Telian SA. Electrical stimulation of the auditory system after labyrinthectomy. *Am J Otol* 1991;12:7–10.

Kennedy DW. Multichannel intracochlear electrodes: mechanism of insertion trauma. *Laryngoscope* 1987; 97:42–49.

Kerr A, Schuknecht HF. The spiral ganglion in profound deafness. *Acta Otolaryngol (Stockh)* 1968;65:586–598.

Kerr GS, Hoffman GS. Fluoride therapy for otosclerosis. *ENT J* 1989;68:427–429.

Khetarpal U, Schuknecht HF, Gacek RR, Holmes LB. Autosomal dominant sensorineural hearing loss. Pedigrees, audiologic findings, and temporal bone findings in two kindreds. *Arch Otolaryngol Head Neck Surg* 1991;117:1032–1041.

Kimura RS. Experimental blockage of the endolymphatic duct and sac and its effect on the inner ear of the guinea pig. *Ann Otol Rhinol Laryngol* 1967; 76:664–687.

Koitchev K, Guilhaume A, Cazals Y, Aran JM. Spiral ganglion changes after massive aminoglycoside treatment in the guinea pig: counts and ultrastructure. *Acta Otolaryngol (Stockh)* 1982;94:431–438.

Konigsmark BW, Gorlin RJ. *Genetic and metabolic deafness.* Philadelphia: WB Saunders, 1976.

Kotzias SA, Linthicum FH Jr. Labyrinthine ossification:

differences between two types of ectopic bone. *Am J Otol* 1985;6:490–494.

Leake-Jones PA, Vivion MC. Cochlear pathology in cats following administration of neomycin sulfate. *Scanning Electron Microsc* 1979;3:983–991.

Lehnhardt E. Plotzliche Horstorungen, auf beiden Seiten gleichzeitig oder nacheinander aufgetreten. *Z Laryngol Rhinol Otol* 1958;37:1.

Levenson MJ, Parisier SC, Jacobs M, Edelstein DR. The large vestibular aqueduct syndrome in children: a review of 12 cases and the description of a new clinical entity. *Arch Otolaryngol Head Neck Surg* 1989;115:54–58.

Lindsay JR, Caruthers DG, Hemenway WG, Harrison S. Inner ear pathology following maternal rubella. *Ann Otol Rhinol Laryngol* 1953;62:1201–1218.

Lindsay JR. Histopathology of deafness due to postnatal viral disease. *Arch Otolaryngol* 1973;98:258–264.

Linthicum FH Jr, Fayad J, Ottor SR, Galey FR, House WF. Cochlear implant histopathology. *Am J Otol* 1991;12:245–311.

Linthicum FH Jr. Viral causes of sensorineural hearing loss. *Otolaryngol Clin North Am* 1978;11:29–33.

Liu X-Z, Newton VE. Waardenburg syndrome type II: phenotypic findings and diagnostic criteria. *Am J Med Genet* 1995;55:95–100.

Liu X-Z, Walsh J, Mburu P, *et al.* Mutations in the myosin VIIA gene cause non-syndromic recessive deafness. *Nat Genet* 1997;16:188–190.

Lowry LD, May M, Pastore P. Acute histopathologic inner ear changes in deafness due to neomycin: a case report. *Ann Otol Rhinol Laryngol* 1973;82:876–880.

Lu C-B, Schuknecht HF. Pathology of pre-lingual profound deafness: magnitude of labyrinthitis fibo-ossificans. *Am J Otol* 1994;15:74–85.

Lurie MH, Davis H, Hawkins JE Jr. Acoustic trauma of the organ of Corti in the guinea pig. *Laryngoscope* 1944;54:375–386.

Magaro M, Zoli A, Altornonte A, *et al.* Sensorineural hearing loss in rheumatoid arthritis. *Clin Exp Rheum* 1990;8:487–490.

Mayot D, Bene MC, Dron K, Perrin C, Faure GC. Immunologic alterations in patients with sensorineural hearing disorders. *Clin Immunol Immunopathol* 1993;68:41–45.

McCabe BF. Autoimmune sensorineural hearing loss. *Ann Otol Rhinol Laryngol* 1979;88:585–589.

McGill TJI, Schuknecht HF. Human cochlear changes in noise induced hearing loss. *Laryngoscope* 1976; 86:1293–1302.

Merchant SN, Gopen Q. A human temporal bone study of acute bacterial meningogenic labyrinthitis. *Am J Otol* 1996;17:375–385.

Myers GJ, Tyler HR. The etiology of deafness in Alport's syndrome. *Arch Otolaryngol* 1972;96:333–340.

Nadol JB Jr, Burgess B. Cochleosaccular degeneration of the inner ear and progressive cataracts inherited as an autosomal dominant trait. *Laryngoscope* 1982;92:1028–1037.

Nadol JB Jr, Hsu W. Histopathologic correlation of spiral ganglion cell count and new bone formation in the cochlea following meningogenic labyrinthitis and deafness. *Ann Otol Rhinol Laryngol* 1991;100: 712–716.

Nadol JB Jr, Ketten DR, Burgess BJ. Otopathology in a case of multichannel cochlear implantation. *Laryngoscope* 1994;104:299–303.

Nadol JB Jr. Patterns of neural degeneration in the human cochlea and auditory nerve: implications for cochlear implantation. *Otolaryngol Head Neck Surg* 1997;117:220–228.

Nadol JB, Thornton AR. Ultrastructural findings in a case of Meniere's disease. *Ann Otol Rhinol Laryngol* 1987;96:449–454.

Nadol JB, Young Y-S, Glynn RJ. Survival of spiral ganglion cells in profound sensorineural hearing loss: implications for cochlear implantation. *Ann Otol Rhinol Laryngol* 1989;98:411–416.

Nadol JB. Degeneration of cochlear neurons as seen in the spiral ganglion of man. *Hear Res* 1990;49:141–154.

Nadol JB. Electron microscopic findings in presbycusic degeneration of the basal turn of the human cochlea. *Otolaryngol Head Neck Surg* 1979;87:818–836.

Nadol JB. Histological considerations in implant patients. *Arch Otolaryngol* 1984;110:160–163.

Nager FR. Histologische Ohruntersuchungen bei Kindern nach mütterlicher Rubella. *Pract Otorhinolaryngol* 1952;14:337–359.

Nakai Y, Konishi K, Chang KC, *et al.* Ototoxicity of the anticancer drug cisplatin: an experimental study. *Acta Otolaryngol (Stockh)* 1982;93:227–232.

Nomura Y. Lipidosis of the basilar membrane. *Acta Otolaryngol (Stockh)* 1970;69:352–357.

Orozco CR, Niparko JK, Richardson BC, Dolan DF, Ptok MU, Altschuler RA. Experimental model of immune-mediated hearing loss using cross-species immunization. *Laryngoscope* 1990;100:941–947.

Otte J, Schuknecht HG, Kerr A. Ganglion cell populations in normal and pathological human cochleae: implications for cochlear implantation. *Laryngoscope* 1978;88:1231–1246.

Palaskas CW, Dobie RA, Snyder JM. Progression of hearing loss in bilateral Meniere's disease. *Laryngoscope* 1988;98:287–290.

Paparella MM, Morizono T, Le CT, *et al.* Sensorineural hearing loss in otitis media. *Ann Otol Rhinol Laryngol* 1984;93:623–629.

Paparella MM, Oda M, Hiraide F, Brady D. Pathology of sensorineural hearing loss in otitis media. *Ann Otol Rhinol Laryngol* 1972;81:632–647.

Paparella MM, Sugiura S. The pathology of suppurative labyrinthitis. *Ann Otol Rhinol Laryngol* 1967; 76:554–586.

Quick CA, Hoppe W. Permanent deafness associated with furosemide administration. *Ann Otol Rhinol Laryngol* 1975;84:94–101.

Rarey KE, Davis LE. Inner ear anomalies in Waardenburg's syndrome associated with Hirschsprung's disease. *Int J Pediatr Otorhinolaryngol* 1984;8:181–89.

Rask-Andersen H, Stahle J. Immunodefence of the inner ear? *Acta Otolaryngol (Stockh)* 1980;89:283–294.

Schachern PA, Paparella MM, Hybertson R, Sano S, Duval AJ III. Bacterial tympanogenic labyrinthitis, meningitis, and sensorineural damage. *Arch Otolaryngol Head Neck Surg* 1992;118:53–57.

Schaefer SD, Post JD, Close LG, Wright CG. Ototoxicity of low- and moderate-dose cisplatin. *Cancer* 1985;56:1934–1939.

Schmidt JM. Cochlear neuronal populations in developmental defects of the inner ear: implications for cochlear implantation. *Acta Otolaryngol (Stockh)* 1985;99:14–20.

Schuknecht HF, Nadol JB Jr. Temporal bone pathology

in a case of Cogan's syndrome. *Laryngoscope* 1994; 104:1135–1142.

Schuknecht HF. Correlation of pathology with symptoms of Meniere's disease. *Otolaryngol Clin North Am* 1968;1:433–440.

Schuknecht HF. Further observations on the pathology of presbycusis. *Arch Otolaryngol* 1964;80:369–382.

Schuknecht HF. Meniere's disease: a correlation of symptomatology and pathology. *Laryngoscope* 1963; 73:651–665.

Schuknecht HF. *Pathology of the ear.* Cambridge, MA: Harvard University Press, 1974.

Schweitzer VG, Hawkins JE, Lilly DJ, *et al.* Ototoxic and nephrotoxic effects of combined treatment with *cis*-diamminedichloroplatinum and kanamycin in the guinea pig. *Otolaryngol Head Neck Surg* 1984;92: 38–49.

Shambaugh GE Jr, Causse J. Ten years' experience with fluoride in otosclerotic (otospongiotic) patients. *Ann Otol Rhinol Laryngol* 1974;83:635–642.

Shambaugh GE Jr, Scott A. Sodium fluoride for arrest of otosclerosis. *Arch Otolaryngol* 1964;80:263–270.

Shojaku H, Watanabe Y, Mizukoshi K, *et al.* Epidemiological study of severe cases of Meniere's disease in Japan. *Acta Otolaryngol (Stockh)* 1995;520[Suppl 520 Pt 2]:415–418.

Silverstein H, Smouha E, Morgan N. Multichannel cochlear implantation in a patient with bilateral Mondini deformity. *Am J Otol* 1988;9:451–455.

Sismanis A, Thompson T, Willis HE. Methotrexate therapy for autoimmune hearing loss: a preliminary report. *Laryngoscope* 1994;104:932–934.

Smith S, Kokodziej P, Olney AH. Waardenburg syndrome. *ENT J* 1998;77:257–58.

Stahle J. Advanced Meniere's disease: a study of 356 severely disabled patients. *Acta Otolaryngol (Stockh)* 1976;81:113–119.

Strauss M, Towfighi J, Lord S, Lipton A, Harvey HA, Brown B. *Cis*-platinum ototoxicity: clinical experience and temporal bone histopathology. *Laryngoscope* 1983;93:1554–1559.

Suga F, Lindsay JR. Histopathological observations of presbycusis. *Ann Otol* 1976;85:169–184.

Suzuka Y, Schuknecht HF. Retrograde cochlear neuronal degeneration in human subjects. *Acta Otolaryngol (Stockh)* 1988;450:1–20.

Suzuki C, Sando I, Fagan JJ, Kamerer DB, Knisely B. Histopathological features of a cochlear implant and otogenic meningitis in Mondini dysplasia. *Arch Otolaryngol* 1998;124:462–466.

Suzuki M, Cheng KC, Krug MS, Yoo TJ. Successful prevention of retrocochlear hearing loss in murine experimental allergic encephalomyelitis with T-cell receptor V beta 8-specific antibody. *Ann Otol Rhinol Laryngol* 1998;107:917–927.

Töndury von G. Zum Problem der Embryopathia Rubeolosa. Untersuchungen an menschlichen verschiedener Entwicklungsstadien. *Bull Schweiz Akad Med Wissensch* 1951;7:307–325.

Takeda T, Sudo N, Kitano H, Yoo TJ. Type II collagen-induced autoimmune ear disease in mice: a preliminary report on an epitope of the type II collagen

molecule that induced inner ear lesions. *Am J Otol* 1996;17:68–74.

Tomiyama S, Harris JP. The role of the endolymphatic sac in inner ear immunity. *Acta Otolaryngol (Stockh)* 1987;103:182–188.

Trune DR, Craven JP, Morton JI, Mitchell C. Autoimmune disease and cochlear pathology in the C3H/lpr strain mouse. *Hear Res* 1989;38:57–66.

Turrini M, Orzan E, Gabana M, Genovese E, Arslan E, Fisch U. Cochlear implantation in a bilateral Mondini dysplasia. *Scand Audiol Suppl* 1997;46:78–81.

Valvassori GE, Clemis JD. The large vestibular aqueduct syndrome. *Laryngoscope* 1978;88:723–728.

Walby AP, Barrera A, Schuknecht HF. Cochlear pathology in chronic suppurative otitis media. *Ann Otol Rhinol Laryngol* 1983;92[Suppl]:1–19.

Ward PH, Honrubia V, Moore BS. Inner ear pathology in deafness due to maternal rubella. *Arch Otolaryngol* 1968;87:22–28.

Watanabe T, Cheng K-C, Krug MS, Yoo T-J. Brain stem auditory-evoked potentials of mice with experimental allergic encephalomyelitis. *Ann Otol Rhinol Laryngol* 1996;105:905–915.

Welling DB, Hinojosa R, Gantz BJ, Lee J. Insertional trauma of multichannel cochlear implants. *Laryngoscope* 1993;103:995–1001.

Woolf NK, Harris JP. Cochlear pathophysiology associated with inner ear immune responses. *Acta Otolaryngol (Stockh)* 1986;102:353–364.

Wright CG, Schaefer SD. Inner ear histopathology in patients treated with *cis*-platinum. *Laryngoscope* 1982;92:1408–1413.

Ylikoski J, Savolainen S. The cochlear nerve in various forms of deafness. *Acta Otolaryngol (Stockh)* 1984; 98:418–427.

Yoo TJ, Cremer MA, Tomoda K, Townes AS, Stuart JM, Kang AH. Type II collagen-induced autoimmune sensorineural hearing loss and vestibular dysfunction in rats. *Ann Otol Rhinol Laryngol* 1983;92:267–271.

Young NM, Johnson JC, Mets MB, Hain TC. Cochlear implants in young children with Usher's syndrome. *Ann Otol Rhinol Laryngol Suppl* 1995;166:342–345.

Zappia JJ, Niparko JK, Oviatt DL, Kemink JL, Altschuler RA. Evaluation of the temporal bones of a multichannel cochlear implant patient. *Ann Otol Rhinol Laryngol* 1991;100:914–921.

Zwolan TA, Shepard NT, Niparko JK. Labyrinthectomy with cochlear implantation. *Am J Otol* 1993;14:220–224.

SELECTED READINGS

Johnsen T, Jorgensen MB, Johnsen S. Mondini cochlea in Pendred's syndrome: a histological study. *Acta Otolaryngol (Stockh)* 1986;102:239–247.

Nakashima S, Sando I, Takahashi H, Hashida Y. Temporal bone histopathologic findings of Waardenburg's syndrome: a case report. *Laryngoscope* 1992;102:563–567.

Schuknecht HF. Pathophysiology of Meniere's disease. *Otolaryngol Clin North Am* 1975;8:507–514.

Appendix 3A

The Epidemiology of Hearing Loss:
How Prevalent Is Hearing Loss?

John K. Niparko

Hearing loss is widely recognized as one of the most common human disorders. Several factors may confound determination of the precise extent of hearing loss in modern society. Given its insidious onset and progressive nature, hearing loss is probably best accounted for by determining its *prevalence*. In contrast to incidence figures (that reflect the rates of onset of new cases of a disorder in a population of a given size), the prevalence of a disorder represents its presence over an interval of time in a given population. The prevalence of hearing loss has been the subject of several large epidemiologic studies.

An accurate determination of the number of affected individuals is hampered by several factors. First, there is great variability in the prevalence of hearing loss across age groups. Lack of heterogeneity among subjects of the population under study can thus introduce bias and reduce the ability to generalize findings to other populations. For example, unscreened cohorts of adults are likely to include various percentages of subjects with significant exposures to occupational and nonoccupational noise. For this reason, the socioeconomic status and ethnic composition of the population under study are likely to affect prevalence rates (Davis *et al.*, 1997). Second, because hearing loss cannot be detected with accuracy by casual means, an individual's lack of awareness or

J. K. Niparko: Department of Otolaryngology—Head and Neck Surgery, The Listening Center at Johns Hopkins, The Johns Hopkins University, Baltimore, Maryland 21205-1809.

denial (Eastwood *et al.*, 1985) of a hearing loss results in underreporting. Formal audiologic testing provides the only means of accurately detecting significant hearing loss (Gates *et al.*, 1990). Third, defining what constitutes a hearing problem is a challenge. Because hearing loss represents a continuum, the criteria used to define hearing loss and testing methods should be given careful consideration. There is no clear dividing line beyond which a hearing loss represents disability (Dobie, 1993), and the definition of a hearing problem is highly individualized, often reflecting a person's communicative lifestyle (Sandor, 1994). A decibel definition of hearing loss is needed to compare results of epidemiologic studies.

CHILDREN

Prevalence rates of permanent hearing loss have been examined in detail for newborns. Although the importance of early detection seems intuitive, governmental interest in such studies relates to whether hearing loss in young children represents a serious public health concern and is therefore a good target for programs of early screening.

Severe to profound losses that are congenital or acquired before the development of speech and language occur in 0.5 to 3 per 1,000 live births (Riko *et al.*, 1985; Prager *et al.*, 1987; Augustsson *et al.*, 1990; Morgan, 1991; Smith *et al.*, 1992; Fortnum *et al.*, 1997). The large range in prevalence figures reflects differences in testing methods, differences in the cohort of children under study, and the length of follow-up of the cohort. One of the most carefully performed epidemiologic studies performed assessed the annual prevalence rate of hearing impairment in children between the ages of 3 and 10 years (Van Naarden *et al.*, 1999). The overall prevalence rate of serious hearing impairment was 1.1 cases per 1,000 children in this age range. The prevalence rate was lowest among 3 year olds (0.67/1,000) and increased steadily to the highest prevalence (1.38/1,000) in 10 year olds. The prevalence rates were higher among males (1.23/1,000) than females (0.95/1000) and higher among black children (1.21/1,000) than white children (1.01/1,000). Approximately 90% of all cases were attributable to a sensorineural hearing loss.

In general, these study results suggest that a set of "60-40" rules apply to permanent hearing losses in children younger than the age of 10 years. Mild to moderate hearing loss (between 40 and 80 dB at frequencies of 0.5, 1, 2, and 4 kHz) occurs more frequently (about 60%) than severe to profound losses (about 40%). Congenital onset is more common (about 60%) than acquired losses (about 40%).

Studies of prevalence that test for the presence of permanent hearing loss over a short period underestimate the number of children ultimately affected. Children with hearing losses that are progressive or delayed in onset are missed by survey methods that track the population for too short of a period. Factors that increase the risk for congenital or delayed-onset sensorineural hearing impairment include a family history of hearing impairment, congenital or central nervous system infections, ototoxic drug exposure, congenital deformities involving the head and neck, birth trauma, minority ethnicity, lower socioeconomic status, and other conditions often related to prematurity that prompt admission to an intensive care nursery (Davis *et al.*, 1997). Approximately 60% of children with significant (>50 dB) hearing loss exhibit one or more of these risk factors.

Large-scale population studies of child-

hood hearing loss are invariably complicated by the prevalence of temporary losses. Ear infections that are chronic and recurrent commonly produce temporary hearing loss. Eighty percent of children younger than 3 years experience an episode of otitis media, and point prevalence rates for otitis media are 12% for children in this age group (Daly, 1991). Prevalence rates of otitis generally decline as children mature: 11% for ages 4 to 5 and 6% for ages 6 to 9 years. At any given time, about 6% of children between the ages of 5 and 8 years have a 25-dB hearing loss, usually a self-limited complication of otitis media with fluid accumulation. The uncertainties of the population occurrence rates and causes of infant and childhood hearing loss have been emphasized.

The detection of a permanent hearing loss may be related to whether it manifests difficulties in scholastic performance and psychosocial development in childhood and adolescence. Even the most rigorous epidemiologic studies have been based on the number of children receiving special services (Van Naarden *et al.*, 1999). For example, the prevalence of unilateral or bilateral hearing loss among children between 6 and 19 years of age was found to be almost 15% using a criterion of 16 dB or more in the high or the low frequencies (Niskar *et al.*, 1998). Depending on the nature and extent of the hearing loss, these children were identified on the basis of deficient or delayed speech and language skills, poorer academic accomplishments, and more problematic psychosocial adjustment. These effects not only occur with children who have moderate, severe, or profound hearing loss, but they may also be present in children with unilateral, minimal, and fluctuating conductive problems. However, because individual children with lesser degrees of hearing losses may not display any apparent communication or academic problems (*i.e.*, they apparently hear and respond appropriately in face-to-face situations), the academic and linguistic "risk" status of such children tends to be overlooked. Moreover, the hearing loss may be completely missed until, on average, the age of 3 years (Van Naarden *et al.*, 1999).

It is only when group performance is considered or when a detailed evaluation is conducted that hearing-related deficiencies in areas related to psychosocial development may become apparent. This was shown in study conducted by Bess *et al.* (1998) that examined the academic achievement and functional status of children with minimal sensorineural hearing loss (MSHL), although the overall incidence of hearing loss in a public school setting was also determined. The investigators took great pains to ensure a representative sample of children in their study, and it is likely that their results can be generalized to other school systems.

The overall prevalence rate of a hearing loss in their study population was 11.3%, and 5.4% of these children exhibited MSHL. The other children had conductive and mixed hearing losses. Three categories of children with MSHL were identified: unilateral hearing loss (*i.e.*, one ear was normal), bilateral losses averaging between 20 and 40 dB, and a hearing loss of 25 dB or more in either ear at frequencies above 2,000 Hz (*i.e.*, high-frequency hearing loss). When the academic and functional status of the MSHL children was compared with hearing peers, 37% had failed at least one grade, compared with a 2% failure rate by their normally hearing peers. Other academic achievement problems were identified, particularly for the children in the lower elementary grades. For the higher-grade MSHL children, functional comparisons revealed poorer ratings for stress, self-esteem, and social support than that observed for normally hearing peers. These results are not unique to this study. Other studies reveal the negative impact of unilateral and mild hearing losses on school-age children (Bess *et al.*, 1998).

ADULTS

Hearing loss is generally regarded as one of the most common clinical conditions affecting adults. One widely quoted study of age-related disability revealed that hearing loss was the third-most self-reported health problem (30%) of individuals 65 years of age or older, listed after arthritis (47%) and elevated blood pressure (39%) (Havlik, 1986).

In virtually all adult populations studied, the highest frequencies of hearing are initially and most severely affected. Hearing loss acquired between adolescence and age 50 may be caused by relatively uncommon causes such as Meniere's disease, temporal bone trauma, otosclerosis, ototoxic drug exposure, and eighth cranial nerve tumors; noise damage is the most common cause in this population. The prevalence of hearing impairment then accelerates dramatically after the age of 50 years, with age-related hair cell degeneration within the cochlea contributing the most to this increase. Approximately 25% of patients between the ages of 51 and 65 years have hearing thresholds greater than 30 dB (normal range is 0 to 20 dB) in at least one ear (Davis *et al.*, 1992). Self-reported hearing loss can be identified in more than one-third of persons 65 years of age or older and in one-half of those 85 years of age and older (Mulrow and Lichenstein, 1991; Havlik, 1986). However, screening by hearing test identifies a significantly larger percentage (by roughly 15%) of individuals with significant hearing loss in these age groups (Gates *et al.*, 1990).

Surveys indicate that more than 28 million Americans are deaf or hearing impaired (National Institute on Deafness and Other Communication Disorders, 1996). This number is expected to increase significantly over the next 2 decades. Based on population projections alone, the overall number of hearing impaired will reach 40 million by the year 2020.

Separate surveys conducted by the National Center for Health Statistics (NCHS, 1991) in 1971 and 1991 revealed a 53% increase in the number of Americans who experienced trouble with their hearing. In addition to an increase in the absolute number of Americans with hearing problems, the prevalence rate of hearing loss had increased by 25%. A prevalence rate controls for changes in population size by reflecting numbers of affected individuals per 1,000 persons in the population, for example.

A portion of this striking increase results from aging of the U.S. population, and prevalence rates will continue to increase as our population continues to age. When National Center for Health Statistics researchers controlled the results for changes in age structure during 20 years, results still revealed an increase of 14%. Moreover, increases in hearing problems have occurred despite dramatic reductions in the incidence of many childhood diseases once responsible for early-onset hearing impairment.

Many experts attribute the rise to environmental noise, which is thought to be at higher levels today than in the past. Occupational and nonoccupational noise are associated with significant sensorineural hearing loss and are known to interact in an additive fashion with age and other contributors to hearing loss (Dobie, 1993). Although the connection between noise and hearing loss has been documented since the late 1800s, it was not until the late 1960s that laws were passed to provide compensation for noise-induced hearing loss and mandates for hearing protection were enacted.

Noise-induced hearing loss is a common cause of sensorineural hearing impairment in individuals younger than 50 years of age. This is particularly true for the estimated 5 million Americans with occupational exposure to hazardous noise levels (Department of Labor, OSHA, 1981). Farming, trucking, and work in heavy industry are the most common ear-damaging vocations. Most of the workers in these professions are men. This observation helps to explain why men of working age constitute the fastest growing population of hearing-impaired individuals.

Investigators face further difficulties in performing epidemiologic studies of hearing loss when attempting to determine prevalence rates of profound hearing loss. In the absence of field testing, precise detection of an individual's inability to benefit from am-

plification is impractical. The criterion of an inability to benefit from amplification is also difficult to apply to existing studies of the prevalence of hearing loss. The National Center for Health Statistics (NCHS, 1991) characterized advanced hearing losses as those in which the individual could under best conditions understand words only when shouted in their ear or could not hear or understand any speech. Approximately 10% of the hearing-impaired population was found to be within this range of impairment.

Taken together, these data indicate that approximately 10% of the American population experiences a noticeable deficit in hearing conversational speech. Of this population, approximately 10% appear to experience a deficit that is severe enough to hamper effective use of amplification. However, existing studies of the prevalence of hearing loss should be generalized to the entire population with caution because rigorous epidemiologic studies of the entire population are not available.

REFERENCES

Augustsson I, Nilson C, Ensgrand I. The preventive value of audiometric screening of preschool and young school-children. *Int J Pediatr Otorhinolaryngol* 1990;20:51–62.

Bess F, Dodd-Murphy J, Parker R. Children with minimal sensorineural hearing loss: prevalence, educational performance, and functional status. *Ear Hear* 1998;19:339–354.

Daly K. Epidemiology of otitis media. *Otolaryngol Clin North Am* 1991;24:775–786.

Davis A, Bamford J, Wilson I, Ramkalawan T, Forshaw M, Wright S. A critical review of the role of neonatal hearing screening in the detection of congenital hearing impairment. *Health Tech Assess* 1997;1:1–177.

Davis A, Stephens D, Rayment A. Hearing impairments in middle age: the acceptability, benefit, and cost of detection (ABCD). *Br J Audiol* 1992;26:1–14.

Department of Labor, Occupational Safety and Health Administration. Occupational noise exposure: hearing conservation amendment. *Federal Register* 1981;46:4078–4180.

Dobie R. *Medical-legal evaluation of hearing loss*. New York: Van Nostrand Reinhold, 1993.

Eastwood M, Corbin S, Reed M, Nobbs H, Kedward H. Acquired hearing loss and psychiatric illness: An estimate of prevalence and comorbidity in a geriatric setting. *Br J Psychiatry* 1985;147:552–556.

Fortnum H, Davis A, Butler A, Stevens J. Health service

implications of changes in aetiology and referral patterns of hearing impaired children in Trent, 1985–1993: report to Trent Health. Nottingham/Sheffield: MRC institute of Hearing Research and Trent Health, 1997.

Gates G, Cooper J, Kannel D, Miller N. Hearing in the elderly the Framingham Cohort, 1983–1985: Part I. Basic audiometric test results. *Ear Hear* 1990;11:247–256.

Havlik R. Aging in the eighties: impaired senses for sound and light in persons age 65 years and over. Preliminary data from the supplement on aging to the National Health Interview Survey: United States, January–June 1984. Advance data from vital and health statistics. DHHS (PHS) publication no. 125. Hyattsville, MD: National Center for Health Statistics, 1986;86–1250.

Morgan D, Canalis R. Auditory screening of infants. *Otolaryngol Clin North Am* 1991;24:277–284.

Mulrow C, Lichtenstein M. Screening for hearing impairment in the elderly: rationale and strategy. *J Gen Intern Med* 1991;6:249–258.

National Center for Health Statistics. Prevalence and characteristics of persons with hearing trouble: US: 1990–1991, series 10, no. 188. Washington, DC: U.S. Government Printing Office, 1991.

National Institute on Deafness and Other Communication Disorders. National strategic research plan. Bethesda: National Institutes of Health, U.S. Department of Health and Human Services, Public Health Services, 1996:5.

Niskar A, Kieszak S, Holmes A, Esteban E, Rubin C, Brody D. Prevalence of hearing loss among children 6 to 19 years of age. *JAMA* 1998;279:1071–1075.

Prager D, Stone D, Rose D. Hearing loss screening in the neonatal intensive care unit: auditory brain stem response versus crib-o-gram; a cost-effectiveness analysis. *Ear Hear* 1987;8:213–216.

Riko K, Hyde ML, Alberti PW. Hearing loss in early infancy: incidence, detection and assessment. *Laryngoscope* 1985;95:137–145.

Sandor G. Hearing a new market. *Am Demogr* 1994;11:48–55.

Smith RJH, Zimmerman B, Connolly PK, *et al.* Screening audiometry using the high-risk register in a level III nursery. *Arch Otolaryngol* 1992;118:1306–1311.

Van Naarden K, Decoufle P, Caldwell K. Prevalence and characteristics of children with serious hearing impairment in metropolitan Atlanta, 1991–1993. *Pediatrics* 1999;103:570–575.

SELECTED READING

National Institutes of Health Consensus Statement Early identification of hearing impairment in infants and young children. NIH Consensus Statement 1993;11:1–24.

Cochlear Implants: Principles & Practices, edited by John K. Niparko, Karen Iler Kirk, Nancy K. Mellon, Amy McConkey Robbins, Debara L. Tucci, and Blake S. Wilson. Lippincott Williams & Wilkins, Philadelphia © 2000.

4

Effects of Deafness on the Human Central Auditory System

Jean K. Moore and John K. Niparko

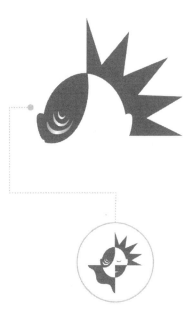

Optimal performance of a cochlear implant requires viable and responsive neuronal elements within the auditory pathway.

- How well do neurons in the central auditory pathway withstand (deafness-associated) loss or reduction of the sensory stimulation that normally drives them?
- How can we detect changes caused by reduced sensory input in the postmortem brain material that is available for study?

One approach is commonly used in looking for structural changes in central neurons as a consequence of severe hearing impairment: measurement of cell size. Cell size is biologically significant in that a larger cell reflects greater branching of the dendritic and axonal extensions from the cell body (Ramón y Cajal, 1909). Larger size also reflects a greater accumulation of the subcellular machinery needed to support higher levels of activity.

J. K. Moore: Department of Neuroanatomy, House Ear Institute; Adjunct faculty, Department of Otolaryngology, University of Southern California, Los Angeles, California 90089.

J. K. Niparko: Department of Otolaryngology—Head and Neck Surgery, The Listening Center at Johns Hopkins, The Johns Hopkins University, Baltimore, Maryland 21205-1809.

There are many examples of reduction in neuronal size in response to sensory deprivation. For example, marked changes in the size of visual neurons occur in response to eyelid closure (Chow and Stewart, 1972). It is not surprising that cell size is often measured in studies of subjects with hearing loss to compare their neural centers with those of normal-hearing subjects.

Published reports on the condition of the human central auditory pathway in deafness are relatively scarce. Early brain studies of adult humans with hearing loss include evaluations of the brain stem auditory centers in elderly subjects with various degrees of presbycusis (Kirkae *et al.*, 1964; Hensen and Reske-Nielsen, 1965). These studies describe markedly smaller cells in the deaf subjects than in control subjects with normal hearing. A more extensive set of descriptions of pathologic change within the human auditory pathway were provided by Dublin (1974, 1976, 1978). His work includes analysis of pathologic changes in cases of tumors of the cochlear nerve, multiple sclerosis, presbycusis, anoxia and severe cases of hyperbilirubinemia (*i.e.*, kernicterus) in newborns. Many of his brain specimens showed evidence of degenerative change in all of the central auditory centers, including the cere-

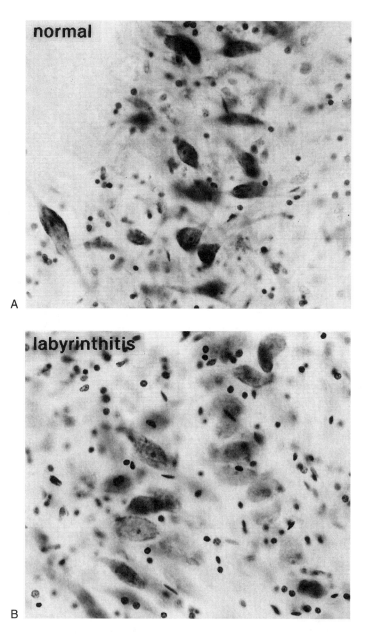

FIG. 4.1. Neurons in the medial superior olivary nucleus (Nissl stain): neurons in a normal, hearing, 62-year-old subject *(upper panel)*; neurons in a subject with idiopathic (possibly viral) labyrinthitis who was deaf for 1 year and was 42 years old when he died *(middle panel)*; and neurons in patient with bacterial meningitis who had been deaf for 31 years and was 54 years old when he died *(lower panel).*

bral cortex. Although the severity of damage to structures of the auditory pathway varied, a consistent finding was a pronounced pathologic response in certain classes of cells (*i.e.*, spherical and globular cells) within the co- chlear nucleus. These cells serve as conduits of relatively high levels of impulse activity within the central auditory pathway and may be more sensitive to reduced levels of stimulation.

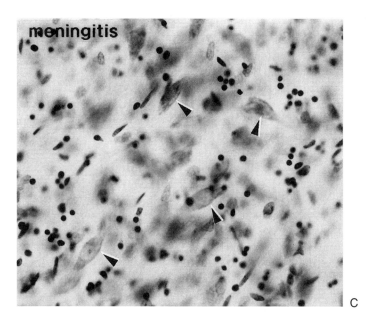

FIG. 4.1. (*Continued*)

Some studies have used computer-assisted morphometry to provide a quantitative picture of the effects of hearing loss. Moore *et al.* (1994, 1997) evaluated brain material from donors with well-documented histories and hearing assessments. The subjects included seven subjects with bilateral profound deafness and five persons of equivalent ages with normal hearing. Background information included the cause of deafness, age of onset and duration of deafness, and number of surviving cochlear ganglion cells. In each subject, the cross-sectional area (silhouette) was measured in a population of cells in the cochlear nuclei, in one of the superior olivary nuclei, and in the inferior colliculus. The results of the study indicted that cells were reduced in size in all cases of profound deafness but that there was considerable variation across the deaf subjects; the average cell size varied from near normal to only 50% of normal size. This variation is illustrated in Fig. 4.1, which shows some of the best preserved neurons in the case of labyrinthitis and some of the most affected in the case of meningitis. The reduction in size of human auditory neurons is similar to what is seen in experimental animal studies of sensory deprivation (Pasic and Rubel, 1989; Sie and Rubel, 1992) and is assumed to reflect down-regulation of metabolic and synthetic activity.

In addition to reduction in cell size, neurons in the profoundly deaf subjects showed marked changes in their pattern of staining. Because the commonly used neuronal stains, cresyl violet and toluidine blue, are basic dyes that bind to nucleic acids (DNA and RNA), staining intensity reflects the status of protein synthetic activity within cells. It can be seen in Fig. 4.1 that the neurons in the two deaf subjects are less intensely stained than those in the subject with normal hearing. The general pallor of the auditory neurons is particularly evident in the subject with meningitis. This is additional evidence for a fundamental change in cellular activity, particularly in regard to protein synthesis. Animals experimental studies have also provided evidence of reduction in intracellular protein production beginning shortly after loss of auditory input (Sie and Rubel, 1988; Born and Rubel 1992).

- What factors could account for the observed intersubject variability?

The best preservation of central neurons was observed in the case of labyrinthitis in which the duration of deafness was only 1 year and the population of cochlear ganglion cells was near normal. Cell size was more reduced in the subjects who had been profoundly deaf for 10 to 30 years, suggesting that degenerative changes occurs progressively rather than immediately after hearing loss. Among the subjects with long-term hearing loss, cell shrinkage was greatest in those with severely reduced populations of cochlear ganglion cells subsequent to meningitis and genetically induced deafness (*i.e.*, Scheibe degeneration). However, it is not possible to identify the most significant single factor in central degenerative change because the factors covary (*i.e.*, earlier onset and longer duration of profound hearing loss are associated with fewer remaining cochlear nerve neurons).

It seems intuitive to expect that maintenance of the presence and activity of cochlear nerve fibers would have a beneficial effect on the central nervous system and that loss of nerve fibers or reduction in their activity would lead to negative changes. The negative effect of hearing loss on the central auditory system is generally attributed to the reduced nerve firing and less release of chemical transmitters onto target neurons within the cochlear nuclei. However, Moore *et al.* (1994, 1997) showed that all of the auditory centers within any given subject were affected equally; the same degree of size loss was seen in neurons of the cochlear nucleus that are directly innervated by the cochlear nerve and in higher centers that are synaptic stations in the pathway. This indicates that the factors that produce cellular degeneration in the central nervous are capable of operating across synapses in the central pathway to propagate changes at higher levels.

The brain material evaluated by Moore *et al.* included specimens from cochlear implant users. Though we would expect the cells in the stimulated cochlear nucleus to be larger than those on the nonstimulated size, the cell measurements showed no observable differ-ence between the two sides. Figure 4.1 shows there is a range of cell size within each single auditory center, making it more difficult to statistically demonstrate consistent size differences between two populations of neurons. It may also be true that the stimulation provided by cochlear implants, though physiologically useful, does not fully restore auditory neurons to the state associated with normal hearing.

These study results provide a framework in which to consider neural factors in performance of a cochlear implant. Profound deafness can induce degenerative changes within the auditory pathway, but there is considerable variation in the degree of this degeneration across subjects. This variability may be one explanation of differences in performance among implant users. These studies also suggest that prosthetic restoration of input need not be immediate, but that it is probably more beneficial when provided within a few years. Clinical studies of congenital deafness (Gandolfi *et al.*, 1981, 1984) and experimental studies in young animals (Trune and Kiessling, 1988; Hashakasaki and Rubel, 1989) indicate that young auditory centers are more sensitive to loss of stimulation than those of adults, and it is possible that a greater degree of cell loss and cell degeneration occurs in early-onset deafness. For adults, however, there is reason for optimism in that even the most severely affected cases maintain a population of viable neurons that should be responsive to stimulation from a cochlear implant.

REFERENCES

Born D, Rubel E. Afferent influences on brain stem auditory nuclei of the chicken: presynaptic action potentials regulate protein synthesis in nucleus magnocellularis neurons. *J Neurosci* 1988;8:901–911.

Chow K, Stewart D. Reversal of structural and functional effects of long-term visual deprivation in cats. *Exp Neurol* 1972;34:409–433.

Dublin W. Cytoarchitecture of the cochlear nuclei. *Arch Otolaryngol* 1974;100:355–359.

Dublin W. Fundamentals of sensorineural auditory pathology. Springfield, IL: Charles C Thomas, 1976.

Dublin W. The cochlear nuclei revisited. *Otolaryngol Head Neck Surg* 1982;90:744–750.

Gandolfi A, Horoupian D, Rapin J, De Teresa RM, Hyams V. Deafness in Cockayne's syndrome: morphological, morphometric and quantitative study of the auditory pathway. *Ann Neurol* 11984;5:135–143.

Gandolfi A, Horoupian DS, De Teresa RM. Pathology of the auditory system in autosomal trisomies with morphometric and quantitative study of the ventral cochlear nucleus. *J Neurol Sci* 1981;81:43–50.

Hashisaki G, Rubel W. Effects of unilateral cochlear removal on anteroventral cochlear nucleus neurons in developing gerbils. *J Comp Neurol* 1989;283:465–473.

Hensen C, Reske-Nielsen E. Pathological studies in presbycusis. *Arch Otol* 1965;32:115–132.

Kirikae L, Sato T, Shitara T. A study of hearing in advanced age. *Laryngoscope* 1964;74:205–220.

Moore J, Niparko J, Miller M, Linthicum F. The effect of profound hearing loss on a central auditory nucleus. *Am J Otol* 1994;15:588–595.

Moore J, Niparko J, Miller M, Perazzo L, Linthicum F. Effect of adult-onset deafness on the human central auditory system. *Ann Otol Rhinol Laryngol* 1997; 106:385–390.

Pasic T, Rubel E. Rapid changes in cochlear nucleus cell size following blockade of auditory nerve electrical activity in gerbils. *J Comp Neurol* 1989;83:474–480.

Ramón y Cajal S. Histologie du système nerveux de l homme et des vertèbres, vol I. Madrid: Instituto Ramón y Cajal, 1952:754–838 [originally published in 1909].

Sie K, Rubel E. Rapid changes in protein synthesis and cell size in the cochlear nucleus following eighth nerve activity blockage or cochlear ablation. *J Comp Neurol* 1992;320:501–508.

Trune D, Kiessling A. Decreased protein synthesis in cochlear nucleus following developmental auditory deprivation. *Hear Res* 1988;35:259–264.

Appendix 4A

Central Auditory System Effects of Cochlear Implantation:
Animal Studies

Debara L. Tucci

Auditory system activity plays a critical role in the development and maintenance of normal central auditory system (CAS) function. Animal studies demonstrate that the effects of profound hearing loss are greatest in the developing auditory system but are also significant in adult subjects. The absence of auditory nerve activation in the profoundly hearing-impaired ear is thought to be responsible for the associated transneuronal degenerative changes observed in the CAS (see Chapter 2). It has been hypothesized that the timely introduction or reintroduction of auditory nerve activity may reverse early degenerative changes observed in adults and may facilitate more normal CAS function in the developing animal.

D. L. Tucci: Division of Orolaryngology, Duke University Medical Center, Durham, North Carolina 27710.

To the extent that animal studies can be used to model human deafness and the CAS response to restored activity, such studies are critical to our ability to optimize benefits of cochlear implantation in humans. Some important questions can be addressed with such studies:

- What are the effects of cochlear implantation in the mature vs. the developing CAS?
- What is the optimal time for cochlear implantation with respect to the onset of profound hearing loss?
- What are the implications of delaying implantation after the onset of hearing loss?
- What parameters of stimulation best facilitate maintenance of CAS neurons?

These questions have been only partially addressed in the literature reviewed in this chapter.

The most frequently used outcome measures reported in these studies include the survival (*i.e.*, number or packing density) of first nerve fibers within the auditory nerve (*i.e.*, spiral ganglion cells [SGCs]) and the volume and mean neuron area in CAS nuclei. More global measures of CAS function have been accomplished using markers of metabolic activity such as the oxidative enzyme cytochrome oxidase and the glucose analogue 2-deoxyglucose. Most investigators have used cat and guinea pig models, although many other species have been studied.

Wong-Riley *et al.* (1981) used cytochrome oxidase, which is usually found in high levels in the CAS, as a measure of neuronal activity or reactivation of neurons in two unilaterally deafened cats. Five to six months after deafening, the cochleas were electrically stimulated 8 or 15 days before brain tissue was processed for measurement of cytochrome oxidase in CAS nuclei. Although quantitative data and statistical analyses were not provided, the investigators reported that cytochrome oxidase levels were significantly higher in the stimulated compared with the nonstimulated ears and approached that of normal auditory neurons. El-Kashlan *et al.* (1993) reported evidence of metabolic activity in the CAS after prolonged deafness in the guinea pig with the use of the 2-deoxyglucose technique. They demonstrated a response to electrical stimulation of the cochlear nucleus (CN) throughout at least 16 weeks after deafening. Although there was a trend toward decreased metabolic activity over time, some response to electrical stimulation of the CN was evident as long as 15 months after deafening.

Effects of electrical auditory nerve stimulation on survival of first-order neurons was first investigated by Lousteau (1987). He found that the density (number) of SGCs was significantly greater in the stimulated than in the nonstimulated ear of bilaterally deafened guinea pigs. Modest amounts of stimulation were used in this study animals were stimulated at 100 μA for 1 hour daily, 6 days per week, for a 45-day period. Several subsequent investigations confirmed and ex-

panded on this finding. Hartshorn *et al.* (1991) also demonstrated increased SGC survival in the stimulated as compared with the nonstimulated ear of deafened guinea pigs. This effect was most pronounced in the basal regions of the cochlea, which was nearest the electrode. Stimulation in this study was limited to 2 hours per day, 5 days per week, for a total of 9 weeks and was delivered at current levels ranging up to 400 μA by an implanted intracochlear electrode.

Studies performed by Leake *et al.* (1991, 1992) in neonatally deafened cats (*n*=4) show that chronic intracochlear stimulation, begun at 9 to 17 weeks of age and lasting for 3 months, resulted in preservation of near-normal SGC numbers in Rosenthal's canal. Unilateral stimulation of two animals was limited to 4 weeks, without any apparent beneficial effects. Similar to the findings by Hartshorn *et al.* (1991), survival was most enhanced in the basal portion of the cochlea. Differences in SGC survival between the stimulated and nonstimulated ears ranged from 5% to 35% in different cochlear sectors. Stimulation level for all conditions was 6 dB above the electrical auditory brain stem evoked response (EABR) threshold. Although the finding that electrical stimulation enhances SGC survival is not uniform (Shepard *et al.*, 1994), most studies support this conclusion.

Several investigators have evaluated the effect of chronic auditory nerve stimulation on morphology of CAS nuclei. Chouard *et al.* (1983) reported CN volume measurements and cell areas for octopus cells in the CN and neurons in the medial nucleus of the trapezoid body and the lateral superior olive. Electrical intracochlear stimulation driven by a hearing aid was presented to eight neonatally deafened guinea pigs. Nuclear volume was larger for stimulated than for nonstimulated deaf ears, and mean octopus cell size measurements were larger for stimulated than nonstimulated ears.

Hultcrantz *et al.* (1991), in a companion paper to the Leake *et al.* (1991) study, reported an analysis of the CN in those same deafened stimulated animals. Analysis included cell counts from three consecutive sections of the anteroventral portion of the CN (AVCN) within a superimposed 0.3- by 0.3-mm grid, cross-sectional cell areas of 30 AVCN spherical cells, and volume of the CN complex. No significant differences were detected between the stimulated and non-stimulated sides of the brain for the four animals studied. However, the restricted sample size, particularly for the measurements of cell area, may be inadequate to detect changes. In a follow-up investigation, Lustig et al. (1994) studied a separate group of five neonatally deafened cats that were stimulated 4 hours daily at 2 dB above the EABR threshold for 3 months. Outcome measures included CN volume, area of spherical cells in the AVCN, and spherical cell density in the AVCN. In deafened nonstimulated ears, the spherical cell area was reduced by 20% to 26% compared with normal ears. After stimulation, area of spherical cells was increased 6% compared with the contralateral, unstimulated CN. No other statistically significant effects of stimulation were found. Thus, beneficial effects of stimulation were observed, but these effects were slight.

Similar findings were reported by Tucci et al. (1992) in the avian. Four-week-old chicks underwent bilateral cochlea removal, followed by unilateral intracochlear stimulation (200 μA biphasic pulse, 200 μA phase at 16.3/second for 12 hours/day for 4 weeks), commencing immediately ($n=11$) or after a 4-week delay ($n=4$). The area of second-order neurons was significantly larger (7.5%) on the stimulated than the unstimulated side of the brain for the immediate and delayed stimulation groups.

Matsushima et al. (1991) also reported significantly larger neuron areas in the AVCN and the posteroventral portion of the CN (PVCN) of deafened stimulated ears in cats. In this study, neonatally deafened kittens were stimulated with a biphasic pulse at a rate of 100/second at a current level halfway between the threshold and that of an aversive stimulus (range, 8 to 12 dB above EABR threshold) for 16 hours each day over a 3- to 4-month period. Data were collected on approximately 5,000 stimulated and 5,000 unstimulated cells in the AVCN (all cell types), spherical cells only in the AVCN, and smaller numbers of cells in the PVCN and dorsal CN (DCN). Findings were most robust in the AVCN, where neurons on the stimulated side were an average 28% larger than on the unstimulated side for deafened cats. No significant effects were observed for the spherical cells measured. Results for the PVCN were of borderline significance, and measurements in the DCN revealed no effect of stimulation. Compared with the Leake studies, it is possible that the longer-duration, higher-intensity stimulus and more extensive data analysis in the Matsushima et al. (1991) study may account for the apparent greater effect of electrical stimulation in the AVCN.

One explanation for the failure of electrical stimulation to completely reverse the CAS effects of deafness may involve the nature of the stimulus used in these studies. Although chronic, repetitive stimuli may replicate the effects of spontaneous activity in these structures, they allow for no stimulation of sound-evoked activity or for any alteration in the pattern of activity. Snyder et al. (1990) evaluated frequency resolution in the central nucleus of the inferior colliculus (IC) of cats that underwent chronic electrical stimulation as described for the Leake et al. (1991) experiment. The IC is characterized by a well-organized spatial tonotopic gradient. Spatial tuning curves were generated from single-unit and multiunit data by determining the threshold for an electrical stimulus generated by a particular intracochlear electrode pair at all levels in an IC electrode penetration. Results for chronically stimulated deaf cats were compared with results for deaf, implanted, unstimulated cats. Although tuning curves obtained from deaf, unstimulated cats were similar to those obtained from normal animals, those obtained from chronically stimulated animals were significantly broader, indicating that the volume of IC stimulated by activation of an electrode pair is significantly expanded or less finely tuned. It is possible that any type of electrical stimulation entrains an expanded neural population in the IC compared with acoustic stimulation and contributes to a loss of frequency specificity in this nucleus. It is also possible that the effects observed in this study are related to the repetitive nature of the stimulus used, which is not typical of the normal physiologic situation in which neural activity is spontaneous and sound evoked.

The studies previously summarized demonstrate that electrical stimulation of the deafened ear results in effective activation of CAS structures and at least partial conservation of these structures or partial reversal of degenerative changes. Many questions remain to be answered regarding mechanisms of these effects. Most of the reported studies have been performed in young animals over relatively short periods, and the effects of subject age and delay between onset of deafness and implantation have not been adequately investigated. Variations in the pattern, type, level, duration, and intracochlear location of stimulation are likely to be important parameters, as is the method of measuring outcome. Further studies are needed, particularly to document the effects of delayed implantation and stimulation.

REFERENCES

Chouard CH, Meyer B, Josset P, Buche JF. The effect of the acoustic nerve chronic electric stimulation upon the guinea pig cochlear nucleus development. *Acta Otolaryngol (Stockh)* 1983;95:639–645.

el-Kashlan HK, Noorily AD, Niparko JK, Miller JM. Metabolic activity of the central auditory structures following prolonged deafferentation. *Laryngoscope* 1993;103:399–405.

Hartshorn DO, Miller JF, Altschuler RA. Protective effect of electrical stimulation in the deafened guinea pig cochlea. *Otolaryngol Head Neck Surg* 1991;104: 311–319.

Hultcrantz M, Synder R, Rebscher S, Leake P. Effects of neonatal deafening and chronic intracochlear electrical stimulation on the cochlear nucleus in cats. *Hear Res* 1991;54:272–280.

Leake PA, Hradek GT, Rebscher SJ, Synder RL. Chronic intracochlear electrical stimulation induces selective survival of spiral ganglion neurons in neonatally deafened cats. *Hear Res* 1991;54:251–271.

Leake PA, Snyder RL, Hradek GT, Rebscher SJ. Chronic intracochlear electrical stimulation in neonatally deafened cats: effects of intensity and simulating electrode location. *Hear Res* 1992;64:99–117.

Lousteau RJ. Increased spiral ganglion cell survival in electrically stimulated, deafened guinea pig cochleae. *Laryngoscope* 1987;97:836–842.

Lustig LR, Leake PA, Synder RL, Rebscher SJ. Changes in the cat cochlear nucleus following neonatal deafening and chronic intracochlear electrical stimulation. *Hear Res* 1994;74:29–37.

Matsushima JJ, Shepherd RK, Seldon HL, Xu SA, Clark GM. Electrical stimulation of the auditory nerve in deal kittens: effects on cochlear nucleus morphology. *Hear Res* 1991;56:133–142.

Shepard RK, Matsushima J, Martin RL, Clark GM. Cochlear pathology following chronic electrical stimulation of the auditory nerve: II. Deafened kittens. *Hear Res* 1994;81:150–166.

Synder RL, Rebscher SJ, Cao K, Leake A, Kelly K. Chronic intracochlear electrical stimulation I the neonatally deafened cat. I: Expansion of central representation. *Hear Res* 1990;50:7.

Tucci DL, Rubel EW. Central auditory system development and disorders. *Neurotology* 1992;344:567–617.

Wong-Riley MT, Leake-Jones PA, Walsh SM, Merzenich MM. Maintenance of neuronal activity by electrical stimulation of unilaterally deafened cats demonstrable with cytochrome oxidase technique. *Ann Otol Rhinol Laryngol* 1981;90[Suppl 82]:30–32.

Cochlear Implant Technology

5

History of Cochlear Implants

John K. Niparko and Blake S. Wilson

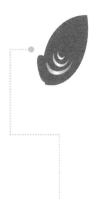

J. K. Niparko: Department of Otolaryngology—Head & Neck Surgery, The Listening Center at John Hopkins, The Johns Hopkins University, Baltimore, Maryland 21205-1809.

B. S. Wilson: Research Triangle Institute, Research Triangle Park, North Carolina 27709.

The biologic application of electricity has driven the development of a wide range of medical treatments, past and present, use electricity. Typically applied to disorders involving the nervous system and to heart and skeletal muscles, electrical stimulation provides well-accepted treatment strategies for disorders as diverse as endogenous depression, paralysis of voluntary muscles, and cardiac arrhythmias. Interest in the biologic application of electricity is centuries old. However, interest has often exceeded the level of understanding the mechanisms of action, and historical descriptions often express a mix of fear and mystique.

In the late 1700s, Luigi Galvani noticed that two different metals (zinc and copper), when placed in an aqueous bath, were capable of producing contractions in the leg muscles of the frog. The notion that electrical current generated by combining nonorganic materials could generate biologic activity was soon applied to the ear. Electrical stimulation of the auditory pathway as an alternative to deafness similarly extends to the late 18th century. Alessandro Volta (1800) is credited with the first observation that electrical current applied to metal rods at a voltage approximating 50 V created a sensation of "une recousse dans la tete" ("a boom within the head"), followed by a sound similar to that of boiling, thick soup (Fig. 5.1).

Subsequently, several crude applications of electrical stimulation to the ear for a range of indications were described through the 18th and 19th century in Paris (l'Academie des Sciences), Amsterdam (Dermann), London (Cavallo and Blezard), and Berlin (Selle) (Simmons, 1965; Luxford and Brackmann, 1985; Vestberg, 1998). Vestberg (1998) found that the optimism surrounding initial bioelectrical approaches to cure deafness was followed by skepticism; such applications appeared to be invasive and provided an important cautionary tale in that prosthetic approaches to solving human problems as complex as deafness require ongoing, critical evaluation.

In the 1930s and 1940s, verbal reports circulated in Europe that battery-supplied electrical current could stimulate the auditory nerve to evoke auditory sensations. Djourno and Eyries (1957) provided the first detailed

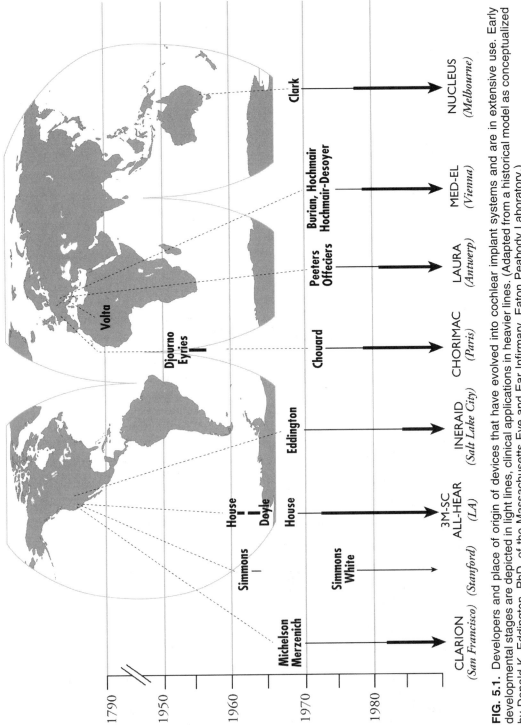

FIG. 5.1. Developers and place of origin of devices that have evolved into cochlear implant systems and are in extensive use. Early developmental stages are depicted in light lines, clinical applications in heavier lines. (Adapted from a historical model as conceptualized by Donald K. Eddington, PhD, of the Massachusetts Eye and Ear Infirmary, Eaton Peabody Laboratory.)

description of effects of directly stimulating the auditory nerve in deafness (Fig 5.2). After a formal proposal to stimulate the auditory nerve directly with a monopolar electrode in 1953, they placed a wire on the auditory nerve of a patient undergoing surgery for facial nerve paralysis that had resulted from previous cholesteatoma surgery in February of 1957. Prior opening of the cochlea provided access to the auditory nerve, and the implantation procedure did not require surgical invasion of the ear. When current was applied to the wire, the patient described generally high-frequency, sounds reminiscent of a "roulette wheel of the casino" and a "cricket." With a signal generator that pro-

vided up to 1,000-Hz pulses (frequencies higher than this failed to elicit discriminable changes in the stimulus), the patient eventually developed limited recognition of common words and improved speech reading capabilities. Although the safety of direct neural stimulation for hearing rehabilitation remained in doubt and continued to spark controversy at this early stage, the experience reported by Djourno and Eyries (1957) is considered the seminal observation suggesting that activation of the auditory periphery through an electrified device was practical and capable of providing physiologic useful information to the central auditory pathway.

Based on a sense of optimism generated

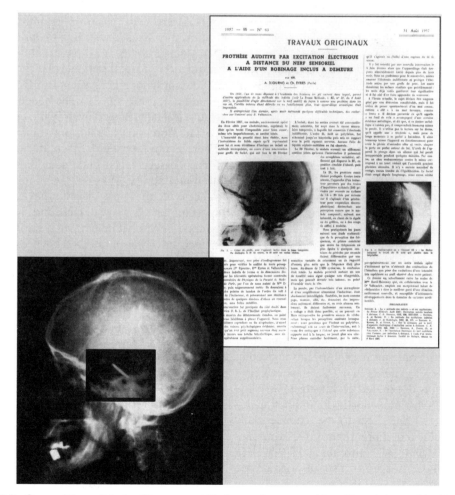

FIG. 5.2. Copy of the article by Djourno and Eyries as it appeared in a French journal in 1957.

by the French case report, attempts at stimulating the auditory nerve for clinical benefit began in the United States. House (1976) and Doyle *et al.* (1964) described approaching the auditory nerve through scala tympani electrode implantation in 1961. Their approach was to simulate patterns of electrical activity within the auditory nerve that they had observed in direct nerve recordings obtained during exposure of the auditory and vestibular nerve during Meniere's disease. Two patients underwent a series of extracochlear and intracochlear stimulus trials in January through March of 1961. Both subjects reported a greater sensation of loudness as stimulating voltage was increased and higher pitch with increments in stimulus rate. Neither patient tolerated the implanted hardware, because reduced responsiveness over several weeks suggested implant rejection, and both patients were explanted. Nonetheless, these reports of hearing sensation that were "pleasant and useful" lent impetus to further development of cochlear implant systems.

In 1964, Simmons (1966) placed an electrode through the promontory and vestibule directly into the modiolar segment of the auditory nerve. The subject demonstrated that, in addition to being able to discern the length of signal duration, some degree of tonality could be achieved.

House (1976) and Michelson (1971) refined clinical applications of electrical stimulation of the auditory nerve through scala tympani implantation of electrodes driven by implantable receiver-stimulators. These devices were evidence of the growing capabilities for microcircuit fabrication that stemmed from space exploration and computer development. In 1972, a speech processor was developed to interface with the House 3M single-electrode implant. This device was the first to be commercially marketed, and more than 1,000 were implanted from 1972 into the mid-1980s. In 1980, age criteria for use of this device were lowered from 18 to 2 years. By the mid-1980s, several hundred children had been implanted with the House 3M single-channel device.

Multiple-channel devices were introduced in 1984, and they supplanted single-channel devices based on enhanced spectral perception and enhanced speech recognition capabilities, as reported in large adult clinical trials (Gantz *et al.*, 1988; Cohen *et al.*, 1993). In the 1990s, clinical and basic science investigation produced changes in implant technology and in clinical approaches to cochlear implantation. Electrode and speech processor designs have evolved to produce encoding strategies that are associated with successively higher performance levels.

In parallel with device development and observations of safety and durability has come an emphasis on earlier implantation of children. There is now recognition of the required services for children to optimize implant performance and the structure of the interaction needed among the implanted child, family members, school staff, and implant team professionals. The benefits of cochlear implants placed in early life appear to be far more predictable (see Chapter xx). There is now substantially greater potential for open-set speech understanding in children and adults. Moreover, technologic advances of the past decade have refined speech encoding strategies and have expanded implant candidacy that have altered speech encoding strategies have expanded implant candidacy (Wilson *et al.*, 1991; Skinner, 1994; NIH Consensus Statement, 1995).

REFERENCES

Burian K, Hochmair E, Hochmair-Desoyer I, Lessel MR. Electrical stimulation with multichannel electrodes in deaf patients. *Audiology* 1980;19:128–36.

Chouard CH, MacLeod P, Meyer B, Pialoux P. Appareillage electronique implante chirurgicalement pour la rehabilitation des surdites totales et des surdi-mutites. *Ann Otolaryngol Chir Cervicofac* 1977;94:353–363.

Clark GM, *et al.* A mulitple-electrode hearing prosthesis for cochlear implantation in deaf patients. *Med Prog Technol* 1977;5:127.

Clark GM, Hallworth RJ. A multiple electrode array for a cochlear implant. *J Laryngol Otol* 1976;90:623–627.

Clark GM. The University of Melbourne Nucleus multi-electrode cochlear implant. *Adv Otol Rhinol Laryngol* 1987;38:V–IX, 1–181.

Cohen NL, Waltzman SB, Fisher SG, the VAH Cochlear Implant Cooperative Study Group: Prospective, randomized study of cochlear implants. The Department of Veterans Affairs Cochlear Implant Study Group. *N Engl J Med* 1993;328:233–237.

Djourno A, Eyries C. Prosthèse auditive par excitation électrique à distance du nerf sensoriel àl'aid d'un bobinage inclus á demeure. [Auditory prosthesis by means of a distant electrical stimulation of the sensory nerve with the use of an indwelling coil.] *Presse Med* 1957;65:1417.

Doyle J, Doyle D, House W. Electrical stimulation of the nerve deafness. Bulletin of the Los Angeles Neurological Society 1963;28:148–150.

Eddington DK. Auditory prostheses research in multi-channel intracochlear stimulation in man. *Ann Otol Rhinol Laryngol* 1983;87:1.

Gantz BJ, Tyler RS, Knutson JF, *et al.* Evaluation of five different cochlear implant designs: audiologic assessment and predictors of performance. *Laryngoscope* 1988;10:1100–1106.

House WF, Urban J. Long-term results of electrode implantation and electronic stimulation of the cochlea of man. *Ann Otol Rhinol Laryngol* 1973;85:504.

House WF. Cochlear implants: beginnings (1957–1961). *Ann Otol Rhinol Laryngol* 1976;85[Suppl 27]:3–6.

House WF. Goals of the cochlear implant. *Laryngoscope* 1974;84:1883–1887.

Luxford W, Brackmann D. The history of cochlear implants. In: Gray R, ed. *Cochlear implants.* San Diego: College Hill Press, 1985:1–26.

Michelson RP, Merzenich MM, Pettit CR, Schindler RA. A cochlear prosthesis; further clinical observations; preliminary results of physiologic studies. *Laryngoscope* 1973;83:1116–1122.

Michelson RP. Electrical stimulation of the human cochlea: a preliminary report. *Arch Otolaryngol* 1971;93:317–323.

Michelson RP. The results of electrical stimulation of the cochlea in human sensory deafness. *Ann Otol Rhinol Laryngol* 1971;80:914–919.

NIH consensus Statement, 1995.

Peeters S, Marquet J, Offeciers FE, Bosiers W, Kinsbergen J, Van Durme M. Cochlear implants: the Laura prosthesis. *J Med Eng Technol* 1989;13:76–80.

Simmons FB, Mathews RG, Walker MG, White RL. A functional multichannel auditory nerve stimulator: a preliminary report on two human volunteers. *Acta Otolaryngol* 1979;87:170.

Simmons FB, White RL, Walker MG, Mathew RG. Pitch correlates of direct auditory nerve electrical stimulation. *Ann Otol Rhinol Laryngol* 1981;90[Suppl]:15–18.

Simmons FB. Auditory nerve: electrical stimulation in man. *Science* 1965;148:104–106.

Simmons FB. Electrical stimulation of the auditory nerve in man. *Arch Otolaryngol* 1966;84:2–54.

Skinner MW, Clark GM, Whitford LA, *et al.* Evaluation of a new spectral peak coding strategy for the Nucleus 22 Channel Cochlear Implant System. *Am J Otol* 1994;15[Suppl 2]:15–27.

Vestberg P. Early experiments with electrical stimulation of hearing. Solvgade 87, St.v. 1307 Copenhagen. 1994.

Volta A. Historical records documenting the first galvanic battery, "The Volta Column." Circa 1800. Asimov's Biographical Encyclopedia of Science and Technology. Garden City, New York: Doubleday & Company 1982.

White RL. Stanford cochlear prosthesis system. In: Schindler R, Merzenich M, eds. *Cochlear implants.* New York: Raven Press, 1985.

Wilson BS, Finley CC, Lawson DT, Wolford RD, Eddington DK, Rabinowitz WM. Better speech recognition with cochlear implants. *Nature* 1991;352:236–238.

Cochlear Implants: Principles & Practices, edited by John K. Niparko, Karen Iler Kirk, Nancy K. Mellon, Amy McConkey Robbins, Debara L. Tucci, and Blake S. Wilson. Lippincott Williams & Wilkins, Philadelphia © 2000.

6

Cochlear Implant Technology

Blake S. Wilson

The catalog of cochlear implant systems developed over the past 15 years includes more than 30 different devices (Gantz, 1987). The differences among designs reflect the wide range of choices for implementing the major building blocks of implant systems. Advances in integrated circuit technology have been used in most of the recent designs. Such use has allowed the reductions in size and substantial increases in processing capabilities that characterize current devices.

In most cases, deafness is caused by the absence or degeneration of sensory hair cells in the cochlea. The situation is illustrated in Fig. 6.1, which shows anatomic structures in the normal and deafened ears. In the deafened ear, the hair cells are largely or completely absent, severing the connection between the peripheral and central auditory systems. The function of a cochlear prosthesis is to bypass the hair cells by stimulating directly surviving neurons in the auditory nerve. In general, at least some neurons survive even in cases of prolonged deafness and even in cases of virulent causes such as meningitis (Hinojosa and Marion, 1983).

The essential components of implant systems are identified in Fig. 6.2. A microphone senses pressure variations in a sound field and converts them into electrical variations. The electrical signal from the microphone is processed to produce stimuli for an electrode or array of electrodes implanted in the cochlea, usually within the scala tympani (ST). The stimuli are sent to the electrodes through a transcutaneous link *(top panel)* or through a percutaneous connector *(bottom panel)*. A typical transcutaneous link includes encoding of the stimulus information for efficient radiofrequency transmission from an external transmitting coil to an internal (implanted) receiving coil. The signal received at the internal coil is decoded to specify stimuli for the electrodes. A cable connects the internal receiver/stimulator package to the implanted electrodes. In the case of the percutaneous connector, a cable connects pins in the connector to the electrodes.

These components are shown in a different way in Fig. 6.3, which is a functional diagram of a current implant system that uses a transcutaneous link. In this system, a speech processor is worn on the belt or in a pocket. It is relatively light and small. A cable connects the output of the speech processor to a head-level unit that is worn behind the ear. A

B. S. Wilson: Research Triangle Institute, Research Triangle Park, North Carolina 27709.

Normal

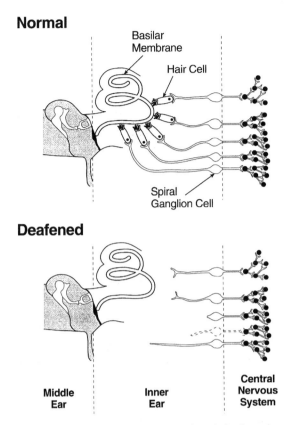

Deafened

FIG. 6.1. Illustrations of anatomic structures in the normal and deafened ears. Notice the absence of sensory hair cells in the deafened ear and the incomplete survival of spiral ganglion cells and of neural processes peripheral to cells that are still viable. Drawings do not reflect the details of the structures and are not to scale.

standard behind-the-ear (BTE) housing is used. A microphone is included within the BTE housing, and its signal is amplified and then transmitted to the speech processor through one of the wires in the cable connecting the processor to the head-level unit. The external transmitting coil is connected to the base of the BTE housing with a separate cable. The external coil is held in place over the internal receiver/stimulator package (which includes the internal coil) with a pair of external and internal magnets. The receiver/stimulator package is implanted in a flattened or recessed portion of the skull, posterior to and slightly above the pinna. The ground electrode is implanted at a location remote from the cochlea, usually in the temporalis muscle. For some implant systems,

a metallic band around the outside of the receiver/stimulator package serves as the ground, or reference, electrode. An array of active electrodes is inserted into the ST through the round window membrane or through a larger fenestration at or near the round window.

Photographs of the components illustrated in Fig. 6.3 are presented in Fig. 6.4. The speech processor, BTE headset, and transmitting antenna are shown in the right panel, and the receiver/stimulator package and electrode array are shown in the lower panel. The left panel shows an x-ray image of the implanted electrode array. The locations of the external coil, implanted receiver/stimulator, and implanted electrode array are indicated in Fig. 6.2B. An internal

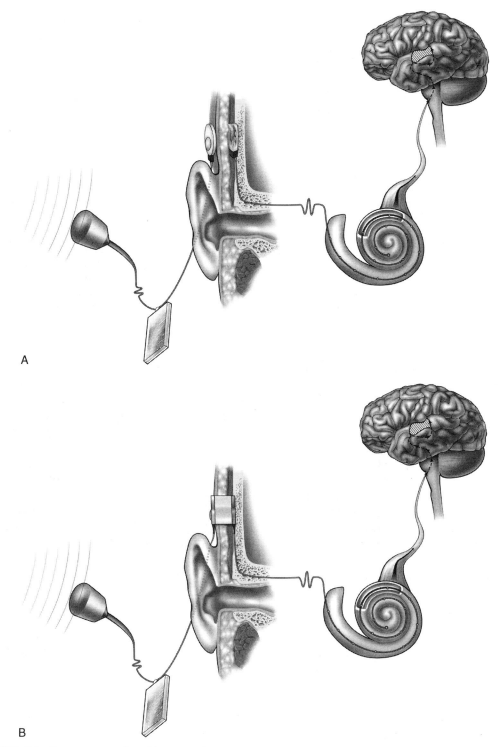

A

B

FIG. 6.2. Components of cochlear prosthesis systems. **A:** A system with a transcutaneous transmission link is illustrated. **B:** A system with a percutaneous connector is shown.

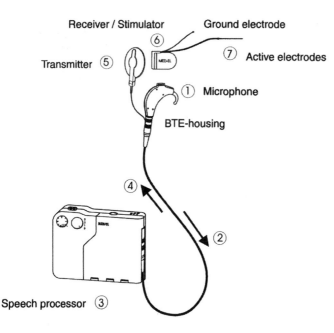

Receiver / Stimulator   Ground electrode

⑥

Transmitter ⑤   ⑦ Active electrodes

① Microphone

BTE-housing

④

②

Speech processor ③

FIG. 6.3. Schematic drawing of the Med El cochlear implant system, with the major elements indicated in Fig. 6.2. The microphone is mounted in a behind-the-ear (BTE) headset. (Courtesy of Med El GmbH, Innsbruck, Austria.)

cable connects the receiver/stimulator and electrode array.

An expanded view of the implanted cochlea is presented in Fig. 6.5. This shows a cutaway drawing of an electrode array inserted into the first turn and part of the second turn of the ST. Different electrodes or closely spaced bipolar pairs of electrodes ideally stimulate different subpopulations of cochlear neurons. Neurons near the base of the cochlea (first turn and lower part of drawing) respond to high-frequency sounds in normal hearing, and neurons near the apex of the cochlea respond to low frequency sounds. Most implant systems attempt to mimic this tonotopic encoding by stimulating basal electrodes to indicate the presence and amplitude of high frequency sounds and by stimulating apical electrodes to indicate the presence and amplitude of low frequency sounds.

Figure 6.5 indicates a partial insertion of the electrode array. This is a characteristic of all available scala-tympani implants; no electrode array has been inserted further than about 30 mm from the round window membrane (at the very base of cochlea)

and typical insertion depths are much less than that. The figure also shows a pristine survival of cochlear neurons. However, survival of neural processes beyond the ganglion cells (the dendrites) is rare in the deafened cochlea. Survival of the ganglion cells and central processes (axons) usually is not uniform within and among deafened cochleas.

Figures 6.3 and 6.4 show components of the Med El (COMBI 40) cochlear implant system. Other systems share the same basic components but are different in detail. For example, systems just introduced by Cochlear Ltd. and by Med El GmbH include the speech processor within a BTE housing, eliminating the separate and much larger speech processor of prior systems and the cable connecting the processor to the BTE housing. The details of processing and of techniques for the transmission of stimulus information across the skin differ widely among implant systems. The details of the electrode design also vary widely across systems.

Some of the choices and unknowns faced by designers of implant systems are summa-

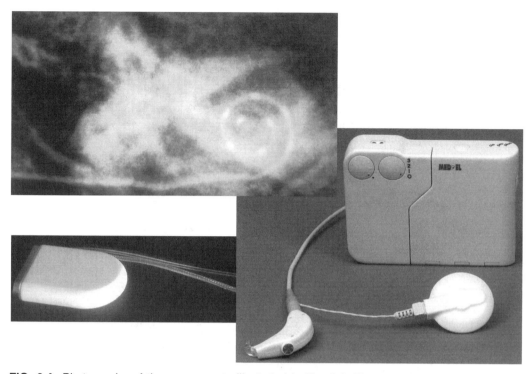

FIG. 6.4. Photographs of the components illustrated in Fig. 6.3. The speech processor, behind-the-ear (BTE) headset, and transmitting antenna are shown in the right panel, and the implanted components are shown in the lower left panel. An X-ray image of the implanted electrode array is shown in the upper left panel. (Courtesy of Med El GmbH, Innsbruck, Austria.)

rized in Table 6.1. Each choice may affect performance, and each choice may interact with other choices. The variability imposed by the patient may be even more important than the particulars of implant design (Wilson *et al.*, 1993). Although any of several implant devices can support high levels of speech reception for some patients, other patients have poor outcomes with each of those same devices. Factors contributing to this variability may include differences among patients in the survival of neural elements in the implanted cochlea, proximity of the electrodes to the target neurons, integrity of the central auditory pathways, and cognitive skills.

In the remainder of this chapter, we describe in greater detail the hardware of implant systems. Further discussion of processing strategies for transforming acoustic inputs into patterns of electrical stimulation is presented in Chapter 7. Likely sources of variability among patients also are discussed in that chapter.

MICROPHONE

The microphone for an implant system typically is housed within a BTE unit (Figs. 6.3 and 6.4) or in the speech processor enclosure. A separate "tie tack" or "clip on" microphone also can be placed remotely and connected to the speech processor with a thin cable. A good microphone for an implant system has a broad frequency response but can minimize responses to low-frequency vibrations that can be produced by head movements and walking.

A directional microphone can help in listening to speech in under adverse conditions,

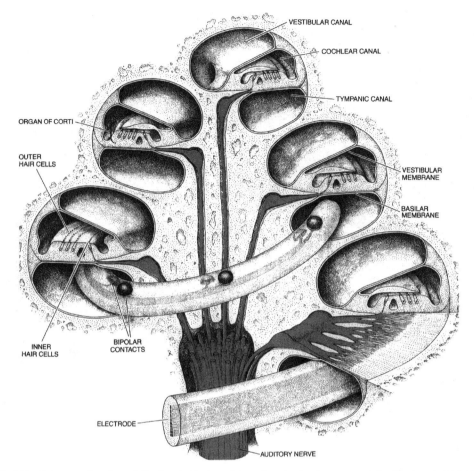

FIG. 6.5. Cutaway drawing of the implanted cochlea. An electrode array originally developed at the University of California at San Francisco is depicted. This array was the progenitor of arrays used with the Clarion device, manufactured by Advanced Bionics, Inc. (Reproduced with permission from Loeb, 1985.)

such as attending to one speaker in competition with other speakers or in competition with background noise (*e.g.*, cafeteria noise). The directional pattern of sensitivity for a single microphone is determined largely by its housing and placement on the body. For example, the head can act as a baffle for high-frequency sounds from the contralateral side when the microphone is mounted at the side of the head (in a BTE unit). The length and orientation of a tube in front of the microphone can affect its frequency response and directional pattern.

The selectivity of the directional pattern can be increased substantially with the use of multiple microphones. With two microphones, for example, sounds originating between and in front of the microphones produce microphone outputs that are in phase with each other, whereas sounds originating at other locations produce microphone outputs that are not. Summation of such microphone outputs produces larger signals for the in-phase conditions, emphasizing sounds in front of the microphones and suppressing sounds emanating from other locations. Use of two microphones with a cochlear implant system has been evaluated by Feinman *et*

TABLE 6.1. *Principal options and considerations in the design of cochlear implant systems*

Processing strategy	Transmission link

Number of channels
Number of electrodes and channel-to-electrode
  assignments
Stimulus waveform
  Pulsatile
  Analog
Approach to speech analysis
  Filterbank representation
  Feature extraction
	Percutaneous
	Transcutaneous
	  Maximum stimulus update rate, within and across
	    channels
	  Back telemetry of implant status, electrode imped-
	    ances, and/or intracochlear evoked potentials

Electrodes	Patient

Placement
  Extracochlear
  Intracochlear
  Within the modiolus
  Cochlear nucleus
  Bilateral
Number and spacing of contacts
Orientation with respect to excitable tissue
	Survival of neurons in the cochlea and auditory nerve
	Proximity of electrodes to target neurons
	Function of central auditory pathways
	Cognitive and language skills

Adapted with permission from Wilson *et al.*, 1995.

al. (1997). The results indicate that speech reception performance under conditions of reduced signal-to-noise ratios can be improved with the addition of a second microphone.

SPEECH PROCESSOR

The function of the speech processor is to convert a microphone or other input (*e.g.*, direct inputs from a telephone, TV, or FM system) into patterns of electrical stimulation. Ideally, the outputs of the speech processor represent the information-bearing aspects of speech in way that can be perceived by implant patients. Strategies for achieving this objective are described in Chapter 7.

The processor is powered with batteries. Hearing aid batteries are used for the head-level processors, and larger batteries (*e.g.*, two to four AA batteries) are used for the body-worn processors. Battery life typically exceeds 12 to 16 hours, allowing patients to use their devices during the waking hours without the need for recharging or replacing the batteries.

Adequate battery life for the head-level processors is made possible through use of low-power integrated circuit technology, particularly low-power digital signal processing (DSP) chips that have become available. The head-level processors in some cases have reduced capabilities or reduced options for changes in processing strategies or processor parameters to save space and to reduce power consumption. Such tradeoffs may reduce the speech reception performance for users. In those cases, a body-worn processor may be preferable to a head-level processor, even though the latter is more cosmetic and convenient.

Advances in battery, integrated circuit, and DSP chip technologies have been driven by huge commercial markets for mobile phones, portable computers, and other hand-held or portable instruments. The economic incentives to develop better batteries and power-efficient chips are enormous.

Recipients of cochlear implants have benefited from such developments, in that the developments have made possible progressively smaller and more capable speech processors and implanted receiver/stimulators. We expect this trend to continue. Even greater capabilities may be available in head-level processors in the near future. Fully implantable systems, with the speech processor placed in the middle ear cavity, may be available in 5 to 10 years.

TRANSMISSION LINK

A percutaneous connector or transcutaneous link is used to convey stimuli or stimulus information from the external speech processor to the implanted electrodes. A principal advantage of a percutaneous connector is signal transparency; the specification of stimuli is in no way constrained by the limitations imposed with any practical design of a transcutaneous transmission link. Also, the percutaneous connector allows high-fidelity recordings of intracochlear evoked potentials, which may prove to be quite useful in assessing the physiologic condition of the auditory nerve on a sector-by-sector basis and for programming the speech processor (Abbas and Brown, in press; Brown *et al.*, 1990; Wilson *et al.*, 1997).

An important advantage of transcutaneous links is that the skin is closed over the implanted components, which may reduce the risk of infection compared with systems using a percutaneous connector. A disadvantage is that only a limited amount of information can be transmitted across the skin with a transcutaneous link. This usually means that the rates at which stimuli can be updated are limited and that the repertoire of stimulus waveforms is limited (*e.g.*, restricted to biphasic pulses only for some systems).

All commercially available implant systems use a transcutaneous link. In some cases, the link is bidirectional, allowing transmission of data from the implanted components out to the external coil and speech processor or speech processor interface, as well as transmission of data from the speech processor to the implanted receiver/stimulator and electrode array. The data sent from the implanted components to the external components can include:

• information about the status of the receiver/stimulator, such as measures of critical voltages;
• impedances of the implanted electrodes;
• voltages at unstimulated electrodes; *and*
• neural evoked potentials, as recorded using unstimulated electrodes.

Rates of transmission required for the first three measures are relatively low and well within the capabilities of the current technology. High-fidelity recordings of intracochlear evoked potentials require high sampling rates (*e.g.*, 50k samples/second), high resolution (at least 12 bits of analog-to-digital converter resolution), and rapid recovery of the recording amplifiers from the saturation produced by the presentation of stimulus pulses (Wilson, 1997). The new CI24M implant system, manufactured by Cochlear Ltd., has a capability to record intracochlear evoked potentials and to send the results from the internal receiver/stimulator to the external coil and speech processor interface (Brown *et al.*, 1998). The arrangement for recording intracochlear evoked potentials in this system is shown in Fig. 6.6. A separate computer is used in conjunction with the speech processor interface and transcutaneous link to specify and transmit the stimuli to the selected stimulus electrodes through the forward path of the link. After delivery of the stimulus pulses, voltages recorded at the selected (unstimulated) electrodes are encoded for transmission from the implanted receiver/stimulator back out to the external coil and speech processor interface. The computer then is used to reconstruct and plot the data received from the internal components.

The "neural response telemetry" feature of the CI24M implant does not fulfill the requirements for high-fidelity recordings described previously, and the types of stimuli that can be specified are highly limited. However, the data obtained with its use may be helpful in assessing the status of the nerve and for the fitting of speech processors (Brown *et al.*, 1998).

New and better transmission links are be-

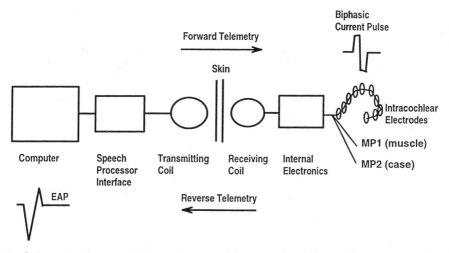

FIG. 6.6. Schematic diagram of the system used for recording intracochlear evoked potentials in the CI24M device. (Courtesy of Cochlear Corporation, Englewood, CO.)

ing developed by several manufacturers of implant systems. Such links may be available within the next several years, and they will support higher rates of information transmission in both directions compared with current transcutaneous links. One or more of them also may support high-fidelity recordings of intracochlear evoked potentials for a wide range of stimuli.

ELECTRODES

The electrodes for most implant systems are placed in the ST. The ST offers an accessible site that is relatively close to the spiral ganglion, which is not readily accessible with current surgical techniques. The electrodes and electrode carrier (together called the electrode array) must be biocompatible and remain so over the lifespan of the patient. The array must also be mechanically stable and facilitate atraumatic insertion. Surgical handling of the array is determined by its stiffness and cross sectional area. In general, flexible arrays and narrow cross-sectional areas facilitate insertion. Use of biocompatible lubricants such as hyaluronic acid also can facilitate insertion.

Intracochlear electrodes can be stimulated in a monopolar or bipolar configuration. In the monopolar configuration, each intracochlear electrode is stimulated with reference to a remote electrode, usually in the temporalis muscle or outside of the case of the implanted receiver/stimulator. In the bipolar configuration, one intracochlear electrode is stimulated with reference to another (nearby) intracochlear electrode. Different pairs of electrodes are used to stimulate different sites along the electrode array.

The spatial specificity of stimulation for selective activation of different populations of cochlear neurons depends on many factors, including:

- whether neural processes peripheral to the ganglion cells are present or absent;
- the number and distribution of surviving ganglion cells;
- the proximity of the electrodes to the target neurons; *and*
- the electrode coupling configuration.

These factors can interact in ways that produce selective excitation fields for monopolar or bipolar stimulation and in ways that produce broad excitation fields for either type of stimulation. For example, highly selective fields can be produced with bipolar electrodes oriented along the length of surviving neural processes peripheral to the ganglion cells (van den Honert and Stypulkowski, 1987). Highly selective fields also can be produced with close apposition of monopolar electrodes to the target neurons (Ranck, 1975). In addition, broad fields become more likely with increasing distance between electrodes and target neurons for either coupling configuration. Broad fields (produced by high stimulus levels) may be required for adequate stimulation of cochleas with sparse nerve survival.

An important goal of implant design is to maximize the number of largely nonoverlapping populations of neurons that can be addressed with the electrode array. This may be accomplished through use of a bipolar coupling configuration for some situations or through positioning of electrode contacts immediately adjacent to the inner wall of the ST. Such positioning would minimize the distance between the contacts and the ganglion cells.

Current electrode arrays do not include any special provisions for positioning the electrodes within the cross section of the ST. The arrays are flexible, and at least the Nucleus and Med El arrays tend to "rail out" against the lateral wall of the ST at the time of insertion (Gstöettner et al., 1998; Shepherd et al., 1985, 1993). Placements close to the inner wall can increase the spatial specificity of stimulation and produce reductions in threshold and increases in the dynamic range of stimulation (Cohen et al., 1998; Ranck, 1975; Shepherd et al., 1993).

Major efforts are underway at several companies and at cooperating universities to develop electrode arrays that place the electrode contacts close to the inner wall of the ST (Cohen et al., 1998; Jolly et al., 1998; Kuzma, 1996, 1998; Spelman et al., 1997). Such designs may increase the number of effective channels with unilateral implants. They also may increase battery life through reductions in stimulus levels required for threshold and comfortably loud percepts.

Although close placement next to the inner wall is likely to improve spatial selectivity, it is important to note that the inner wall is not always close to the spiral ganglion (SG) throughout the length of the ST (Ariyasu et

al., 1989; Ketten et al., 1997). Inasmuch as the spiral ganglion cells or the first central node of Ranvier are the most likely sites of stimulation with implants (Klinke and Hartmann, 1997), electrodes next to the inner wall may not be the ideal placement, particularly in regions where the distance between the inner wall and the SG is relatively large. The SG has $1\frac{3}{4}$ turns, whereas the ST has $2\frac{3}{4}$ turns. The SG reaches no higher than the middle of the second turn of the ST. The distance between the inner wall of the ST and the closest turn of the SG increases with increasing distance from the round window (toward the apex). These differences in the anatomic courses of the ST and SG preclude the possibility of close apposition of the structures throughout the length of the cochlea. The closest apposition is available along the basal turn.

Although placements of electrodes next to the inner wall of the ST may not be a panacea, such placements may be much better than placements with current electrode arrays. Resulting improvements in the spatial specificity and dynamic range of stimulation may improve the speech reception performance of implant systems.

REFERENCES

Abbas PJ, Brown CJ. Electrophysiology and device telemetry. In: Waltzman SB, Cohen N, eds. *Cochlear implants*. New York: Thieme Medical and Scientific Publishers, in press.

Ariyasu L, Galey FR, Hilsinger R Jr, Byl FM. Computer-generated three-dimensional reconstruction of the cochlea. *Otolaryngol Head Neck Surg* 1989; 100:87–91.

Brown CJ, Abbas PJ, Gantz B. Electrically evoked whole-nerve action potentials: data from human cochlear implant users. *J Acoust Soc Am* 1990;88:1385–1391.

Brown CJ, Abbas PJ, Gantz BJ. Preliminary experience with neural response telemetry in the Nucleus CI24M cochlear implant. *Am J Otol* 1998;19:320–327.

Cohen LT, Saunders E, Treaba C, Pyman BC, Clark GM. The development of a precurved cochlear implant electrode array and its preliminary psychophysical evaluation [Abstract 53]. Presented at the *Fourth European Symposium on Paediatric Cochlear Implantation;* s'Hertogenbosch, The Netherlands, June, 1998.

Feinman G, LeMay M, Staller S, *et al.* Audallion beam forming clinical trial results. Abstracts for the *5th Cochlear Implant Conference*; New York, NY May 1997, p 116.

Gantz BJ. Cochlear implants: an overview. *Adv Otolaryngol Head Neck Surg* 1987;1:171–200.

Gstöettner W, Baumgartner W-D, Jafar H, Jolly CN, Hochmair-Desoyer IJ. Perimodiolar electrode insertion process [Abstract 20]. Presented at the *Fourth European Symposium on Paediatric Cochlear Implantation;* s'Hertogenbosch, The Netherlands, June, 1998.

Hinojosa R, Marion M. Histopathology of profound sensorineural deafness. *Ann NY Acad Sci* 1983; 405:459–484.

Jolly CN, Gstöettner W, Baumgartner W-D, Jafar H. Breakthrough in perimodiolar concepts [Abstract 51]. Presented at the *Fourth European Symposium on Paediatric Cochlear Implantation;* s'Hertogenbosch, The Netherlands, June, 1998.

Ketten DR, Skinner MW, Gates GA, Nadol JB Jr, Neely JG. *In vivo* measures of intracochlear electrode position and Greenwood frequency approximations. *Abstracts for the 1997 Conference on Implantable Auditory Prostheses.* Los Angeles: House Ear Institute, 1997:33.

Klinke R, Hartmann R. Basic neurophysiology of cochlear implants. *Am J Otol* 1997;18:S7–10.

Kuzma JA. Cochlear electrode implant assemblies with positioning system therefor. US patent 5545219. *Am J Otol* [Suppl]:S7–S10. 1996.

Kuzma JA. Evaluation of new modiolus-hugging electrode concepts in a transparent model of the cochlea [Abstract 52]. Presented at the *Fourth European Symposium on Paediatric Cochlear Implantation;* s'Hertogenbosch, The Netherlands, June, 1998.

Loeb GE. The functional replacement of the ear. *Sci Am* 1985;252:104–111.

Ranck JB Jr. Which elements are excited in electrical stimulation of the mammalian central nervous system: a review. *Brain Res* 1975;98:417–440.

Shepherd RK, Clark GM, Pyman BC, Webb RL. Banded intracochlear electrode array: evaluation of insertion trauma in human temporal bones. *Acta Otolaryngol Suppl* 1985;399:19–31.

Shepherd RK, Hatsushika S, Clark GM. Electrical stimulation of the auditory nerve: the effect of electrode position on neural excitation. *Hear Res* 1993;66: 108–120.

Spelman FA, Clopton BM, Lineaweaver SK, Voie A. Focusing fields for cochlear implants: concepts, design, and tests of a high-density cochlear electrode array. *Abstracts for the 1997 Conference on Implantable Auditory Prostheses.* Los Angeles: House Ear Institute, 1997:37.

van den Honert C, Stypulkowski PH. Single fiber mapping of spatial excitation patterns in the electrically stimulated auditory nerve. *Hear Res* 1987;29:195–205.

Wilson BS. Signal processing. In: R Tyler, ed. *Cochlear implants: audiological foundations.* San Diego: Singular Publishing Group, 1993:35–85.

Wilson BS, Finley CC, Lawson DT, Zerbi M. Temporal representations with cochlear implants. *Am J Otol* 1997;18:S30–34.

Wilson BS, Lawson DT, Finley CC, Wolford RD. Importance of patient and processor variables in determining outcomes with cochlear implants. *J Speech Hear Res* 1993;36:373–379.

Wilson BS, Lawson DT, Zerbi M. Advances in coding strategies for cochlear implants. *Adv Otolaryngol Head Neck Surg* 1995;9:105–129.

SELECTED READING

Wilson BS. The future of cochlear implants. *Br J Audiol* 1997;31:205–225.

Appendix 6A

Microcircuitry in Cochlear Implants

John K. Niparko

Human interest in tiny machines can be traced back to the clockwork toys of the 16th century, but it was not until the 20th century that making things smaller and smaller conferred military and economic advantage. With the cold war and the space race combining to provide a strong stimulus, U.S. scientists in the 1950s sought to miniaturize the electronic circuits necessary to guide missiles, creating small, lightweight devices for launch into space. In Japan, the value of applying inexpensive, miniaturized technology to the consumer market was first realized. In his book *Made in Japan*, Akio Morita records his experience of showing Sony's $29.95 transistor radio to U.S. retailers in 1955. He was repeatedly asked, "Who needs these tiny things?"

The development of cochlear implants was

J. K. Niparko: Department of Otolaryngology—Head and Neck Surgery, The Listening Center at Johns Hopkins, The Johns Hopkins University, Baltimore, Maryland 21205-1809.

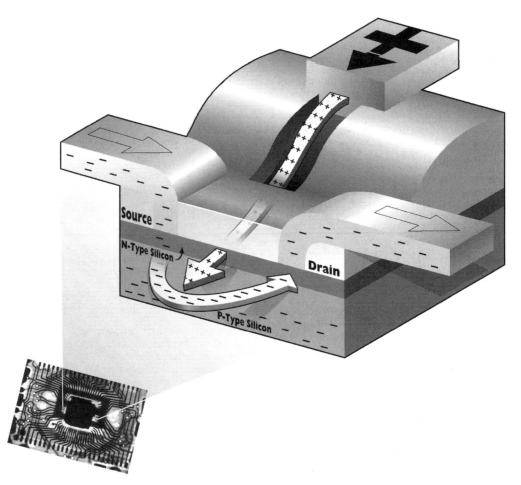

FIG. 6A.1. The speech processor and implanted receiver in a cochlear implant system use modern integrated circuits to perform their functions. The basic building blocks of integrated circuits are transistors, which act as switches to indicate a logical 1 (true) or illogical 0 (false) response at the outputs. The processing of information in this digital domain uses Boolean logic to implement rules for decisions. A typical integrated circuit contains thousands of transistors, interconnected in a way to implement to implement a particular processing function. Many such functions are implemented in microcomputers and digital signal processing (DSP) chips, which typically include millions of transistors. Most implant systems use a microcomputer or DSP chip in the speech processor and a custom integrated circuit in the implanted receiver. A transistor acts as a gating device that admits or resists current flow, depending on a small triggering current. A transistor makes it possible for small current to control a second, stronger current. The source of the small current is a positive ion flow that, when activated, slides into a current pool within the N-type silicon later to attract negative ions from the pool contained within the P-type silicon. This completes a circuit by opening the gate between the primary source and drain. In digital computations, this is a "1" bit in 0-versus-1 binary notation. If the small triggering current is not activated, the positive charge fails to slide into the current pool. Negative ions in the pool remain repelled, and the circuit remains open. Under this condition, no current from this particular transistor is sent for analysis. In digital computations, this is a "0" bit in 0-versus-1 binary notation. (After White R. How Computers Work. Emeryville, Ziff-Davis Press, 1997.)

made possible by the ability to rapidly transfer and process sound-based information and to store significant amounts of information in an easily portable unit. Such processing and storage are made possible by combinations of microscopic electronic circuits. Transistors, microchips, and a processor make up the critical components that enable an implant to process sound. This hardware requires instructions about how to perform. Software makes the hardware perform a range of functions as carried out by the processing unit.

The miniaturization of technology has made extraordinary progress in the decades since the invention of the transistor. The transistor is an electronic switch. Transistors make it possible for a small amount of electricity to trigger a second, much stronger electrical current, just as wall-mounted switch can produce the needed current to light a room. The capacity for switching on an electrical current lies in a transistor's component materials, typically different forms of silicon that serve as semiconductors. Different forms of silicon, because of their unique electronic behaviors, offer different resistances to conducting electricity. A small electrical charge can induce a layer of silicon to become less resistive to flow, enabling a surge of electricity to flow only when activated.

The transistor is a basic building block for the microchip. The microchip is a Lilliputian-like library of thousands of transistors connected together on a slice of silicon. Information flows in, and processed information flows from the microchip to other components of the implant system. This design enables decisions to be made about when and how to activate an electrode contact within an implanted array within the cochlea (Fig. 6A.1). Microchips are combined to fabricate the powerful and complex data-processing device known as the microprocessor. Operations of a microprocessor are performed by turning on or off combinations of transistors contained within a microchip. The microprocessor acts as the important decision-maker

within an implant system by using preprogrammed instructions. Components of the microprocessor are designed to extract specific components from the flow of incoming information as guided by instructions and then turn out processed information. The processor is capable of manipulating information gathered by the microphone to generate the electrical code called for by a system's processing strategy.

Faster processing speeds have come about as a result of integrating millions of transistors into areas of less than a couple square inches. Manufacturers of microchips have continued to increase the number of transistors that can be incorporated in a single integrated circuit. State-of-the-art microprocessors in 1980 contained about 30,000 transistors linked together. By 1990, microprocessors were developed containing more than 1 million transistors. Today, commonly used processors hold over 7 million transistors. Ever-larger numbers of components will be fitted onto the microchip in the future.

Larger numbers of transistors enable processing routines to go on simultaneously, rather than successively. Increasing speed is also gained by freeing chips from the need to go into an idle mode, increasing the capacity to store and manipulate data.

Microprocessors are capable of integrating specialized circuits. For example, analog circuits are used to generate time delays and compare the phase relationship of two different incoming signals. Operational amplifiers are used in comparing the magnitude of two signals and indicating which is larger, providing the basis for extracting and prioritizing sound signals.

REFERENCES

Barna A, Porat D. *Integrated circuits in digital electronics,* 2nd ed. New York, John Wiley & Sons, Inc. 1987.

Holland R. *Integrated circuits and microprocessing.* Oxford, Butterworth-Heineman, 1986.

Marks MH. *Basic integrated circuits.* Blue Ridge Summit, Pennsylvania: Tab Books, 1986).

Zaks R, Wolfe A. *From chips to systems,* 2nd ed. San Francisco, Sybex, 1987.

Appendix 6B

Food and Drug Administration Approval Process for Cochlear Implants

Harry R. Sauberman

The Food and Drug Administration (FDA) oversees the process of assessing new medical devices for the American market. In the process of screening new devices, FDA representatives attempt to determine the degree to which risk offsets the opportunities afforded by innovation. The screening process is not simple but should not be burdensome. The FDA aims to provide a level of assurance of safety and effectiveness and perhaps refine the assessment of a new device without impeding progress. Effective communications between the device manufacturer, clinical investigators, institutional review boards (IRBs), and the FDA are crucial to this process.

Clinical studies compile safety and effectiveness information and are the cornerstone of the approval process for new devices such as the cochlear implant. Authority to mandate clinical studies was granted to the FDA by the Federal Food, Drug, and Cosmetic Act (ACT), amended by the Medical Device Amendments of 1976, the Safe Medical Device Act of 1990, and the Food and Drug Administration Modernization Act (FDAMA) of 1997.

An FDA study approval permits an implant to be lawfully investigated in human subjects. This part of the chapter examines the approval process as it applies to devices such as the cochlear implant.

STUDIES IN THE REGULATORY PROCESS

Investigational studies in the regulatory process follow a standard sequence:

H. R. Sauberman: ENT Branch, Food and Drug Administration, Rockville, Maryland 20850.

I. Prototype is developed
II. Feasibility study (5 to 10 patients)
III. Pivotal study to determine safety and effectiveness (requiring adequate sample size to ensure statistical confidence of 95% with power of 80% that reflects a substantiation of claims in the device labeling)
IV. Submission of a premarket approval (PMA) application

For PMA applications that are deemed suitable for filing, FDA decisions of approval, or denial, are provided within 180 days.

Definitions

The FDA has defined *implant* to mean any device that is placed into a surgically or naturally formed cavity of the human body if it is intended to remain there for a period of 30 days or more.

Clinical device studies are designated as being significant risk (SR) or nonsignificant risk (NSR). *SR studies* generally involve implants and include devices used to support or sustain human life; are of substantial importance in diagnosing, curing, mitigating, or treating disease; or otherwise present a potential for serious risk to the health, safety, or welfare of a patient. *NSR studies* are those that do not meet the SR criteria. SR studies must have FDA approval before starting.

CLASSIFICATION OF IMPLANTS USED IN OTOLARYNGOLOGY

The ACT of 1976 recognized the need for clinical studies of certain devices and devised a scheme wherein all medical devices intended for human use were placed in a regulatory category that would ensure their safety and effectiveness. This process, known as *classification*, places all medical devices into one of three regulatory categories, based on risk:

- Class I: This is the lowest level of regulation to which all devices are subject. These requirements consist of general controls, which include manufacturer registration, product listing, the keeping of specified records and reports, and following good manufacturing practices.
- Class II: It is in this category that certain implants, such as commonly used tympanostomy tubes (*e.g.*, those without semipermeable membranes or antimicrobial biomaterials) and partial or total ossicular replacement prostheses have been placed. Class II is designated for devices wherein general controls alone are not sufficient and special controls, such as postmarket surveillance, performance standards, and patient registries are deemed necessary.
- Class III: Most of the implants used in the head and neck region are class III devices that require individual assessment of their safety and effectiveness through a premarket approval process before they gain entry to the market.

INVESTIGATIONAL DEVICE EXEMPTION

Regulation for the Conduct of Clinical Studies

Based on requirements of the ACT, the FDA implemented regulations for protecting human subjects in clinical investigations of medical devices. The investigational device exemption (IDE) regulation (21 CFR Part 812) sets forth the procedures and requirements under which clinical studies of medical devices are conducted.

Overview of Investigational Device Exemption Studies

Cochlear implants, by virtue of the privileged anatomic space that they occupy and their interaction with the delicate structures of the inner ear, are deemed SR devices for which IDE studies are necessary. Four key participants are critical to the conduct of IDE studies:

1. The sponsor, who is responsible for initiating, coordinating and managing the study
2. The investigators, who carry out the study
3. The IRB, which approves and oversees the study
4. The subjects (patients), who give their informed consent and agree to participate in the study

The roles and responsibilities of the sponsor, the investigators, and the IRB are critical to the success of an implant study. An investigation involving significant risk must be approved by the FDA and an IRB before the clinical study can begin.

FDA approval to conduct a clinical investigation after a determination of a significant risk implant device requires the sponsor submit a complete IDE application for FDA review. The application should contain the following items:

- A detailed investigational plan with citations of reports of prior investigations (including a description of literature sources and any related clinical studies)
- A complete description of the device and its intended use
- Names of qualified clinical investigators who have agreed to participate in the study
- The patient informed consent form
- Confirmation that all necessary background information regarding the investigational plan has been provided to the investigators and that a signed agreement has been obtained from each
- Identification of the investigational sites where the study is to be conducted

After receipt of an IDE application, a timely schedule of agency review is set into motion. Within 30 days from the date of receipt of the application, FDA will approve, conditionally approve, or disapprove an IDE application.

If an IDE application is disapproved or conditionally approved, the sponsor is given the opportunity to respond to the deficiencies cited by FDA and may request a regulatory hearing.

After a clinical implant study has begun, the sponsor is responsible for ensuring that it is properly monitored and that the required reports are sent to FDA and the IRB. It is the sponsor's responsibility to maintain a current history of all pertinent records and reports and to ensure during the course of the study that the implant device is not otherwise promoted, advertised to the general public, or in any other way commercialized. Limited advertising is permitted for the purpose of recruiting qualified investigators and study subjects.

Valid Scientific Evidence in an Investigational Study

An investigational study should be intended to obtain valid scientific evidence that supports the safety and effectiveness of the device. The most effective way to accomplish this is through a properly designed and controlled clinical investigation. The approved clinical protocol should be strictly followed, the patient data should be thoroughly analyzed, and the scientific and statistical integrity of the data collected should be rigorously examined and verified. Adherence to sound design principles, such as single- or double-blind controlled studies, randomization, and the observance of strict procedures to eliminate or minimize bias, is essential.

Design of the Clinical Protocol

The clinical protocol that is formulated by a sponsor is critical to the value of an investigational study. Protocol design concepts include formulation of the research questions about whether an implant offers safety and effectiveness in its intended use. The research question then leads to a determination of what the desired end points of the study should be. Other criteria also require determination and analysis, such as the location and duration of the study, subject population, subject inclusion and exclusion criteria, and the study design itself (*e.g.*, blinding, randomization, controls).

Statistical criteria must be established. These involve selecting an adequate sample size, choosing proper comparability methods to assess data from treatment and control groups, selecting optimal statistical procedures for evaluating short-term and long-term safety and effectiveness, establishing confidence limits, and defining procedures for follow-up and monitoring. Clinical protocols and assessments of results need to substantiate a manufacturer's claims (or labeling) of the device's indications and expected results.

Conducting the Study

The investigator is pledged to follow the specific investigational protocol approved by the FDA and to work within the guidelines of the IRB. This pledge is reflected in the signed agreement that every investigator must have with the study sponsor. Deviations from the protocol require the express approval of the sponsor, the FDA, and the responsible IRB.

Modifications of the study plan can easily undermine the quality and objectivity of a clinical study and the validity of the results. However, an investigator may wish to modify a study plan to accommodate a family's wishes or a particular request of a subject. Modifications can be made only after convincing rationale has been presented and the sponsor, the FDA, and the IRB have given their approval. Strict adherence to a clinical study protocol is crucial to a study's validity and the ability to produce conclusions that can be generalized to larger populations of potential recipients.

In cases of emergency, such as to protect the physical well-being of an implanted subject, an investigator may have no choice but to deviate from an approved protocol. Deviation must be reported to the sponsor, the FDA, and the IRB involved. On the basis of its assessment of the nature of the emergency and prior similar events, the FDA may request that the sponsor undertake appropriate measures.

The investigator should agree to abide by all applicable FDA and IRB requirements, including the requirement not to begin a study until FDA and IRB approvals have been received. The investigator has special duties, apart from those of the sponsor. He or she must see that:

- The subjects intended for enrollment in an implant study or their legally authorized representative are provided with and complete an informed consent statement before enrollment
- The informed consent statements are presented in a manner that provides sufficient opportunity to consider whether to participate in a study in a manner that is free from the possibility of coercion or undue influence
- The intended subjects give assurance that they fully understand the implant procedure and have received an assessment of the potential risks and benefits of the surgical procedure
- The safety and health of the enrolled subjects are adequately followed during the course of the study
- There are no unapproved departures from the clinical protocol
- There is no advertising, promotion, or commercialization of the clinical study by the investigator to the public
- Factual and complete records of the study are maintained and periodic reports are given to the sponsor and to the IRB
- There is responsibility for timely reporting of any and all unanticipated complications or adverse effects that may occur during the study

Evaluating and Monitoring an Implant Study: Role of the Institutional Review Board

A committee of individuals designated by an institution as an IRB has the delegated authority from the FDA to evaluate the perceived risks and benefits of an investigational study and to oversee the conduct of the study. IRBs are a part of the organization of nearly all major and many smaller hospital and medical centers. Their responsibility is to ensure the protection of the rights, safety, and welfare of human subjects. IRBs apply ethical considerations and standards in their review of clinical studies. Their interests are such that they are generally sensitive to local and regional community conditions and attitudes.

IRB committees are usually composed of members who represent medical, scientific, and community attitudes. Their purpose is to determine the acceptability of a study at their institution in view of institutional commitments and regulations, applicable laws, community interests, and standards of professional conduct.

An IRB reviews the intended use of the implant and ascertains whether the risks to subjects are minimized in accordance with the protocol design. The IRB further determine whether the risks to subjects are reasonable in relation to the anticipated benefits and the importance of the knowledge that may result from a study. The IRB also determines whether:

- The selection of patients is equitable and the manner in which consent will be obtained and documented from each prospective patient or legally authorized representative
- The clinical protocol contains adequate provision for monitoring data collection to ensure the safety of the patients
- Adequate provision is in place for protecting the privacy of patients and the confidentiality of the data

After this review, the IRB recommends approval, revision, or disapproval of the study. An IRB may also offer an opinion on significant and nonsignificant risks.

Although not directly responsible for obtaining informed consent (which is the responsibility of the investigator), one of the significant obligations of an IRB is its role with respect to protection of the patient. IRBs ensure that information given to prospective study patients is in accordance with the required elements of fully informed consent. IRBs may require that information above and beyond that provided by the sponsor or an investigator be provided to study patients when, in the judgment of the IRB committee, such information would add meaningfully to the protection of a patient's rights and welfare.

An IRB has the authority to suspend or terminate a study that is not being conducted in accordance with requirements or that has been associated with harm to patients. Suspension or termination action must include a statement in writing of the reasons for the IRB's action and must be reported in a timely manner to the sponsor, the FDA, and resident investigators.

PRESENTATION OF DATA IN A PREMARKET APPROVAL APPLICATION

After completion of an implant study, safety and effectiveness data are thoroughly analyzed and reviewed by the sponsor and investigators. Analysis is for the determination of an implant's safety and effectiveness and may require biocompatibility review, toxicology review, medical review, engineering review, and statistical review. This information may then be presented to the FDA in the form of a premarket approval (PMA) application. The key feature inherent in the PMA application is that the data are representative of a sound clinical study; this feature implies a study has a sufficient number of subjects to demonstrate statistical and clinical significance.

The review and approval of a PMA application, as with the IDE application, requires that:

• There must be a complete summary, analysis, and discussion of the safety and effectiveness data presented by the sponsor
• There must be a formal review, analysis,

and discussion of the entire application, including the summary of safety and effectiveness data by FDA staff and possibly by the FDA advisory panel charged with reviewing the application
• If the application is considered by an advisory panel, a positive recommendation by the panel must be corroborated by the FDA.

FDA MODERNIZATION ACT OF 1997 AS IT RELATES TO COCHLEAR IMPLANTS

With the passage of the FDAMA in 1997, sponsors engaged in clinical studies of cochlear implants are afforded the opportunity for early collaboration with the FDA regarding the data requirements for relevant studies. Meetings with FDA staff are encouraged before submitting a formal application for an IDE or a PMA. At pre-IDE meetings, the sponsors may present and discuss their investigational plans and clinical protocols. Sponsors may seek to exchange medical and scientific information in a determination meeting, or they may seek to reach a formal agreement with the FDA on the investigational plan to be followed and the data to be collected in a clinical study.

A determination meeting with the FDA would normally precede an aggrement meeting. Specific topics that may be discussed at these meetings include review of the investigational plan, the type of study to be performed, and the statistical controls for the study. A request from a sponsor for an aggrement meeting should include a detailed description of the device, the proposed conditions of use, and the proposed investigational plan, including the clinical protocol. After receipt of this information, the FDA will meet with the sponsor within 30 days. The objective is to reach aggrement on the details of the clinical study.

A record is kept of any agreement that is reached between the sponsor and the FDA. This agreement is binding on both parties. An exception is made, however, if the sponsor is notified by the FDA of a substantial scientific issue that was not included in the original agreement. The sponsor is then given the opportunity to discuss the scientific matter before issuance of an FDA decision.

Before submission of a PMA, sponsors are also encouraged to meet with the FDA. The purpose of these meetings is to discuss the type of data in terms of valid scientific evidence that must be submitted to substantiate the effectiveness claims that have been made for a specific cochlear implant. A pre-PMA meeting request should include a detailed description of the device, proposed conditions of use, a copy of the investigational plan, and whatever information is available concerning the expected performance of the device. After receipt of this information, the FDA will meet with the sponsor. Within 30 days after this meeting, the FDA will determine the type of data that is believed necessary to substantiate device effectiveness. The FDA's decision is binding unless the agency determines, by way of new information, that its decision is not in the best interest of the patient or that it is contrary to public health.

On receipt of a PMA application, the document is first reviewed for administrative completeness. If all of the required sections are contained in the submission, the PMA is filed and presented to a selected FDA review team, under a lead reviewer, for scientific review. On request, the FDA will meet with the sponsor within 100 days of receipt of the filed PMA application to review the status of the application. Before this meeting, however, the FDA will inform the sponsor of any deficiencies, major or minor, that the review team has found in the course of its scientific review. As part of this process, the FDA apprises the sponsor about information that is required to correct those deficiencies.

SUMMARY

Cochlear implants are significant risk devices for which investigational studies are necessary. The regulatory process of introducing these implants to the market follows sound principles in the application of good science. The procedural steps in filing IDE and PMA applications requires a careful understanding of the need for rigor in clinical trials. A device's sponsor, the clinical investigators, the IRB, and the FDA all have a role in seeing that the device a patient receives does not pose an unreasonable risk to the safety or welfare of the patient. The results of clinical trials enable appraisals that assist FDA in determining device safety and effectiveness. Given these conditions, the regulatory approval process should proceed in a straightforward and efficient manner.

Cochlear Implants: Principles & Practices, edited by John K. Niparko, Karen Iler Kirk, Nancy K. Mellon, Amy McConkey Robbins, Debara L. Tucci, and Blake S. Wilson. Lippincott Williams & Wilkins, Philadelphia © 2000.

7

Strategies for Representing Speech Information with Cochlear Implants

Blake S. Wilson

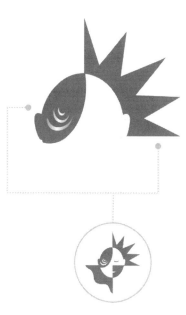

Remarkable progress has been made in the design and application of speech-processing strategies for cochlear implants. In particular, use of the new *continuous interleaved sampling* (CIS) and *spectral peak* (SPEAK) strategies have produced large improvements in speech reception performance compared with prior strategies (Skinner *et al.*, 1994; Wilson *et al.*, 1991a). All major manufacturers of multichannel implant systems now offer CIS or CIS-like strategies in their speech processors, with one offering both SPEAK and CIS. According to the 1995 National Institutes of Health Consensus Statement on Cochlear Implants in Adults and Children, "A majority of those individuals with the latest speech processors for their implants will score above 80-percent correct on high-context sentences, even without visual cues." Additional information on levels of performance is presented later in this chapter and in Chapter 10.

Although great progress has been made, much remains to be done. Patients with the best performance still do not hear as well as people with normal hearing, especially in adverse acoustic environments, and many

patients do not enjoy high levels of performance even with the new processing strategies. The range of performance across patients is large with any of the current multichannel implant systems.

The purpose of the speech processor is to transform microphone inputs into patterns of electrical stimulation that convey the information content of speech and other sounds (see Chapter 6). This chapter describes how information is encoded in the production of speech and how such information can represented or partially represented with cochlear implants.

ELEMENTS OF SPEECH

A simple but useful model of speech production is shown in Fig. 7.1. This source-filter model (Flanagan, 1972) recognizes the first-order independence between excitation of the vocal tract and its resonant response to the excitation. Unvoiced sounds of speech are produced with a source of broadband turbulent noise. This noise is generated by forcing air through a narrow constriction (for production of unvoiced fricatives such as /s/) or by building pressure behind an obstruction and suddenly releasing the pressure with removal of the obstruction. Stop consonants, such as /t/, are produced in this way.

B. S. Wilson: Research Triangle Institute, Research Triangle Park, North Carolina 27709.

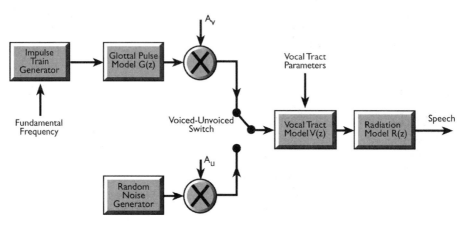

FIG. 7.1. A basic model of speech production. Parameters controlling the model include a binary indication about whether the sound is voiced or unvoiced, the frequency of glottal openings for voiced sounds, and the frequency transfer characteristics of the vocal tract. Parameters typically are updated at 5- to 30-ms intervals. The cross-marked circles indicate multiplier blocks. Speech amplitudes are controlled by the gain factors A_v and A_u for voiced and unvoiced sounds, respectively. (Adapted from O'Shaughnessy, 1987, with permission.)

The spectral characteristics of the broadband noise are altered by transmission though the vocal tract and to a lessor extent by radiation of sound at the lips.

In contrast, voiced sounds in speech are produced by exciting the vocal tract with puffs of air released through the vibrating folds of the glottis. The shape of the vocal tract, as adjusted through positions of the tongue, lip, jaw, and velum, determines how the excitation is filtered in the transmission of sound through the tract. The transfer function of the vocal tract is the *filter* in the source-filter model, and the spectral peaks in this transfer function are called *formants*. The frequencies of the first two formants convey adequate information for identification of vowels and for distinctions among other voiced sounds.

A third class of speech sounds is produced by the combination of periodic glottal excitation and aperiodic (supraglottal) noise sources. Voiced fricatives are produced in this way. For example, the addition of glottal excitation can change an /s/ sound into a /z/ sound.

Experiments with models of the type shown in Fig. 7.1 have demonstrated that a relatively small set of parameters can specify the information content of speech (Flanagan, 1972; O'Shaughnessy, 1987). In general, the parameters must specify the type of excitation (*i.e.*, voiced, unvoiced, or mixed) and the transfer function of the vocal tract. For most voiced speech sounds, the transfer function can be adequately specified by the frequencies of the first two formants. For most unvoiced speech sounds, an indication of overall spectral shape is adequate (*e.g.*, tilting up or down, principal resonance of the vocal tract). Updating such parameters every 5 to 30 milliseconds allows production of intelligible speech with a model such as the one in Fig. 7.1. The parameters specifying the transfer function of the vocal tract may be quantized along rather coarse scales and still preserve intelligibility. The information rate required to transmit these parametric data can be as low as 1,000 bits/s, which is far less than the 30,000 bits/s required for voice transmission over a typical telephone channel (Flanagan, 1972).

Taxonomy of Speech Sounds

Speech sounds can be classified according to the way in which they are produced, their

TABLE 7.1. *Classification of vowels*

Vowel	Place of constriction	Tongue height	Shape of lips	Example
i	Front	High	Spread	b*ee*t
I		High	Neutral	b*i*t
e		Upper-mid		b*ai*t
ε		Lower-mid		b*e*t
æ		Low		b*a*t
ɝ	Central, retroflex	High		b*i*rd
ə	Central	Mid		*a*bout
a		Low		French "l*a*"
u	Back	High	Rounded	b*oo*t
U		High	Slightly rounded	f*oo*t
o		Upper-mid	rounded	c*oa*t
ɔ		Lower-mid		b*ou*ght
Λ		Lower-mid	Neutral	b*u*t
ɑ		Low		h*o*t

acoustic characteristics, or the way in which they are perceived. These are interrelated; for example, the acoustic characteristics are a direct result of the way in which the sounds are produced.

Tables 7.1 and 7.2 present classifications of vowels and consonants, respectively, according to the way in which they are produced. Vowels are produced with an open vocal tract, with relatively large distances between the tongue and the roof of the mouth. Consonants are produced by narrowing or obstructing the vocal tract at some point. Air forced through narrow passages produces turbulent noise, as does the sudden release of air with the removal of an obstruction. Such sources of noise are the excitation signals for the unvoiced speech sounds.

TABLE 7.2. *Classification of consonants*

Consonant	Manner of production	Voicing	Place of constriction	Example
p	Stop	Unvoiced	Bilabial	*p*at
b		Voiced		*b*at
t		Unvoiced	Alveolar	*t*ar
d		Voiced		*d*one
k		Unvoiced	Velar	*k*ite
g		Voiced		*g*ate
f	Fricative	Unvoiced	Labiodental	*f*ar
v		Voiced		*v*iew
θ		Unvoiced	Linguadental	*th*in
ð		Voiced		*th*en
s		Unvoiced	Alveolar	*s*ee
z		Voiced		*z*oo
ʃ		Unvoiced	Palatal	*sh*ow
ʒ		Voiced		a*z*ure
h		Unvoiced	Glottal	*h*at
ʧ	Affricative	Unvoiced	Palatal	*ch*ase
ʤ		Voiced		*j*udge
m	Nasal	Voiced	Bilabial	*m*an
n			Alveolar	*n*ot
ŋ			Velar	si*ng*
l	Liquid		Alveolar	*l*oud
r			Alveolar + velar	*r*oad
w	Glide		Bilabial + velar	*w*ay
j			Palatal	*y*es

Many of the consonants also are characterized by relatively rapid movements of the articulators and consequently relatively rapid changes in the acoustic domain. Stop consonants are produced with a complete obstruction of the vocal tract followed by a sudden release of the obstruction. A noise is produced at the release, and this noise is filtered according to the shapes (principally the lengths and cross-sectional areas) of the vocal tract in front of and behind the initial obstruction.

The time between the release and onset of voicing for the following speech sound (*i.e.*, the voice onset time) is short or even negative for the voiced stop consonants, whereas the time between the release and the onset of voicing is tens of milliseconds for unvoiced stop consonants. Cognate pairs of stop consonants are identical in all respects except for the voiced or unvoiced distinction. These pairs are /p/-/b/, /t/-/d/, and /k/-/g/ in spoken English; the unvoiced members of the pairs are listed first.

Fricative consonants are produced with a narrowing of the vocal tract sufficient to generate turbulent noise. This source of noise may be accompanied by periodic puffs of air from the glottis. Unvoiced fricatives are produced with the noise source only, whereas voiced fricatives are produced with a combination of the noise source and the periodic excitation from the glottis. The voiced and unvoiced consonants also form cognate pairs: /f/-/v/, /θ/-/ð/, /s/-/z/, and /ʃ/-/ʒ/. An additional unvoiced fricative, /h/, does not have a voiced counterpart in spoken English.

Affricative consonants are concatenations of stop and fricative consonants. They can be unvoiced (/ʧ/) or voiced (/ʤ/).

Nasal consonants are produced by opening the velum passage to the nasal tract and closing the vocal tract. Different nasals are produced with different points of closure along the vocal tract. The closed vocal tract acts as a side branch resonator, which affects the spectrum of the sound emerging from the nostrils.

Liquid consonants include the lateral and retroflex consonants. The laterals (/l/ and related sounds) are produced with contact of the tip of the tongue with the roof of the mouth, although with a narrowing of the tongue to allow the passage of air around the sides of the tongue. This alters the resonant properties of the vocal tract compared with those of vowel sounds. The retroflex consonants (/r/ and related sounds) are produced with the tongue tip and tongue dorsum elevated (but not contacting the roof of the mouth), resulting in two points of constriction along the vocal tract. This also alters the resonant properties of the tract compared with the laterals and compared with vowel sounds.

The glide consonants (/w/ and /j/) are produced with closer appositions of the tongue to the roof of the mouth compared with vowels and are characterized by relatively rapid transitions compared with vowels. The appositions are not close enough to produce a separate source of turbulent noise, and all of the glides are voiced.

As indicated in Table 7.2, consonants can be classified according to manner of production and the place of constriction (*i.e.*, place of articulation). Within the broad classes of manner of production are the cognate pairs of voiced and unvoiced consonants for stops, fricatives, and affricatives. Consonants for all other manners of production are voiced.

Vowels often are classified according to the highest point of the tongue along the length of the vocal tract (*i.e.*, front to back) and with respect to the floor of the mouth (*e.g.*, low tongue position versus high tongue position). Vowels also are classified according to lip rounding, which affects the resonant properties of the vocal tract and radiation of sound at the lips.

The degree of constriction in the vocal tract ranges from open for the low and middle vowels to closed for the stops. The continuum from low to complete constriction includes low and mid vowels, high vowels, liquids and glides, fricatives, and stops. The vocal tract is closed for nasals, but the nasal tract is open.

In broad terms, the site of constriction or closure along the vocal tract affects its transfer function and resonant properties. The tract filters the excitation, which may be voiced, unvoiced, or a combination of the two.

Vocoder Theory and Models

Models of the type shown in Fig. 7.1 have been applied in analysis-synthesis or vocoder (for *voice coder*) systems for efficient transmission of speech signals. An example of such an application is the channel vocoder illustrated in Fig. 7.2. The upper panel shows a block diagram of the analysis part of the system at the transmitting end, and the lower panel shows a block diagram of the synthesis part of the system at the receiving end. Only a limited set of parameters, as extracted from the speech input in the analysis part of the system, is transmitted to the receiver. The advantage provided by analysis-synthesis systems is that the information rate required for transmission of the parameters is much less than that required for transmission of the unprocessed speech signal. Such savings allow the transmission of many more conversations through a channel of limited capacity. Extraction of parameters at the transmitting end also can allow encryption of messages for secure communications; encryption of a limited set of parameters is relatively straightforward and more secure compared with encryption of the unprocessed speech waveform.

The development of vocoder systems has a long and illustrious history, beginning with the initial development of the channel vocoder by Dudley in the late 1930s. Excellent reviews of vocoder designs and performance are presented in books by Flanagan (1972), O'Shaughnessy (1987), Papamichalis (1987), and Rabiner and Shafer (1978).

In channel vocoders, information about the excitation of the vocal tract is extracted with a voicing detector and with a pitch (or fundamental frequency) detector. The voicing detector determines whether the current speech sound is voiced or unvoiced, and the pitch detector determines the frequency of glottal openings for voiced speech sounds. Information about the configuration of the vocal tract is extracted with a bank of bandpass filters and envelope detectors. This analysis provides snapshots of the filtering by the vocal tract at 5- to 30-millisecond intervals.

The information transmitted between the analysis and synthesis ends of the system includes a binary indication of whether the sound is voiced or unvoiced, the fundamental frequency of voiced speech sounds, and the smoothed envelopes of energies within multiple bandpass ranges of the speech input. At the receiver, this information is used to reconstruct the speech waveform for the listener. The binary indication of voicing controls a switch that connects a noise source or a source of periodic pulses to the inputs of a set of multiplier blocks. The rate of the periodic pulses for voiced speech sounds is controlled by the parameter specifying the frequency of glottal openings. The other inputs to the multiplier blocks are the envelope signals for each of the bandpass channels. The outputs of the multiplier blocks are directed to a bank of bandpass filters (corresponding to the bank in the analysis portion of the system). A synthesized speech signal is formed by summing the outputs of the bandpass filters.

The performance of channel vocoders is affected by the accuracy of parameter extraction and by many choices in design, including the resolution with which the channel and fundamental frequency parameters are quantized and the number and frequency boundaries of the bandpass filters. In general, performance is improved with increases in resolution and increases in the number of bandpass filters up to points corresponding to limits in the *perception* of speech and other sounds. For example, multiple bandpass filters within critical bands of hearing are no better than one bandpass filter for each of the critical bands. Depending on the selected endpoints, 14 to 19 critical bands span the range of speech frequencies. This has led to

Analysis

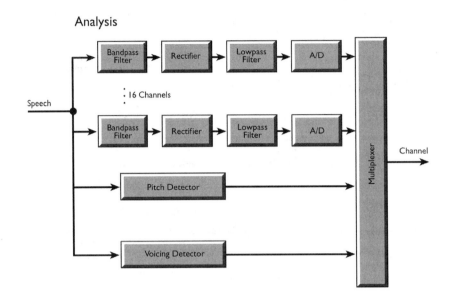

Synthesis

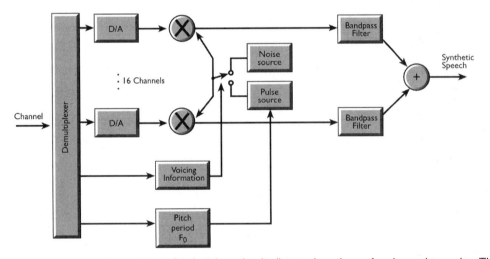

FIG. 7.2. Diagrams of the analysis *(top)* and synthesis *(bottom)* portions of a channel vocoder. The blocks labeled A/D *(top)* correspond to analog-to-digital converters, and the blocks labeled D/A *(bottom)* correspond to digital-to-analog converters. The cross-marked circles indicate multiplier blocks, and the circle with a plus mark indicates a summation block. (Adapted from Papamichalis, 1987, with permission.)

the design of channel vocoder systems with 14 to 19 bandpass channels, with the frequency boundaries for the channels distributed along a logarithmic scale corresponding to the distribution of frequency boundaries for critical bands in hearing. Departures from the logarithmic scale or reductions in the number of channels usually produce decrements in performance.

Synthesized speech produced by a channel

vocoder is not perfectly intelligible even with a high number of bandpass channels and fine quantization of the transmitted parameters. One limitation of channel vocoders is in the binary decision between voiced and unvoiced sounds. Obviously, the binary decision does not recognize mixed excitations of the vocal tract, such as those of the voiced fricatives. This oversimplification eliminates some important distinctions among speech sounds. Also, reliable determination of whether a sound is predominately voiced or unvoiced and reliable determination of the fundamental frequency for voiced speech sounds are difficult speech analysis problems, especially for speech in typical acoustic environments with reverberation and competing speakers or other noise. Unavoidable errors in the extraction of these parameters can produce further decrements in performance.

An improvement in the quality and intelligibility of transmitted speech can be realized with a different approach for representing the excitation of the vocal tract. In this approach, the speech input is filtered to include frequencies below a cutoff frequency in the range of 400 to 1,000 Hz. This filtered or baseband signal then is transmitted without further analysis to the receiver. At the receiver, the baseband signal is used for the source of excitation. No decisions are made about voicing and no analysis is required to determine fundamental frequencies for voiced sounds. Instead, the baseband signal reflects the excitation of the vocal tract. It is periodic for voiced speech sounds, aperiodic for unvoiced speech sounds, and has periodic and aperiodic components for mixed excitation of the vocal tract. The periodicity of the voiced sounds corresponds to the rate of glottal openings.

The bandpass channels of this baseband vocoder are the same as those used in the channel vocoder. Transmission of the baseband signal requires a much higher information rate than that required for the transmission of the voiced or unvoiced and fundamental frequency parameters in the channel vocoder. There is a tradeoff in qual-

ity versus information rate requirements in choosing between channel and baseband vocoders. Baseband vocoders provide higher quality, especially in noisy environments, but at the cost of higher information rate requirements compared with channel vocoders.

The representation of how the vocal tract is excited is far from perfect, even in baseband vocoders. In particular, only a small part of the broad spectrum of noise excitation is represented in the baseband signal, and this can lead to errors in levels of excitation for unvoiced sounds.

Another approach to vocoder design is to extract and transmit parameters to specify the principal resonances and anti-resonaces of the vocal tract, as opposed to the transmission of bandpass envelope signals in the channel vocoder. This approach is based on the observation that peaks in the spectra of voiced speech sounds convey almost as much information as the full spectrum. For vowels and some of the other voiced sounds, a savings in the information rate required for transmission can be realized by sending a reduced set of parameters that specify the frequencies and widths of the first two to four peaks (formants) in speech spectra at 5- to 30-millisecond intervals. A further savings can be realized by specifying the frequencies only, because the widths convey less information than the frequencies and can be fixed for demanding applications.

A block diagram of the synthesis portion of such a formant vocoder is presented in Fig. 7.3. The upper path is used for the synthesis of voiced speech sounds, and the lower path is used for the synthesis of unvoiced speech sounds. The parameters F_1 through F_3 specify the center frequencies of three resonant filters connected in series, and the parameters B_1 through B_3 specify the widths (or bandwidths) of the filters.

Synthesis of unvoiced speech sounds requires an anti-resonance (spectral zero) in addition to a resonance (spectral pole), corresponding the cavities between the source of noise and the lips (resonance) and between the source of noise and the glottis

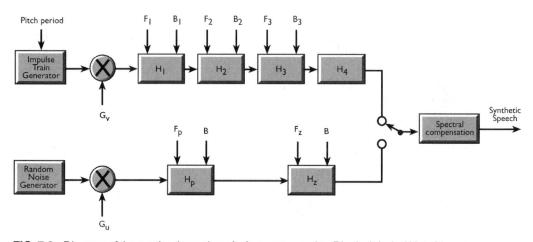

FIG. 7.3. Diagram of the synthesis portion of a formant vocoder. Blocks labeled H_1 to H_3 are resonance filters with center frequencies controlled by the parameters F_1 to F_3 and with bandwidths controlled by the parameters B_1 to B_3. The filters represent the first three formants of voiced speech sounds. Block H_4 is a resonance filter whose parameters are fixed and do not vary with time. This filter represents the relatively invariant fourth formant of voiced speech sounds. Blocks H_p and H_z represent the principal resonance (*i.e.*, spectral pole) and anti-resonance (*i.e.*, spectral zero) of unvoiced speech sounds, respectively. Parameters F_p and F_z control the center frequencies of those filters, and the single parameter B controls the bandwidth for both of the filters. Speech amplitudes are controlled by the gain factors G_v and G_u for voiced and unvoiced sounds, respectively. (Adapted from Papamichalis, 1987, with permission.)

(anti-resonance). The frequencies of the resonance and anti-resonance are specified by the parameters F_p (pole) and F_z (zero), respectively. The selectivity for both filters is specified by the single parameter B.

The formant vocoder offers a reduction in the information rate needed to transmit the extracted parameters. However, this reduction comes at the cost of a great increase in the complexity of the analysis part of the system. Accurate extraction of formant frequencies (and bandwidths) in conversational speech is difficult and highly subject to noise interference.

The formant vocoder also shares some limitations of the channel vocoder previously discussed. In particular, the weaknesses associated with the voiced or unvoiced decision and with extraction of the fundamental frequency for voiced speech sounds apply to both types of vocoder. The formant vocoder also fails to represent nasals well, in that accurate synthesis of nasals requires an anti-resonance (produced by the closed cavity of

the vocal tract) in addition to the resonances of other voiced sounds. The anti-resonance is not included in the path for the synthesis of voiced sounds.

Formant vocoders work best for transmission and synthesis of vowels and work less well for transmission and synthesis of other speech sounds. Formant vocoders also are more complex and more susceptible to noise interference than channel vocoders. Formant vocoders have been used in situations requiring extremely low information rates for transmission of speech parameters. The quality and intelligibility of speech transmitted with formant vocoders is not as high as those with channel vocoders, but the formant vocoder allows lower information rates while maintaining an acceptable intelligibility for some applications.

Implications for Cochlear Implants

The amount of information that can be presented and perceived with a cochlear implant is much less than that for someone with normal hearing listening to an unprocessed acoustic signal. For example, the number of electrodes that can be included in a scala tympani implant is far less than the number of ganglion cells and neurons in normal and probably in most deafened cochleas. The rate at which stimulus information can be sent to the electrodes is further restricted by the properties of transcutaneous links (see Chapter 6). Current implant systems have no more than 22 intracochlear electrodes, which for such closely spaced electrodes address highly overlapping populations of neurons because of the spread of the electric fields across electrode positions. Data from studies manipulating the number of channels and electrodes used with the 22-electrode implant indicate that addition of channels and electrodes beyond four to six does not increase speech reception scores (Fishman *et al.*, 1997; Lawson *et al.*, 1996; Wilson, 1997). This suggests that only four to six sites along the array elicit clearly discriminable percepts. This number may be increased with the use of new electrode designs (see Chapter 6). This number is lower than the number of critical bands in hearing that span the range of speech frequencies (14 to 19 critical bands), much lower than the number of rows of sensory hair cells (approximately 3,000, which probably correspond to the smallest units of frequency resolution according to place of stimulation in the cochlea), and very much lower than the number of auditory neurons (approximately 30,000 in the healthy cochlea).

In addition to the limitations of the implant system, perception of electrical stimuli is different from perception of acoustic stimuli. The dynamic range of stimulus amplitudes from auditory threshold to loud percepts is on the order of 10 to 20 dB for electrical pulses and on the order of 100 dB for acoustical stimuli. The number of discriminable steps in stimulus amplitudes within these ranges is lower in electrical hearing than in normal hearing. Changes in the rate or frequency of stimuli delivered to single electrodes of an implant are perceived as changes in pitch only up to

a pitch saturation limit, typically around 300 pulses/s for electrical pulses or 300 Hz for electrical sinusoids. Higher rates or frequencies do not produce increases in pitch. In normal hearing, different pitches are heard over much wider ranges of rates or frequencies, probably through combinations of rate and place cues to pitch.

A wide range of outcomes is found for any of the current multichannel implants (see Chapter 10). Different patients using identical implant devices may have quite different speech reception scores. This indicates the importance of patient variables in the design and performance of implant systems. Such variables may include differences among patients in the survival of neural elements in the implanted cochlea, proximity of the electrodes to the target neurons, depth of insertion for the electrode array, integrity of the central auditory pathways, and cognitive and language skills.

The various limitations described above suggest a highly impoverished link for the representation and perception of speech information with cochlear implants. Indeed, design of implant systems can be viewed as a problem of squeezing speech through a narrow bottleneck, imposed by the lack of spatial specificity in stimulation and by limitations in perception. Early designs attempted to represent only the most important aspects of speech at the electrodes, and they attempted to match the representations with what could be perceived. This involved transformations of extracted parameters such that the minimum and maximum values of each parameter would span a perceptual dimension, such as from auditory threshold to loud percepts.

Vocoder theory and models played major roles in these early designs, at least for multielectrode implant systems. Vocoder results demonstrated that a small set of parameters could specify the synthesis of intelligible speech at low rates of information transfer. The results also indicated how such parameters could be extracted from continuous speech.

PROCESSING STRATEGIES

The development of cochlear prostheses began with the work of Djourno and Eyries in 1957 and with the separate efforts led by House, Simmons, and Michelson in the 1960s. Many approaches to the design of processing strategies and other components such as electrode arrays have been proposed or used in the 4 decades of work from these beginnings to the present.

Only a few among the many approaches to processor design are described in this chapter. Emphasis is given to the most recent strategies, and to the major steps that led to the development of those strategies. Emphasis also is given to within-subject comparisons of processing strategies, in which effects of processor variables can be separated from effects of patient variables (Wilson *et al.*, 1993). These comparisons include CIS versus a *compressed analog* (CA) strategy and SPEAK versus a *multipeak* (MPEAK) strategy. The comparisons illustrate issues in processor design and show what is possible with the use of the CIS and SPEAK strategies. Descriptions of many more of the approaches to processor design that have been

proposed or used throughout the history of cochlear implants are presented in a number of comprehensive reviews (Dorman, 1993; Gantz, 1987; Loizou, 1998; Millar *et al.*, 1984 and 1990; Moore, 1985; Parkins, 1986; Pfingst, 1986; Tyler and Tye-Murray, 1991; Wilson, 1993).

Interleaved Pulses Strategies

Early designs of processing strategies based on vocoder analogies included the *interleaved pulses* (IP) strategies and a series of feature extraction strategies. An approach similar to that of channel vocoders was used in the IP strategies, and an approach similar to that of formant vocoders was used in the feature extraction strategies.

A block diagram of the IP processor (Wilson *et al.*, 1985 and 1988a) is presented in Fig. 7.4. The "front end" of the processor is nearly identical at the block diagram level to the analysis portion of a channel vocoder. The front end includes a bank of bandpass filters and associated envelope detectors, a voicing detector. The outputs from these blocks then are used to control patterns of electrical stimulation at the electrode array.

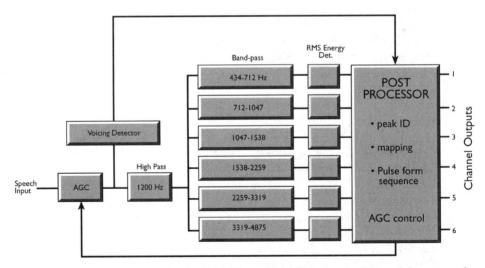

FIG. 7.4. Diagram of an interleaved pulses processor. The initial stages of processing are performed by a voicing detector and a bank of bandpass filters and associated envelope detectors. A postprocessor uses inputs from these stages to control patterns of stimulation at the electrode array. AGC, automatic gain control. (Adapted from Wilson *et al.*, 1988a, with permission.)

A *postprocessor* determines the timing and amplitudes of stimulus pulses delivered to the electrodes. In variation 1 of the IP processor, it presents pulses at the fundamental frequency when the voicing detector indicates the presence of a voiced speech sound, or at a relatively high (*e.g.*, 300 pulses/s/electrode) or randomized rate when the voicing detector indicates the presence of an unvoiced speech sound.

In variation 2 of the IP processor, inputs from the voicing and fundamental frequency detectors are ignored and pulses are presented at fixed interpulse intervals (*e.g.*, 1 millisecond) to a subset of selected electrodes. The electrodes are selected according to the n highest envelope signals among the m bandpass channels for each cycle of stimulation. This variation of the IP processor was the first implementation of an n-of-m strategy for cochlear implants (Wilson *et al.*, 1985 and 1988; McDermott and Vandali, 1997). The basic n-of-m approach is used to this day, as described later in this chapter.

Patterns of stimulation for variation 1 of the IP processor are illustrated in Fig. 7.5. Speech inputs are shown in the top panel, and stimulus pulses are shown for each of four electrodes (and channels) in the bottom panel. The four electrodes are arranged in an apex-to-base order, with electrode 4 being most basal. The amplitudes of the pulses for each of the electrodes are derived from the envelope signals in the corresponding bandpass channels. The envelope signal in the bandpass channel with the lowest center frequency controls the amplitudes of pulses delivered to the apical-most electrode, and the envelope signal in the bandpass channel with the highest center frequency controls the amplitudes of pulses delivered to the basal-most electrode. This arrangement mimics the tonotopic organization of the cochlea in normal hearing, with high-frequency sounds exciting neurons at basal locations and low-frequency sounds exciting neurons at apical locations.

Pulse amplitudes are derived from the envelope signals in both variations of IP processors. A logarithmic transformation is used to map the relatively wide dynamic range of envelope variations onto the narrow dynamic range of electrically evoked hearing. (The effect of such mapping is not shown in Fig. 7.5.)

Variation 1 of the IP processors is a close analog of a channel vocoder. As illustrated in Fig. 7.5, the stimuli produced with this variation indicate voiced versus unvoiced sounds (compare rates of stimulation between the lower panels of the figure, corresponding to the voiced /ɔ/ and the unvoiced /t/) and the fundamental frequency of voiced sounds (*i.e.*, the pulse rate in the lower left panel). Variations in pulse amplitudes across electrodes also indicate the shape and transfer function of the vocal tract; at least some of the principal resonances and anti-resonances of the tract are reflected in the different pulse amplitudes for different electrodes. For example, the high-frequency resonance of the /t/ sound is reflected in the relatively intense stimulation of electrode 4 (lower right panel of Fig. 7.5).

Variation 2 of the IP processors uses the bandpass channel outputs only and represents only a subset of those for each cycle of stimulation across electrodes. The presentation of information is sparse compared with variation 1 of the IP processors. Such a presentation may provide a more optimal match for patients with highly limited perceptual abilities (Wilson *et al.*, 1988a). Information about the excitation of the vocal tract is discarded, but some information about the transfer function of the tract is retained.

An additional aspect of the design of IP processors is the nonsimultaneous presentation of pulses across electrodes. This eliminates direct summation of electric fields from different electrodes produced with simultaneous stimulation. Such summation can greatly reduce the independence of stimulation among electrodes and thereby reduce the salience of channel-related cues.

Comparisons between IP and other processing strategies are described in several reports (Lawson *et al.*, 1993; Wilson, 1993; Wil-

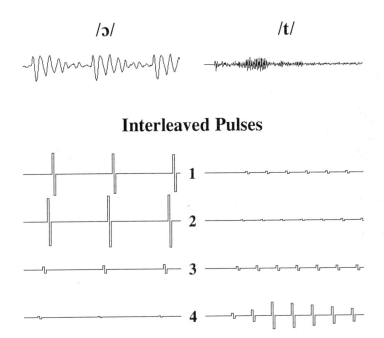

/ɔ/   /t/

Interleaved Pulses

FIG. 7.5. Stimuli produced by a simplified implementation of variation 1 of an interleaved pulses (IP) processor. The top panels show pre-emphasized (6-dB/octave attenuation below 1.2 kHz) speech inputs. An input corresponding to a voiced speech sound (/ɔ/) is shown in the left panel, and an input corresponding to an unvoiced speech sound (/t/) is shown in the right panel. The remaining panels show stimulus pulses produced by an IP processor for these inputs. The numbers indicate the electrodes to which the stimuli are delivered. The lowest number corresponds to the apical-most electrode and the highest number to the basal-most electrode. The pulse amplitudes in the figure reflect the amplitudes of the envelope signals for each channel. In actual implementations, the range of pulse amplitudes is compressed using a logarithmic or power-law transformation of the envelope signal for each channel. Notice that the stimuli are presented nonsimultaneously across electrodes and that the rates of stimulation are different for voiced and for unvoiced segments of speech. The duration of each trace in this figure is 25.4 ms. (From Wilson, 1993, with permission.)

son *et al.*, 1985, 1988a, 1988b, and 1991b). Performance for one subject was remarkably improved with substitution of variation 2 of the IP processors for the CA processor of his clinical device. This subject did not recognize speech as such with the clinical processor. In contrast, speech sounded like speech with the IP processor, and the subject scored well above chance on tests of consonant and vowel identification. The amount of information presented with the IP processor was much less than that presented with the CA processor (discussed later in this chapter), and this may have helped the subject to perceive a limited but important subset of speech information. The nonsimultaneous presentation of stimuli with the IP processor,

as opposed to the simultaneous presentation of analog waveforms with the CA processor, may have enhanced the representation and perception of channel-related cues.

This second variation of IP processors has been developed further in *n*-of-*m* strategies in current use. These designs are described later in this chapter.

Additional comparisons involving IP processors included comparisons of the first variation of the processors with CA processors in groups of six subjects using the USCF/ Storz implant system and two subjects using the Ineraid implant system. All of these subjects had higher levels of speech reception performance with their clinical CA processors compared with the subject described previously. In general, results obtained with IP processors with these groups of subjects were immediately as good on average as results obtained with the CA processor, despite considerable experience with the latter and essentially no experience with the former. Some subjects had better performance with the CA processor, and others had better performance with the IP processor. This finding suggested that availability of multiple strategies might help individual patients to achieve the best possible outcome.

Although the results with variation 1 of the IP processor were promising, its further development was discontinued in favor of a clearly better approach, the CIS strategy, that also was evaluated with the second group of two Ineraid subjects.

Feature Extraction and Multipeak Strategies

Several processing strategies have been used in conjunction the Nucleus electrode array and implanted receivers since 1982, when the first system was introduced for clinical application (Clark, 1987; Clark *et al.*, 1990; Patrick and Clark, 1991). The first three of the strategies were based largely or in part on a formant vocoder model. The SPEAK, CIS, and *advanced combination encoder* (ACE) strategies have superseded these earlier strategies and are the processing options now available

for use with the Nucleus implant. These strategies are described later in this chapter.

The first strategy used with the Nucleus implant was designed to represent voicing information and the frequency and amplitude of the second formant (F2 and A2, respectively). The second strategy added a representation of the first formant (F1 and A1).

Block diagrams of the second strategy are presented in Figs. 7.6 and 7.7. Fig. 7.6 shows a diagram of the entire processor, and Fig. 7.7 shows a more detailed diagram of the front end of the processor. The first processor in the Nucleus series used the components associated with extraction and representation of voicing and second formant information, and the second processor used all of the components shown in Figs. 7.6 and 7.7, including those associated the extraction and representation of first formant information.

In the first strategy, a zero crossings detector was used to estimate the fundamental frequency (F0) of voiced speech sounds from the output of a 270-Hz lowpass filter (Fig. 7.7, upper path). A separate zero crossings detector was used to estimate the spectral centroid (or spectral center of gravity) in the output of a bandpass filter spanning the frequency range of the second formant (1 to 4 kHz in one implementation of the strategy). The amplitude of the second formant was

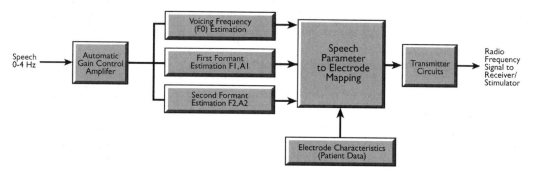

FIG. 7.6. Diagram of the F0/F1/F2 processing strategy. The F0/F2 strategy uses all blocks shown here except for the block labeled First Formant Estimation F1,A1. (Adapted from Patrick *et al.*, 1990, with permission.)

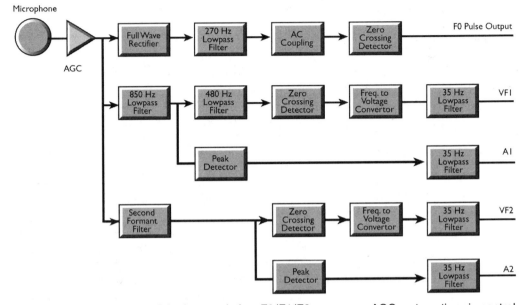

FIG. 7.7. Detailed diagram of the front end of an F0/F1/F2 processor. AGC, automatic gain control. (From Blamey *et al.*, 1987, with permission.)

estimated with an envelope detector at the output of the bandpass filter. The envelope detector included a peak detector and lowpass filter, whose cutoff frequency was set at 35 Hz. These components are shown in the lower path of Fig. 7.7.

This F0/F2 processor represented voicing information by presenting stimulus pulses at the estimated F0 rate during voiced speech sounds and at quasi-random intervals, with an average rate of about 100 pulses/s, during unvoiced speech sounds. The frequency of the spectral centroid in the F2 band was represented by selecting one position along the electrode array for each successive pulse. High frequencies were represented with stimulation of an electrode or a pair of closely-spaced bipolar electrodes near the basal end of the array, and low frequencies were represented with stimulation of an electrode or electrodes near the apical end of the array. The estimated amplitude of the second formant was represented with the amplitude of each pulse, derived with a logarithmic transformation of the envelope sig-

nal, as in the IP processors described previously.

The F0/F2 strategy is a highly reduced analog of a formant vocoder. Only one formant is represented. However, this formant probably confers the greatest information about speech among the formants. Perception of F2 can allow the classification of vowels into groups, and transitions of F2 from vowels into consonants can cue place of articulation for some of the consonants. The aim of the F0/F2 strategy is to extract from speech an irreducible set of parameters and then to represent those parameters in a way that can be perceived and used by implant patients. Performance with this initial strategy was encouraging in that its use allowed some patients to recognize portions of speech with hearing alone (Clark, 1987 and 1995; Clark *et al.*, 1990; Dowell *et al.*, 1986 and 1987a). The average of scores among 13 patients for recognition of monosyllabic Northwestern University Auditory Test 6 (NU-6) words was 4.9% correct (Dowell *et al.*, 1987a).

In late 1985, the F0/F2 strategy was modified to include extraction and representation of information about the first formant. An additional channel of processing was used to derive estimates of the spectral centroid and amplitude in a band of frequencies encompassing the range of F1 (Fig. 7.7, middle path). For each stimulus cycle, a postprocessor (Fig. 7.6) selected two electrode positions for stimulation, one corresponding to the estimated frequency of F1 and the other corresponding to the estimated frequency of F2. As in the F0/F2 processor, the electrodes were stimulated at a rate equal to the estimated F0 during voiced speech and at a quasi-random rate during unvoiced speech. A stimulus cycle included stimulation of the electrode or electrode pair selected to represent F2, followed by stimulation of the electrode or electrode pair selected to represent F1.

Within-subject comparisons of the F0/F2 and F0/F1/F2 strategies demonstrated higher levels of speech reception with the latter (Dowell *et al.*, 1987b; Tye-Murray *et al.*, 1990). All seven subjects in the study of Dowell *et al.*, for instance, obtained higher scores for recognition of key words in the Central Institute for the Deaf (CID) sentences of everyday speech using the F0/F1/F2 processor. The average score for these live-voice presentations of the sentences was 30.4% correct for the F0/F2 processor and 62.9% correct for the F0/F1/F2 processor. The average scores for separate groups of subjects in another study (Dowell *et al.*, 1987a) were 15.9% correct for the F0/F1 processor group ($n = 13$) and 35.4% correct for the F0/F1/F2 processor group ($n = 9$). Scores for recognition of monosyllabic words in this study was 4.9% correct for the F0/F2 group, and 12.4% correct for the F0/F1/F2 group. Test items were presented from recorded material in the second study, and this may have contributed to the lower scores for the CID sentence tests in that study compared with the first study. Scores with the F0/F1/F2 processor were significantly higher than scores with the F0/F2 processor in both studies.

Although performance with the F0/F1/F2 strategy was better than that with the F0/F2 strategy, patients using the F0/F2 strategy for an extended period in their daily lives initially rejected the F0/F1/F2 strategy as inferior (Dowell *et al.*, 1987b). Ultimately, the patients preferred and performed better with the F0/F1/F2 strategy. This, along with similar observations by others, suggests that preference is an unreliable guide at best in selecting processing strategies for implants. In addition, a substantial period of experience or learning may be required before asymptotic performance is attained with a new strategy (Dorman and Loizou, 1997; Pelizzone *et al.*, 1995; Tyler *et al.*, 1986).

From 1985 to 1989, Cochlear Ltd. (then a subsidiary of Nucleus Ltd.), in collaboration with investigators at the University of Melbourne, developed new external hardware for use with the Nucleus implant (Patrick and Clark, 1991; Patrick *et al.*, 1990; Skinner *et al.*, 1991). Analog components were replaced with digital components, and various aspects of the signal processing and mapping of envelope levels onto stimulus levels were refined in the new hardware (Skinner *et al.*, 1991; Wilson, 1993). Use of a custom integrated circuit for much of the processing allowed substantial reductions in the size and weight of the new Mini Speech Processor (MSP) compared with the prior Wearable Speech Processor (WSP III). These reductions helped to make the MSP more suitable for use by young children.

The MSP could be programmed to implement versions of the F0/F2 and F0/F1/F2 strategies, with the refinements provided by the MSP hardware. In addition, a new strategy, MPEAK, could be implemented through software choices. The MPEAK strategy was designed to augment the F0/F1/F2 strategy by adding a representation of envelope variations in high-frequency bands of the input speech signal.

As described previously, a formant vocoder approach cannot provide a good representation of many speech sounds, particularly unvoiced sounds and many of the voiced consonants. The high-band channels of the MPEAK strategy are similar in design to the upper channels of the IP processors, which are based on a channel vocoder approach. The MPEAK strategy combines aspects and channel and formant vocoders, with the aim of improving the representation and perception of consonants.

A block diagram of the MPEAK strategy is presented in Fig. 7.8. This diagram is in the style of Fig. 7.6 for the F0/F2 and F0/F1/F2 strategies and shows all components of a MPEAK processor. The principal difference between the F0/F1/F2 and MPEAK strategies is in the addition of the energy indicators for three high-frequency bands. The bands are 2.0 to 2.8 kHz (band 3, as distinguished from the two bands for F1 and F2), 2.8 to 4.0 kHz (band 4), and 4.0 to 7.0 kHz (band 5).

In the MPEAK strategy, four pulses are delivered in each stimulus cycle. During voiced speech, these cycles are presented at a rate equal to the estimated F0 and, during unvoiced speech, at quasi-random intervals but with an average rate in the range of 200 to 300 pulses/s. Fixed electrode positions are reserved at the basal end of the array for representations of the envelope signals in bands 3 through 5, and the remaining (more apical) electrode positions are used for representations of F1 and F2. During voiced speech, the electrodes for bands 4 and 3 and for F2 and F1 are selected for stimulation. During unvoiced speech, the electrodes for bands 5, 4, and 3 and for F2 are selected. Stimulation of the four electrodes (or electrode pairs) selected for each cycle is in a base-to-apex order. Manipulations of pulse amplitude and pulse duration are used to code loudness. (These manipulations produce changes in the charge per phase of stimulus pulses, which is strongly correlated with the loudness of auditory percepts.) Changes in either can be used to code loudness, but the combination allows a reduction in the time required for the transmission of stimulus information through the transcutaneous link of the Nucleus device. In particular, transmission of high-amplitude, short-duration pulses requires less time than transmission of low-amplitude, long-duration pulses (Crosby *et al.*, 1985; Shannon *et al.*, 1990).

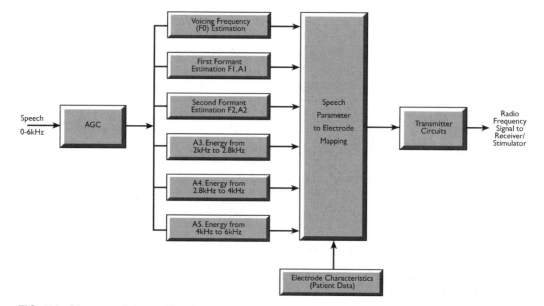

FIG. 7.8. Diagram of the multipeak processing strategy and the hardware components of the Mini Speech Processor (MSP). AGC, automatic gain control. (Adapted from Patrick *et al.*, 1990, with permission.)

Coding loudness with changes in the amplitude of short-duration pulses up to the amplitude (current) limit of the device and then coding further increases in loudness with increases in duration at that highest amplitude minimize the amount of time required to transmit each stimulus pulse. This allows rates of stimulation up to about 400 cycles/s.

Studies have been conducted to compare the F0/F1/F2 strategy as implemented in the WSP III, the F0/F1/F2 strategy as implemented in the MSP or a prototype of the MSP, and the MPEAK strategy as implemented in the MSP (Dowell *et al.*, 1991; Skinner *et al.*, 1991). In within-subject comparisons with five subjects, Dowell *et al.* found significant increases in the recognition of key words in the Bamford-Kowal-Bench (BKB) sentences when the MSP implementation of the F0/F1/F2 strategy was substituted for the WSP III implementation of that strategy, and when the MPEAK strategy was substituted for the F0/F1/F2 strategy in the MSP hardware. The scores increased from approximately 50% correct with the WSP III implementation of the F0/F1/F2 strategy to approximately 80% correct with MPEAK strategy (using the MSP hardware). Results for the MSP implementation of the F0/F1/F2 strategy were almost exactly midway between these.

Skinner *et al.* also observed large improvements in speech reception scores when the MPEAK strategy was substituted for either implementation of the F0/F1/F2 strategy in studies with a separate group of five subjects. Scores for the two implementations of the F0/F1/F2 strategy were not statistically different, however. The MSP implementation used a prototype of the MSP with some differences in design, and those differences may have affected the comparisons. Average scores for recognition of NU-6 monosyllabic words improved from 13.3% to 29.1% correct when the MPEAK strategy was substituted for the WSP III implementation of the F0/F1/F2 strategy, and recognition of key words in the BKB sentences improved from 51.0% to 70.0% correct for the same processor conditions.

Continuous Interleaved Sampling Strategy

The CIS strategy was the direct descendant of the IP strategies described earlier. The design of the CIS strategy was motivated in part by a desire to represent voicing information in a more natural way and to increase the amount of information transmitted and perceived with the implant. With the first variation of the IP processing, in which voicing information was explicitly represented, subjects remarked that changes in their percepts at boundaries between voiced and unvoiced sounds seemed abrupt and unnatural. The chunkiness of the representation did not reflect the smoother transitions in speech and did not reflect mixed excitations of the vocal tract.

These anecdotal comments by subjects were corroborated by voicing errors in tests of consonant identification. The errors may have been produced by an incomplete and distorted representation of voicing information and by errors in the voiced or unvoiced decision. The former errors are inherent to channel and formant vocoder approaches, and the latter errors are difficult or impossible to eliminate for less than ideal speech inputs, even using highly sophisticated algorithms and hardware (Hess, 1983).

A block diagram of the CIS strategy is presented in Fig. 7.9. Inputs from a microphone and optional automatic gain control (AGC) are directed to a pre-emphasis filter, which attenuates frequency components below 1.2 kHz at 6 dB/octave. This pre-emphasis helps relatively weak consonants (with a predominant frequency content above 1.2 kHz) compete with vowels, which are intense compared with most consonants and have strong components below 1.2 kHz.

The output of the pre-emphasis filter is directed to a bank of bandpass channels. Each channel includes stages of bandpass filtering, envelope detection, and compression. Envelope detection is accomplished with a

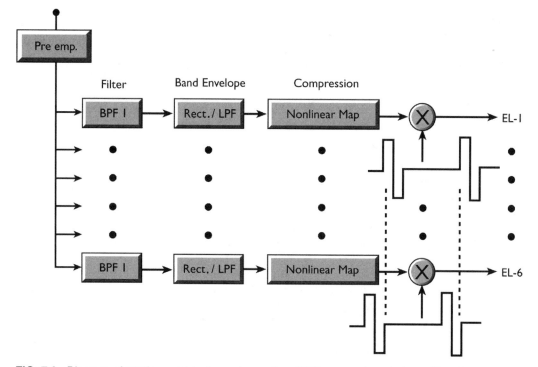

FIG. 7.9. Diagram of continuous interleaved sampling (CIS) processing strategy. The strategy uses a pre-emphasis filter (Preemp) to attenuate strong components in speech below 1.2 kHz. The pre-emphasis filter is followed by multiple channels of processing. Each channel includes stages of bandpass filtering (BPF), envelope detection, compression, and modulation. Carrier waveforms for two of the modulators are shown below the two corresponding multiplier blocks. (Adapted from Wilson *et al.*, 1991a, with permission.)

rectifier, followed by a lowpass filter. The channel outputs are used to modulate trains of biphasic pulses. The modulated pulses for each channel are applied through a percutaneous or transcutaneous link to a corresponding electrode in the cochlea. Stimuli derived from channels with low center frequencies for the bandpass filter are directed to apical electrodes in the implant, and stimuli derived from channels with high center frequencies are directed to basal electrodes in the implant.

As with the IP, F0/F2, F0/F1/F2, and MPEAK processors, stimuli for the CIS strategy are delivered nonsimultaneously across electrodes. This eliminates one component of electrode or channel interactions that otherwise would be produced through direct summation of the electric fields from different (simultaneously stimulated) electrodes.

In contrast to the IP, F0/F2, F0/F1/F2, and MPEAK processors, the CIS strategy does not include an explicit representation of voiced or unvoiced distinctions or of the fundamental frequency of voiced sounds. Instead, voicing information is represented through relatively rapid variations in the modulation waveforms for each of the channels. These variations are included in the modulation waveforms with the use of high cutoff frequencies for the lowpass filters in the envelope detectors. A typical cutoff for CIS processors is in the range of 200 to 400 Hz, whereas a typical cutoff for the other processors is in the range of 20 to 35 Hz. The higher cutoff in CIS processors allows voicing information to pass through each envelope detector. The envelope signal in CIS processors conveys slow variations corresponding to changes in the shape of the vocal tract and the rapid variations corresponding to periodic, aperiodic, or mixed excitation of the tract. For voiced speech, the rapid periodic variations occur in synchrony with the periodic openings of the glottis.

CIS processors use higher rates of stimulation than the processors mentioned previously to represent adequately the rapid variations in the modulation waveforms. Rates for CIS processors typically exceed 500 pulses/s/electrode and often are much higher than that. Stimulus pulses for the other processors are delivered at the F0 rate during voiced speech and at a quasi-random or a somewhat higher fixed rate (*e.g.*, 300 pulses/s/electrode in variation 1 of the IP processor) during unvoiced speech.

The pulse rate for CIS processors must be higher than twice the cutoff frequency of the lowpass filters to avoid digital aliasing effects in the patterns of stimulation on single electrodes (Rabiner and Shafer, 1978; Wilson, 1997). Results from recent recordings of auditory nerve responses to sinusoidally amplitude modulated pulse trains indicate that the pulse rate should be even higher—four to five times the cutoff frequency—to avoid other distortions in the neural representations of modulation waveforms (Wilson, 1997 and 1999). A typical CIS processor might use a pulse rate of 1,000 pulses/s/electrode or higher, in conjunction with a 200-Hz cutoff for the lowpass filters.

The approach used in the CIS strategy departs from the vocoder-based approaches of prior strategies. No specific features of speech are extracted or represented with CIS processors. Instead, envelope variations in each of multiple bands are presented to the electrodes through modulated trains of interleaved pulses. The rate of stimulation for each channel and electrode does not vary between voiced and unvoiced sounds. This waveform or filterbank representation does not make any assumptions about how speech is produced or perceived. Instead, it seeks to represent the *acoustic environment* in a way that uses to the maximum extent possible the perceptual abilities of implant patients. The amount of information presented with CIS processors is much higher than the amounts presented with the prior approaches based on vocoder models. The information is tailored to fit within the perceptual spaces of electrically evoked hearing. The maximum frequency of envelope variations does not exceed the pitch saturation limit of typical patients (200 to 400 Hz), and the stimuli are interlaced to eliminate a principal component of electrode interactions. High pulse rates are used to represent without distortion the highest frequencies in the modulation waveforms. The modulation waveforms reflect rapid transitions in speech, including rapid consonant transitions and voicing information.

Stimuli for a simplified implementation of a four-channel CIS processor are shown in Fig. 7.10. The organization of this figure is the same as that of Fig. 7.5, which shows stimuli for variation 1 of the IP processors. The rate of stimulation is much higher for the CIS processor. The rate does not vary between voiced and unvoiced sounds, and the rate is adequate to represent most or all of the frequency information that can be perceived within channels.

An expanded display of stimuli during a 3.3-millisecond segment of the vowel input is presented in Fig. 7.11. This display shows the pattern of stimulation across electrodes. In this particular implementation of a CIS processor, stimulus pulses are delivered in a nonoverlapping sequence from the basalmost electrode (electrode 4) to the apicalmost electrode (electrode 1). The rate of pulses on each electrode may be varied through manipulations in the duration of the pulses and time between sequential pulses. Any ordering of electrodes may be used in the stimulation sequence, such as an apex-to-base order or a staggered order (*i.e.*, an order designed to produce on average the maximum spatial separation between sequentially stimulated electrodes).

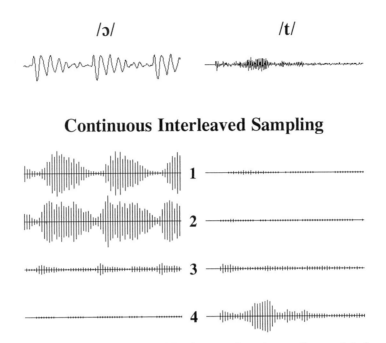

FIG. 7.10. Stimuli produced by a simplified implementation of a continuous interleaved sampling processor. The organization and speech inputs for this figure are the same as those in Fig. 7.5. (Adapted from Wilson *et al.*, 1991a, with permission.)

The first evaluations of the CIS strategy included comparisons among CA, IP (variation 1), and CIS processors for two subjects implanted with the Ineraid device. The percutaneous connector of the Ineraid device allowed high-quality implementations of each of the strategies. The results from tests of open-set recognition of words and sentences are presented in Fig. 7.12. Scores for the CIS processor were higher than the scores for the CA and IP processors for both subjects. For example, subject SR1 scored 8%,

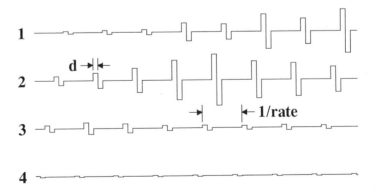

FIG. 7.11. Expanded display of continuous interleaved sampling stimuli. Pulse duration per phase (d) and the period between pulses on each electrode (1/rate) are indicated. The sequence of stimulated electrodes is 4-3-2-1. The duration of each trace is 3.3 ms. Notice that the pulses are nonsimultaneous, eliminating a principal component of electrode interactions due to summation of electric fields from different electrodes. (Adapted from Wilson *et al.*, 1991a, with permission.)

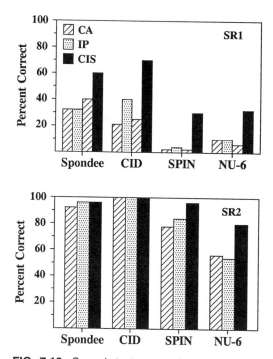

FIG. 7.12. Speech test scores for compressed analog (CA, *striped bars*), interleaved pulses (IP, *stippled bars*), and continuous interleaved sampling (CIS, *solid bars*) processors. Scores for Ineraid subject SR1 are presented in the top panel, and scores for Ineraid subject SR2 are in the bottom panel. The two CA scores for each test for subject SR1 are from separate evaluations of that processor. The first evaluation (4/89) was contemporaneous with the evaluation of the IP processor for this subject, and the second evaluation (8/90, *right-most CA bar for each test*) was contemporaneous with the evaluation of the CIS processor. Separate evaluations of the CA processor were not conducted for subject SR2, because evaluations of the IP and CIS processors were contemporaneous with the (single) evaluation of the CA processor. The tests included recognition of two-syllable words (Spondee), key words in the Central Institute for the Deaf (CID) sentences of everyday speech, the final word in each of 50 high-predictability sentences from the Speech Perception in Noise (SPIN) test (presented in these studies without noise), and monosyllabic words from Northwestern University Auditory Test 6 (NU-6). The CA processors for both subjects used four channels of processing and stimulation, and the IP and CIS processors for both subjects used six channels. The CA processors were used by the subjects in their daily lives. (From Wilson, 1993, with permission.)

10%, and 32% correct in recognizing NU-6 words with the CA, IP, and CIS processors, respectively, and subject SR2 scored 56%, 54%, and 80% correct in recognizing those words for the same processors (Lawson *et al.*, 1993; Wilson, 1993). The subjects had used the CA processor for two or more years in their daily lives at the time of these tests and had had some limited (laboratory) experience with the IP processor. Experience with the CIS processor was no more than several hours for each of the subjects. Despite this relative lack of experience, both subjects achieved their highest scores with CIS for all tests that were sufficiently difficult not to produce scores at or near 100% correct for all three processors. The score of 80% correct for recognition of the NU-6 words was unprecedented at the time of this study. The immediate jumps in scores with these initial implementations of the CIS strategy encouraged its further development and subsequent tests with additional subjects.

Compressed Analog Strategy

The CA strategy was among the first strategies used with multi-electrode implants (Eddington, 1980; Merzenich *et al.*, 1984). Its development was roughly contemporaneous with the development of the F0/F2 strategy and predated the development of the IP strategies.

The CA strategy has been applied in conjunction with the now-discontinued Ineraid and UCSF/Storz implants. A modification of the strategy, *simultaneous analog stimulation* (SAS), is used as one of several strategies that can be selected for the Clarion (Advanced Bionics) implant. The differences between CA and SAS are described in a separate section on SAS.

In contrast to the other strategies described in this chapter, the CA and SAS strategies use analog waveforms for stimuli instead of biphasic pulses. A block diagram of the CA strategy is presented in Fig. 7.13. A microphone or other input is compressed with a fast-acting AGC. The AGC output is

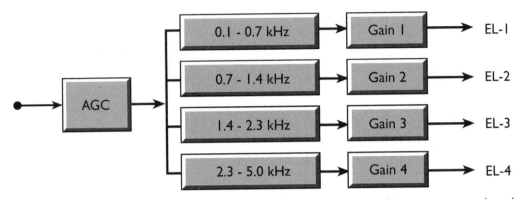

FIG. 7.13. Diagram of the compressed analog processing strategy. The CA strategy uses a broadband automatic gain control (AGC), followed by a bank of bandpass filters. The outputs of the filters can be adjusted with independent gain controls. Compression is achieved through rapid action of the AGC, and high-frequency emphasis and limited mapping to individual electrodes is accomplished through adjustments of the channel gains. (Adapted from Wilson *et al.*, 1991a, with permission.)

filtered into contiguous bands (usually four) that span the range of speech frequencies. The signal from each bandpass filter is amplified and then directed to a corresponding electrode in the implant. The gains of the amplifiers for the different bandpass filters can be adjusted to produce stimuli that do not exceed the upper end of the dynamic range of percepts for each electrode and that provide a high-frequency emphasis (*e.g.*, percepts for high-frequency channel 4 can be made as loud as percepts for low-frequency channel 1 even though high-frequency sounds in speech generally are much less intense than low-frequency sounds).

The compression provided by the AGC reduces the dynamic range of the input to approximate the dynamic range of electrically evoked hearing. The dynamic range of stimulation also can be restricted with a clipping circuit before or after the amplifiers for some or all of the bandpass channels (Merzenich, 1985; Merzenich *et al.*, 1984).

Stimuli produced by a simplified implementation of a CA processor are shown in Fig. 7.14. The format of this figure is the same as that in Figs. 7.5 and 7.10, which show stimuli for IP and CIS processors, respectively. Comparisons of the figures show a highly detailed representation for the CA processor, a somewhat less detailed repre-

sentation for the CIS processor, and a relatively sparse representation for the IP processor. The CA and CIS processors do not extract nor explicitly represent features of speech. The IP processor extracts voiced or unvoiced boundaries and the fundamental frequency of voiced speech sounds. These features are represented by rates of stimulation, which are different between the panels for voiced and unvoiced inputs in Fig. 7.5.

CA stimuli represent a large portion of the information in unprocessed speech input. Spectral and temporal patterns of speech are represented in the relative amplitudes of the stimuli across electrodes and in the temporal variations of the stimuli for each of the electrodes. The approach is to present as much information as possible to the implant and to allow the brain to extract what it can from this minimally processed representation.

Like the CIS strategy, the CA strategy is not based on a vocoder model. Neither strategy extracts features from speech inputs. Both strategies present a range of temporal variations in each channel (and at each electrode) that at least includes the range of voicing information in speech. The ranges of temporal variations within channels for CA and CIS processors are much greater than the range within channels for a typical channel vocoder.

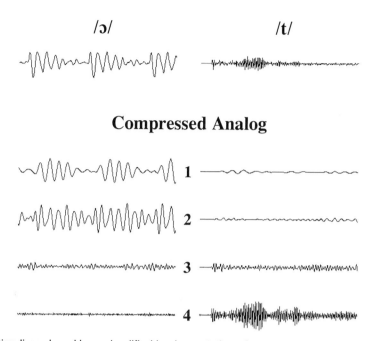

FIG. 7.14. Stimuli produced by a simplified implementation of a compressed analog processor. The organization and speech inputs for this figure are the same as those in Figs. 7.5 and 7.10. (Adapted from Wilson *et al.*, 1991a, with permission.)

Such departures from a vocoder model recognize that the principal goal of vocoder designs is different from the principal goal of implant designs. The goal for vocoders is to minimize the information rate of transmission while still supporting an acceptable intelligibility of the reconstructed speech signal at the receiver. The goal for implants is to maximize the amount of speech information that can be perceived and used by the recipient. This fundamental difference can lead to different choices in design.

Until the advent of the CIS strategy, performance with the CA strategy was at least as good as the performance with any other processing strategy for commercially available multi-electrode implants (Cohen *et al.*, 1993; Dorman, 1993; Dorman *et al.*, 1989; Gantz *et al.*, 1987 and 1988; Tye-Murray and Tyler, 1989; Tyler *et al.*, 1995; Tyler and Moore, 1992). It supported some open-set recognition of speech for a relatively large fraction of patients. In one group of 50 Ineraid patients, for example, recognition of NU-6 words ranged from 0% to 60% correct, with a median score of 14% correct (Dorman *et al.*, 1989). Comparisons of scores for different groups of subjects using the Nucleus implant (with the F0/F2 or F0/F1/F2 processing strategies) or the Ineraid implant (with the CA processing strategy) showed no difference for a wide variety of speech reception tests in quiet. In some studies, scores for tests in noise were significantly higher for the CA strategy (Gantz *et al.*, 1987; Tyler *et al.*, 1995). The relative advantage of the CA strategy in noise may have been a result of the high sensitivity of the feature extraction circuits in the Nucleus processors to noise interference.

Although performance with the CA strategy was among the best before the introduction of CIS, substantial open-set recognition by most patients still had not been achieved. The average user struggled to understand even high-context sentences with hearing alone, and very few patients were able to use the telephone except in constrained situations involving exchanges of previously arranged codes.

Comparisons of Compressed Analog and Continuous Interleaved Sampling Strategies

The CIS strategy was designed to eliminate or at least ameliorate some possible weaknesses in the CA strategy. A major concern with the CA approach is that simultaneous stimulation of multiple electrodes can produce large and uncontrolled interactions through vector summation of the electric fields from each of the electrodes (White *et al.*, 1984). The resulting degradation of independence among electrodes and channels would be expected to reduce the salience of channel-related cues. In particular, the neural response to stimuli presented at one electrode may be significantly distorted or even counteracted by coincident stimuli presented at other electrodes. The pattern of interaction also may vary according to the instantaneous phase relationships among the stimuli for each of the electrodes. Phase is not controlled within or across channels in CA processors, and this may degrade further the representation of the speech spectrum according to place of stimulation.

The problem of electrode interactions is addressed in CIS processors with the use of nonsimultaneous stimuli. This eliminates a principal component of interactions due to of direct summation of electric fields from different electrodes. It does not eliminate another component, often called *temporal channel interactions.* These interactions refer to effects of preceding stimuli on the response to a given stimulus. They may be produced by the refractory properties of neurons or by temporal summation of sequential stimuli at neural membranes. In the first case, a stimulus at one electrode can excite a population of neurons that overlaps the population that would be excited by another electrode, if not preceded by the stimulus at the first electrode. The neurons excited by the

first stimulus may still be in a refractory state at the time of the second stimulus. Neurons in their absolutely refractory period cannot be excited by a second stimulus, and neurons in their relatively refractory period may or may not be excited by a second stimulus. Neurons in their relatively refractory period are less excitable (*i.e.*, have higher thresholds) than neurons in a resting state. Stimulation of neurons by a prior stimulus or prior stimuli can alter the number and distribution of neurons stimulated by a following stimulus when the following stimulus falls within the refractory periods of the previously stimulated neurons (typical auditory neurons have absolute refractory periods of about 0.5 milliseconds and relatively refractory periods with time constants in the range of 0.5 to 4.0 milliseconds).

The number and distribution of neurons excited by a stimulus pulse also can be altered by preceding stimuli through temporal summation effects. In this mechanism, a subthreshold depolarization of a neural membrane can be augmented with a subsequent depolarization if the second stimulus is presented within the temporal integration window of the membrane. The integration window is determined by the time constant of the membrane, which is on the order of 50 to 200 microsecond for myelinated mammalian neurons. An accumulation of subthreshold depolarizations ultimately may excite the neuron that would not have been excited with the final stimulus alone. Refractory effects can reduce the number of neurons excited with a final stimulus compared with the number excited with that stimulus in the absence of preceding stimuli, whereas summation effects can increase the number. Either change distorts the intended pattern of stimulation for a given electrode.

Fortunately, temporal channel interactions appear to be small compared with the interactions produced with simultaneous stimulation of electrodes (Favre and Pelizzone, 1993). The relatively small effects of temporal channel interactions may be reduced further through a staggered order of stimulation across electrodes in CIS and other pulsatile processors. Such orders are designed to produce the maximum possible spatial separation (on average) between sequentially stimulated electrodes (*e.g.*, an order of 6-3-5-2-4-1 for a six-channel CIS processor). In general, a greater spatial separation should reduce the overlaps in the excitation fields between electrodes and thereby reduce the magnitudes of the interactions.

An additional possible weakness of CA processors is that only a small part of the presented information can be perceived. For example, patients cannot perceive differences in frequencies of electrical stimulation on single electrodes above the pitch saturation limit, usually between 200 and 400 Hz. Thus, many of the temporal details in CA stimuli are not likely to be accessible to the typical user. Presentation of information outside the perceptual space does not help the patient and may be destructive if it gets in the way of something else or if it distorts or interferes with the information that can be perceived. Presentation of highly detailed temporal information with analog stimuli, for instance, precludes a reduction in electrode interactions that might otherwise be obtained with nonsimultaneous pulses.

The cutoff frequency of the lowpass filters in the envelope detectors of CIS processors is set to include most or all of the frequencies that can be perceived as different pitches by implant patients (typical cutoffs of 200 to 400 Hz). Rates of stimulation at each electrode are at least high enough to prevent aliasing (twice the cutoff frequency of the lowpass filters) and usually much higher than that to eliminate other distortions in the neural representation of modulation waveforms.

A further concern with the CA strategy is its front-end compression. The signal presented to the bank of bandpass filters is a highly compressed version of the signal at the input to the processor. A typical compression ratio is 6 to 1 (Merzenich *et al.*, 1984). Such high levels of compression produce harmonics and other distortions in the spectrum of the input signal, sometimes called *spectral*

splatter. These distortions are transmitted through the bank of bandpass filters and ultimately to the electrodes (White, 1986). They most likely degrade the representation of across-channel cues to the speech spectrum. For example, spurious components at high frequencies are produced for all speech sounds that have significant energy at low frequencies.

CIS processors do not use an AGC or use one with relatively slow attack and release times and with a low compression ratio. This eliminates or greatly reduces the spectral distortions described above.

Compression in CIS processors is accomplished with the logarithmic or power-law mapping functions for each of the electrodes. This back end compression eliminates the spectral distortions produced with front end compression and allows a precise matching of the full range of envelope signals in each channel to the dynamic range (from threshold to a comfortably loud or loud level) of the corresponding electrode. The logarithmic function produces a normal or near-normal growth of loudness with increases in sound level (Dorman *et al.*, 1993; Eddington *et al.*, 1978; Zeng and Shannon, 1992). The channel-by-channel mapping of acoustical dynamic range onto the electrical dynamic range uses fully the discriminable steps in amplitude available for each electrode.

The CA and CIS strategies have been compared in a number of studies, beginning with a study conducted by Wilson *et al.* in 1989 and 1990 (Wilson *et al.*, 1991a). In that study, a laboratory implementation of the CIS strategy was compared with the clinical CA processor of the Ineraid device. Eleven subjects participated in the study. Seven of the subjects were selected for their high levels of performance with the CA processor and Ineraid implant, and four additional subjects were subsequently selected for their low levels of performance with that processor and implant. The high-performance subjects were representative of the best results in terms of speech reception scores that had been obtained with the Ineraid or any other implant system at the time of the study. All subjects had had at least 1 year of daily experience with the clinical CA processor when the comparisons were conducted, and most had had multiple years of such experience. In contrast, experience with CIS was limited to several days of initial tests to evaluate fitting alternatives. Experience with the CIS processor ultimately compared with the clinical CA processor was no more than several hours.

Results from the study are presented in Fig. 7.15. Lines connect CA scores with CIS scores for each subject. The four panels show results for different open-set tests. Scores for the high-performance subjects are indicated

by the endpoints of the light lines in the upper part of each panel, and scores for the low-performance subjects are indicated by the end points of the thicker lines closer to the bottom of each panel. All tests were conducted with hearing alone, and all tests used single presentations of recorded material without feedback about correct or incorrect responses.

Scores for all 11 subjects were improved with the CIS processor. The average scores across subjects increased from 57% to 80% correct in the spondee tests (*i.e.*, recognition of two-syllable words), from 62% to 84% correct in the CID sentence tests, from 34% to 65% correct in the Speech Perception in

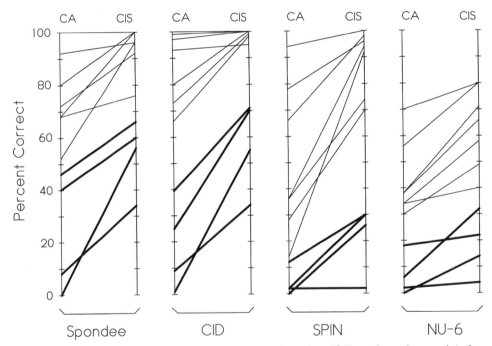

FIG. 7.15. Speech recognition scores for compressed analog (CA) and continuous interleaved sampling (CIS) processors. A line connects the CA and CIS scores for each subject. Light lines correspond to seven subjects selected for their excellent performance with the clinical CA processor of the Ineraid device, and the heavier lines correspond to four subjects selected for relatively poor performance. The CA strategy provided performance that was equal to or better than all clinically available alternatives at the time of these comparisons, which began in 1989. The tests included recognition of two-syllable words (Spondee), key words in the Central Institute for the Deaf (CID) sentences of everyday speech, the final word in each of 50 high-predictability sentences from the Speech Perception in Noise (SPIN) test (presented in these studies without noise), and monosyllabic words from Northwestern University Auditory Test 6 (NU-6). (Adapted from Wilson *et al.*, 1995, with permission.)

Noise (SPIN) sentence tests, and from 30% to 47% correct in the NU-6 word tests. All of these increases were highly significant.

The scores of 80% correct on the NU-6 test for two of the subjects were unprecedented at the time of this study. Perhaps even more important were the improvements produced with CIS for the low-performance subjects. Subject SR1, for instance, achieved scores with the CIS processor that moved him from a low-performance to a high-performance category. His scores improved from 40% to 60% correct for the spondee tests, from 25% to 70% correct for the CID sentence tests, from 2% to 30% correct for the SPIN sentence tests, and from 6% to 32% correct for the NU-6 tests. Similarly, results for subject SR10 demonstrated quite large improvements with CIS. His scores improved from 0% to 56% correct for the spondee tests, from 1% to 55% correct for the CID sentence tests, from 0% to 26% correct for the SPIN sentence tests, and from 0% to 14% correct for the NU-6 tests. This subject went from no open-set recognition of speech to useful open-set recognition with substitution of a CIS processor for the clinical CA processor.

Results from subsequent studies (e.g., Böex et al., 1994 and 1996; Dorman and Loizou, 1997a and 1997b) have replicated and extended these initial findings. Subsequent studies have demonstrated a potential for additional increases in performance with adjustments in the parameters of CIS processors (Wilson et al., 1995) and with further experience in using CIS processors (Dorman and Loizou, 1997a; Lawson et al., 1995; Pelizzone et al., 1995). One of the subjects who scored 80% correct on the NU-6 test using the CIS processor of the initial comparisons scored in the high 90th percentile with his clinical CIS processor. Subject SR10 scores in the 60th percentile with his refined fitting of a CIS processor and with the experience he has gained using the processor in his daily life.

The immediate improvements observed with substitution of a laboratory CIS processor for the clinical CA processor may have been produced by one or more of the differences in design described previously. In addition, five or six channels (and electrodes) were used for the CIS processors, whereas the standard four were used with the clinical CA processor. This increase also might have contributed to the better performance of the CIS processors.

Spectral Maxima Sound Processor Strategy

The progenitor of the SPEAK strategy was the *spectral maxima sound processor* (SMSP) strategy. It and SPEAK mark a departure from the feature extraction approach of prior strategies used in conjunction with the Nucleus implant.

The SMSP strategy is an *n*-of-*m* strategy, as described in the section on IP processors. The patent for the SMSP builds on the variation 2 of IP processors by specifying particular choices for *n* and *m* and by specifying a higher cutoff frequency for the lowpass filters in the envelope detectors (McDermott and Vandali, 1997).

In the SMSP (McDermott *et al.*, 1992; McDermott and Vandali, 1997), the microphone or direct input is directed to an AGC (with long time constants and a low compression ratio), and the AGC output is directed to a bank of 16 bandpass filters spanning the range from 250 to 5,400 Hz. Envelope signals are derived for each of the bandpass outputs with a rectifier and lowpass filter, as in the IP, F0/F2, F0/F1/F2, and MPEAK strategies. In contrast to those strategies, the cutoff frequency for the lowpass filters is set at 200 Hz instead of a much lower value. As with the IP strategies, each bandpass channel is assigned to a position along the electrode array. Channels with low center frequencies deliver their outputs to electrodes at apical positions, and channels with high center frequencies deliver their outputs to electrodes at basal positions. A postprocessor is used to scan the outputs of the bandpass channels (*i.e.*, the envelope signals) for each cycle of stimulation across electrodes. The scan first selects channel outputs above a preset noise threshold, and if more than six channel outputs are selected, it selects the six channel outputs that have greatest amplitudes among the set. The identified channels and associated electrodes (usually six except for quiet conditions or weak sounds of speech) are used for stimulation in that cycle. A logarithmic transformation of the envelope signals is used to determine pulse amplitudes, as in the prior strategies described earlier. The electrodes are stimulated in a nonsimultaneous sequence for each cycle, starting with the electrode or electrode pair assigned to the channel with the highest envelope signal among the selected channals, and ending with the electrode or electrode pair assigned to the channel with the lowest envelope signal among the selected channels. Stimulation cycles are repeated at the rate of 250/s, which approximates the maximum rate possible for stimulation of six electrodes or six electrode pairs in each cycle with the Nucleus transcutaneous link. (A rate of around 400/s can be attained under certain conditions, see Crosby *et al.*, 1985, and Shannon *et al.*, 1990).

As with the CIS strategy, voicing information may be represented with the SMSP strategy through variations in modulation waveforms out to 200 Hz. However, the maximum pulse rate on each electrode with the SMSP strategy is only 250/s, which is below the aliasing rate of 400 pulses/s for a 200-Hz variation in the modulation waveform. The representation of frequencies above 125 Hz is subject to aliasing effects with the SMSP, and the representation of frequencies in the range of one-fourth to one-half the pulse rate probably is distorted to a lessor extent (Busby *et al.*, 1993; McKay *et al.*, 1994; Wilson, 1997). Such aliasing effects and distortions are likely to degrade the representation of voicing information and also produce reversals in judgments of fundamental frequencies when the frequencies exceed one-half the carrier rate (*i.e.*, 125 Hz in the middle part of the F0 range for male talkers and in lower part of the F0 ranges for female and child talkers).

Results from tests with a small number of subjects indicated that the SMSP strategy might offer substantial improvements in speech reception compared with the F0/F1/F2 and MPEAK strategies (McDermott *et al.*, 1992; McKay *et al.*, 1991 and 1992). For example, in studies with four subjects, McKay *et al.* (1992) recorded significant increases in several measures of speech reception when the SMSP was substituted for the MPEAK processor. The measures included identification of vowels and consonants, recognition of consonant-vowel nucleus-consonant (CNC) monosyllabic words, and recognition of BKB sentences in competition with multitalker babble at the speech-to-babble ratio of 10 dB. The average scores across subjects improved from 76.3% to 91.3% correct for vowels, from 59.4% to 74.9% correct for consonants, from 39.9% to 57.4% correct for words, and from 50.0% to 78.7% correct for sentences in noise.

Spectral Peak Strategy

After the encouraging results with the SMSP, Cochlear Ltd. and the University of Melbourne developed the SPEAK strategy, which is a refinement of the SMSP strategy. New hardware also was developed to implement the SPEAK strategy in a smaller package and with more processing options than the MSP (Patrick *et al.*, 1997).

In the SPEAK strategy (Patrick *et al.*, 1997; Skinner *et al.*, 1994), the input is filtered into as many as 20 bands rather than the 16 bands of the SMSP. Envelope signals are derived with a rectifier and lowpass filter, as in the SMSP and prior strategies. The cutoff of the lowpass filters is set at 200 Hz, as in the SMSP. The outputs of the envelope detectors are scanned with a postprocessor in a manner similar to that of the SMSP. The number of bandpass channels selected in each scan depends on the number of envelope signals exceeding a preset noise threshold and on details of the input such as the distribution of energy across frequencies. In many cases, six channels are selected, as in the SMSP strategy. However, the number can range from one to a maximum that can be set as high as

10. Cycles of stimulation, which include the selected channels and associated electrodes, are presented at rates between 180 and 300/s. The amount of time required to complete each cycle depends on the number of electrodes and channels included in the cycle and the pulse amplitudes and durations for each of the electrodes. In general, inclusion of relatively few electrodes in a cycle allows relatively high rates, whereas inclusion of many electrodes reduces the rate.

A diagram illustrating the operation of the SPEAK processor is presented in Fig. 7.16. The speech input is directed to a bank of bandpass filters and envelope detectors, whose outputs are scanned for each cycle of stimulation. In this diagram, six channels are selected in the scan and the corresponding electrodes are stimulated nonsimultaneously in a base-to-apex order. Two such scans are depicted in the figure.

The new hardware, called the Spectra 22 processor, includes a custom integrated circuit to perform the functions of bandpass filtering and envelope detection. The integrated circuit can be programmed to produce changes in the frequency ranges and gains for the bandpass filters. In a typical implementation of the SPEAK strategy, 20 bandpass filters span the range from 150 to 10,823 Hz, with a linear spacing of bandpass frequencies below 1,850 Hz and a logarithmic spacing of bandpass frequencies above 1,850 Hz. (Such linear-logarithmic spacing may provide an even closer match to the distribution of critical bands in normal hearing compared with a strictly logarithmic spacing.) The filter gains normally are all set to a single value. Alternative choices may be specified, such as when fewer than 20 electrode positions are available for a given patient.

Comparisons between Spectral Peak and Multipeak Strategies

Within-subject comparisons of the SPEAK and MPEAK strategies have been conducted with 63 English-speaking patients at various centers in Australia, the United States, Can-

ada, and England (Skinner *et al.*, 1994). Some of the principal results and key processing steps in the SPEAK strategy are presented in Fig. 7.17. Subjects were tested using an ABAB crossover design, in which subjects used their clinical MPEAK processor during an initial 3-week period, then used the SPEAK processor for 6 weeks, then returned to the MPEAK processor for 3 weeks, and then used the SPEAK processor during a final 3-week period. The processors were tested at the end of each period. All subjects had had at least 8 months of daily experience with the MPEAK processor before the study.

The subjects participating in the study all had scores of 5% correct or better for recognition of key words in the CID or BKB sentences. This group of subjects represented approximately 75% of the population using the Nucleus device at that time. (The remaining 25% of the population had little or no open-set recognition of speech, even for relatively easy tests such as the sentence tests described earlier.)

Averages of the scores for each subject and processor are presented in the middle and bottom panels of Fig. 7.17. The middle panel shows scores for the recognition of key words in the City University of New York (CUNY) sentences or in the Speech Intelligibility Test for Deaf Children (SIT) sentences presented in quiet. The bottom panel shows scores for the sentences presented in competition with multitalker speech babble at the speech-to-babble ratio of 10 dB. Two of the 63 subjects were excluded from the tests of sentence recognition in quiet, and 5 were excluded from the tests of sentence recognition in noise because of their low scores in preliminary tests using the CID sentences; the excluded subjects scored below 35% correct on the CID test.

Among the 61 subjects who were tested with sentences in quiet, 24 had significantly higher scores with the SPEAK processor, and 2 had significantly higher scores with the MPEAK processor. Many of the subjects obtained high scores on this relatively easy test and therefore possible differences be-

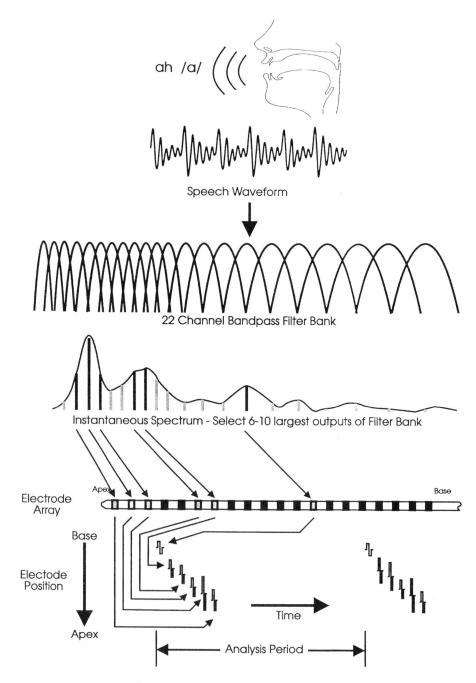

FIG. 7.16. Key steps in the spectral peak processing strategy. Speech inputs are directed to a bank of up to 20 bandpass filters and envelope detectors. A postprocessor scans the envelope signals for each cycle of stimulation across electrodes. Between 1 and 10 of the highest-amplitude signals are selected in each scan, depending on characteristics of the input (*i.e.*, overall level and spectral composition). Electrodes associated with the selected envelope signals and bandpass channels are stimulated in a base-to-apex order. (From Patrick *et al.*, 1997, with permission.)

Spectral Peak Strategy

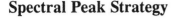

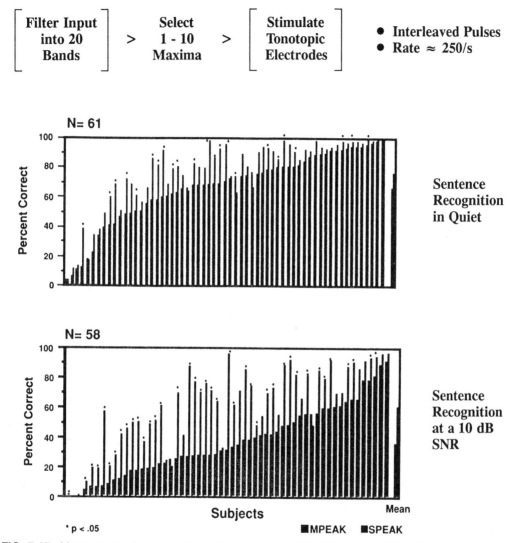

FIG. 7.17. Mean scores for recognition of key words in City University of New York sentences or in the Speech Intelligibility Test for Deaf Children sentences with multipeak (MPEAK) and spectral peak (SPEAK) processors. The top panel indicates the design of the SPEAK strategy. The MPEAK strategy was used in the clinical Nucleus processor at the time of these comparisons. The MPEAK strategy operated in a fundamentally different way from SPEAK, extracting and representing specific features of the speech input, such as formant frequencies and amplitudes. The middle panel shows scores for each of 61 subjects listening to the sentences in a condition without interfering noise, and the bottom panel shows scores for each of 58 subjects listening to the sentences in competition with multitalker-babble noise at the speech-to-babble ratio of 10 dB. (Adapted from Wilson *et al.*, 1995, with permission; data from Skinner *et al.*, 1994)

tween processors may have been masked by ceiling effects. Among the 58 subjects who were tested with sentences in noise (for the 10 dB speech-to-babble condition), 41 had significantly higher scores with the SPEAK processor, and none had a significantly higher score with the MPEAK processor.

The principal advantage of the SPEAK processor, as demonstrated by these and other tests (Skinner *et al.*, 1994), is in better recognition of speech in noise. This advantage may be a result of the filterbank approach used in the SPEAK processor. It also may be a result of the high sensitivity of the feature extraction portions of the MPEAK processor to noise. The accuracy of such extraction can be severely degraded by even small amounts of noise. Zero crossings analysis in particular is susceptible to deleterious effects of noise interference (Rabiner and Shafer, 1978).

Comparisons between Spectral Peak and Continuous Interleaved Sampling Strategies

Comparisons of SPEAK and CIS strategies indicate that both support high levels of speech reception in quiet conditions (Aubert *et al.*, 1998; Kiefer *et al.*, 1996; Lawson *et al.*, 1996; Loizou *et al.*, 1997). Comparisons with matched groups of patients in the study of Kiefer *et al.* (1996) produced significantly higher scores with CIS (as implemented in the Med El COMBI 40 device) for recognition of key words in the Göttingen sentences at the two tested speech-to-noise ratios of 15 and 10 dB. Scores for recognition of key words in the easier Innsbruck sentences were not significantly higher with CIS for presentation of the sentences in quiet and at the tested speech-to-noise ratios of 15 and 10 dB. Scores for the Innsbruck sentences were high for the CIS strategy for the three test conditions, and therefore the comparisons between the two strategies with those sentences may have been limited by possible ceiling effects. The average scores for the CIS strategy were 88%, 81%, and 72% correct for the

quiet, 15 dB and 10 dB conditions, respectively, and the average scores for the SPEAK strategy were 79%, 66%, and 56% correct for those same conditions.

Comparisons with separate matched groups of patients in the study of Loizou *et al.* (1997) also indicated an advantage of CIS (as implemented in the CIS-Link processor developed by Med El for use with the Ineraid implant) for speech reception in noise. The tests included identification of 16 consonants in an /a/-consonant-/a/ context, identification of 8 vowels in an /h/-vowel-/d/ context, and recognition of key words in sentences from the Hearing in Noise Test (HINT) database. Each of the tests was administered without noise and at the speech-to-noise ratios of 15, 10 and 5 dB. The scores from the tests of consonant identification were significantly higher with CIS for all conditions. The score from the test of vowel identification for the most adverse speech-to-noise ratio (5 dB) also was significantly higher with CIS. Scores from the remaining tests were not significantly higher with CIS. Loizou *et al.* suggested that the results from the sentence tests were consistent with those reported by Kiefer *et al.*, in that the HINT sentences are comparable in difficulty to the Innsbruck sentences. Tests with more difficult material may have provided a greater sensitivity for demonstrating possible differences between the two strategies.

Lawson *et al.* (1996) evaluated CIS, *n*-of-*m*, and SPEAK processors in within-subject comparisons with five subjects. The tests included identification of 16 or 24 consonants in an /a/-consonant-/a/ context, presented without noise; the 24 consonant test was used for the two subjects with the highest levels of performance among processors to avoid possible ceiling effects. The results indicated an equivalence or superiority of six-channel CIS processors (as implemented with a laboratory system) compared with the clinical SPEAK processor used by the subjects in their daily lives. The CIS and SPEAK strategies produced scores that were not statistically different when the range of frequencies spanned by the bandpass filters in the CIS processors was from 350 to 5,500 Hz. The CIS strategy produced significantly higher scores when the upper end of the range was extended to 9,500 Hz, approximating the upper end of the range in the SPEAK processors.

In a separate study with 41 subjects, Aubert *et al.* compared the clinical SPEAK processor used by the subjects with a CIS processor, as implemented in the new Sprint hardware of the Cochlear Ltd. CI24M implant system. Some subjects obtained higher speech reception scores with the SPEAK strategy, and other subjects obtained higher scores with the CIS strategy. The remaining subjects had similar scores with the two strategies.

Comparisons of the CIS and SPEAK strategies have indicated an approximate equivalence of the two for some tests, such as the Innsbruck and HINT sentences, and a superiority of CIS for other tests, such as identification of consonants. CIS appears to provide an advantage for listening to speech in noise, particularly for consonants and difficult sentences.

N-of-*M* Strategies

Variation 2 of the IP strategy was the first *n*-of-*m* processor for cochlear implants. Since that beginning, the SMSP and SPEAK strategies have been developed for use with the Cochlear Ltd. implant, and an *n*-of-*m* strategy using much higher rates of stimulation than the SMSP or SPEAK strategies has been developed for use with the Med El COMBI 40 and COMBI 40+ implants. An *n*-of-*m* strategy using similarly high rates of stimulation has been developed as a processing option for use with the new Cochlear Ltd. CI24M device. This last implementation is called the ACE strategy.

The *n*-of-*m* approach may help in making more prominent the highest amplitude envelope signals among many. Results from early vocoder studies (Flanagan, 1972) indicated that envelope signals 30 dB below the peak signal can be discarded without damaging the intelligibility of speech transmitted and reconstructed with a channel vocoder and that a modest further reduction in the number of selected envelope signals still can support high levels of intelligibility while allowing a reduction in the information rate of transmission. The latter observation led to the development of peak-picker vocoders that applied various rules to select the peaks from among the envelope signals that would maximize intelligibility for a given number of peaks or minimize the transmission rate for a given target intelligibility. In general, the most effective rules did not involve simple selection of the *n* greatest envelope signals, but instead selected signals that would convey the essential spectral information without redundancy. (The performance of *n*-of-*m* strategies for cochlear implants may be improved with the use of such rules, but this possibility has not yet been evaluated.)

Lawson *et al.* (1996) compared processors implementing an *n*-of-*m* strategy along with other strategies in tests with five subjects implanted with the Nucleus electrode array and with percutaneous access to that array. The percutaneous access allowed implementations of strategies that combined relatively high rates of stimulation with a relatively large number of addressed electrodes. The *n*-of-*m* processors selected the six highest envelope signals from among 18. In one implementation, the cycles of stimulation across electrodes were repeated at 250/s (approximating the rates of the SMSP and SPEAK strategies), and in another implementation the cycles were repeated at 833/s. The cutoff frequency of the lowpass filters in the envelope detectors was 200 Hz for both implementations. This choice matched the cutoff frequency used in the SMSP and SPEAK strategies. The additional processors evaluated with these subjects included the clinical SPEAK processor used by the subjects in their daily lives and several implementations of CIS processors using different rates of stimulation, different numbers of channels, different polarities of stimulus pulses, different update orders, and different ranges of frequencies spanned by the bandpass filters. (The *n*-of-*m* variations also included processors with a 350- to 5,500-Hz or a 350- to 9,500-Hz range for the bandpass filters.) The tests included identification of consonants in an /a/-consonant-/a/ context for recorded male and female speakers.

In broad terms, the results indicated significantly better performance with the higher-rate *n*-of-*m* processor using the extended frequency range than with the clinical SPEAK processor. This better performance was obtained with no more than a few hours of experience with the *n*-of-*m* processor compared with more than a year of daily use of the SPEAK processor by each of the subjects. The *n*-of-*m* processor also produced the best performance among the tested processors for one of the subjects and the female speaker. Scores across subjects and speakers with the high-rate, extended-frequency range *n*-of-*m* processor were not significantly different from the scores for a six-channel CIS processor also using the extended frequency range and a stimulus rate of 833 pulses/s/electrode. Scores for these two processors were significantly higher than the SPEAK processor or a six-channel CIS processor using the narrower frequency range for the bandpass filters. Scores for these latter two processors were not significantly different.

These comparisons indicate the value of relatively high rates of stimulation and of an extended frequency range for the bandpass filters. They also indicate that *n*-of-*m* processors can be competitive with or better than CIS or SPEAK processors, particularly for certain subjects and speakers.

The *n*-of-*m* approach may allow the representation of spectral detail through use of *m* sites of stimulation, without exceeding the transmission rate limits of transcutaneous links. For example, a 6-of-18 *n*-of-*m* processor may convey more spectral information than a 6-of-6 CIS processor if more than six electrodes (or six bipolar pairs of electrodes) are perceptually separable. In addition, for the same *m* and stimulus rate, an

n-of-*m* processor is likely to have lower electrode interactions than an *m*-of-*m* (CIS) processor, especially for large values of *m* or close spacing of the intracochlear electrodes. So long as *n* is not too low, the *n*-of-*m* approach may be the best among the available options for some patients, possibly including patients with limited transcutaneous links or relatively high temporal interactions among electrodes.

The ACE implementation of the *n*-of-*m* strategy has been described as combining the best aspects of the SPEAK strategy with the best aspects of the CIS strategy. In particular, CIS has been described as a strategy that emphasizes the representation of temporal variations in speech through relatively rapid rates of stimulation, whereas SPEAK has been described as a strategy that emphasizes the representation of channel or spectral cues through use of a relatively large number of electrodes. The combination of an *n*-of-*m* approach, as in SPEAK, with relatively high rates of stimulation, as typically used in CIS processors, may support especially high levels of speech reception.

Although relatively rapid rates of stimulation can produce improvements in the performance of *n*-of-*m* processors, as demonstrated in the study of Lawson *et al.* and elsewhere (studies cited in Patrick, 1997), the characterization of CIS as using high rates and relatively few electrodes is at least somewhat simplistic. CIS processors may use all of the electrodes available for a particular implant. The first CIS processors were implemented for use with the Ineraid implant and its six electrodes. However, subsequent implementations have addressed 21 of the 22 available electrodes in the Nucleus implant (in the study of Lawson *et al.*) and all 12 of the available electrodes in the Med El COMBI 40+ implant. CIS also may combine rapid rates of stimulation with a large number of electrodes. However, such combinations have been no more effective than combinations of rapid rates with four to six electrodes, as described earlier. This may change with new electrode designs, which may increase the number of perceptually distinct sites of stimulation compared with the number available with the current designs. CIS processors coupled with selective electrodes may well support significant gains in performance with the addition of channels and electrodes beyond six.

The options among SPEAK, high-rate *n*-of-*m* (ACE), and CIS in the new Cochlear Ltd. CI24M device, and the options between high-rate *n*-of-*m* and CIS in the Med El COMBI 40 and COMBI 40+ devices, may help patients to achieve a better outcome than would be possible with one option only. Results from various studies have established the value of the *n*-of-*m* approach and have demonstrated that it can be superior to SPEAK and CIS for some patients and talkers, at least in quiet conditions. Further improvements in the performance of *n*-of-*m* processors may be produced with different rules for selecting the envelope signals to be represented in each cycle of stimulation or with application of the strategy in conjunction with electrodes that have a greater spatial selectivity of stimulation than current electrodes.

Simultaneous Analog Stimulation Strategy

Advanced Bionics has developed two variations of CA processors for use with its Clarion implant. Both variations use back-end compression, in contrast to the front-end compression of the prior CA implementations in the Ineraid and UCSF/Storz devices. The AGC that feeds the bank of bandpass filters in the Clarion implementations has relatively long attack and release times and a relatively low compression ratio. As in CIS processors that use an AGC, this greatly reduces the spectral distortions produced by the AGC stage in the prior CA implementations. As in the CIS and other strategies, bandpass channel outputs in the CA implementations of the Clarion device are individually mapped onto stimulus amplitudes using a nonlinear compression function. Such channel-by-channel mapping may help to

produce normal or nearly normal growths of loudness within channels and use most or all of the dynamic range of perception available at each electrode position.

In the first CA implementation used with the Clarion, channel outputs were directed to offset radial pairs of bipolar electrodes. As many as eight channels and associated pairs of electrodes could be used. The offset radial electrodes were modeled after the original UCSF design (Loeb *et al.*, 1983), which could support high spatial specificity of stimulation for cochleas with good survival of neural processes peripheral to the ganglion cells and with positioning of the bipolar pairs immediately adjacent to the peripheral processes.

Such selectivity of stimulation could reduce electrode interactions compared with those produced with monopolar stimulation. Unfortunately, survival of processes peripheral to the ganglion cells is rare in the deaf human cochlea (Hinojosa and Marion, 1983) (see Chapter 6). Also, results of recent studies have demonstrated that a mechanical memory for the curvature of the first and second turns in the average cochlea, as implemented in the original UCSF design, is not sufficient to ensure close apposition of the electrodes to the osseous spiral lamina (where surviving peripheral processes would reside) or to the inner wall of the scala tympani. New approaches for placement of electrodes next to the inner wall of the scala tympani are described in Chapter 6.

Although the first CA implementation used with the Clarion addressed the likely problems associated with front-end compression, it probably did not address the likely problems associated with the interactions that can be produced with simultaneous stimulation across electrode positions. Conditions for selective stimulation were not met with the offset radial electrodes. Quite high levels of stimulation often were required to produce auditory percepts with these electrodes, which probably reflected a focused electrical field coupled with a relatively long distance to excitable neurons (in the spiral ganglion or modiolus), along with large shunting currents between the closely spaced electrodes of each bipolar pair. Many patients could not be stimulated at all within the current and charge limits of the device using the offset radial electrodes.

The fact that many patients could not be stimulated with the offset radial electrodes led Advanced Bionics to reassign the outputs of its implanted receiver/stimulator to address monopolar electrodes or "enhanced bipolar" electrodes, which had a greater spacing between the electrodes in each bipolar pair (about 1.7 mm). Seven such enhanced bipolar electrodes could be addressed.

The Clarion device implements a CIS strategy that addresses monopolar electrodes and a variation of a CA strategy that addresses the enhanced bipolar electrodes. To distinguish this variation of a CA strategy from the prior variation (which addressed up to eight pairs of offset radial electrodes), Advanced Bionics has called it the SAS strategy. Like the CIS strategy, the SAS strategy addresses possible weaknesses of the original CA strategy as implemented in the Ineraid and UCSF/Storz devices. In contrast to the CA strategy of the Ineraid device, the SAS strategy uses the enhanced bipolar electrodes, which may be more selective in stimulating neurons along the longitudinal dimension of the cochlea compared with monopolar electrodes. (The enhanced bipolar electrodes also may be more selective than the offset radial electrodes of the UCSF/Storz device, at least for typical neural survival patterns and placements of electrodes.) The use of back-end compression in the SAS strategy addresses the likely problems associated with front-end compression.

The SAS strategy also uses more channels and electrodes than the prior CA processors of the Ineraid and UCSF/Storz devices. In the default condition, SAS outputs are directed to seven pairs of enhanced bipolar electrodes, whereas the CA outputs were directed to four monopolar electrodes in the Ineraid device or to four offset-radial bipolar electrodes in the UCSF/Storz device. If the spatial specificity of enhanced bipolar electrodes is relatively high, the additional channels in SAS may help.

Evaluation of the SAS strategy is just beginning. In preliminary studies, attempts were made to fit SAS in groups of newly implanted patients. The results showed that the dynamic ranges of percepts from threshold to loud sounds could be spanned for most of the patients using analog stimuli and the enhanced bipolar electrodes. Patients who could be fit with SAS and CIS strategies were asked to indicate a preference between the two. Some indicated a preference for SAS, whereas others indicated a preference for CIS. The proportion of patients indicating a preference for SAS was about 50% among a group implanted in Hannover, Germany (Battmer *et al.*, 1997b), and about 30% among a group implanted at various medical centers in the United States (Osberger, 1998; Kessler, 1998).

The patients in these studies were allowed to use their preferred strategy after the initial fittings and then tested periodically with both strategies. The results suggest a relationship between initial preference and performance, but this impression needs to be verified in a crossover study that provides controls for possible order and experience effects. Such a study is in progress, and results from fully controlled comparisons of a SAS strategy using enhanced bipolar electrodes versus a CIS strategy using monopolar electrodes should be available in the near future.

Convergence of Findings

The developments outlined in this chapter are good news for recipients of cochlear implants. Applications of the CIS and SPEAK processing strategies have produced large improvements in speech reception performance compared with prior strategies. Realistic expectations for prospective patients can be higher than was the case before these strategies became available for clinical use.

Progressive improvements in performance

were obtained in the series of strategies developed for the Nucleus implant as more information was added to the representation for the feature-extraction strategies and when the feature-extraction approach was abandoned in favor of a filterbank approach. The strategies in this series included the F0/F2, F0/F1/F2, MPEAK, and SMSP/SPEAK strategies, each with better performance than its predecessor.

In another line of developments, a filterbank approach also was superior to a strategy that was modeled after the analysis portion of a channel vocoder. In particular, the filterbank approach of the CIS strategy was superior to variation 1 of the IP strategy, in which the features of voiced or unvoiced boundaries and the fundamental frequency of voiced speech sounds were extracted and represented.

Assumptions about how speech is produced and perceived, as used in the design of vocoder systems, are not necessary for the design of effective processing strategies for cochlear implants. Strategies based on such assumptions have produced relatively low levels of performance, especially for listening to speech in competition with noise.

The initial comparisons between the CIS and CA strategies demonstrated large improvements in speech reception scores with the former. This better performance may have been produced by one or more of the following: a reduction in electrode interactions through the use of nonsimultaneous stimuli, the use of five or six channels instead of four, representation of rapid envelope variations through relatively high cutoff frequencies for the lowpass filters in the envelope detectors and rates of stimulation at least twice as high as the cutoff frequencies, or preservation of amplitude cues with channel-by-channel compression and logarithmic or power-law mapping functions.

The new analog strategy of SAS also addresses possible weaknesses of the prior CA strategies. It addresses likely problems associated with front-end compression by using back-end compression on an channel-by-channel basis. To the extent that a high spatial specificity of stimulation is achieved with the enhanced bipolar electrodes, it also may address the likely problem of electrode interactions with the prior strategies. Controlled comparisons of SAS with CIS are underway in a crossover study involving multiple medical centers in the United States. The results may show that SAS is competitive with or better than CIS for some patients.

Various *n*-of-*m* strategies available with the Cochlear Ltd. CI24M implant and the Med El COMBI 40 and COMBI 40+ implants may provide higher speech reception scores for some patients than the SPEAK or CIS strategies. The higher stimulus rates used with the *n*-of-*m* implementation in the CI24M device, compared with the rates used with the SPEAK implementation, may prove to be beneficial. The selection of the highest envelope signals (and the rejection of the lowest envelope signals) may help in listening to speech in noise or for patients with relatively large temporal interactions among electrodes. Studies are in progress to evaluate these possibilities.

The available processing strategies for cochlear implants all use a filterbank or waveform approach. Most of the strategies use nonsimultaneous pulses to reduce deleterious effects of electrode interactions. One of the strategies uses simultaneous stimulation across electrodes but does this in conjunction with bipolar electrodes that may provide a greater spatial specificity of stimulation than other configurations of electrodes. All strategies use back-end, channel-by-channel compression. None of the strategies extracts nor represents specific features of speech.

ADDITIONAL CONSIDERATIONS

Importance of Fitting

Large improvements in the speech reception performance of implant systems can be obtained through informed choices of parameters within a particular processing strategy.

In studies with CIS processors, for example, quite large gains in performance have been produced through choices of pulse rate, pulse duration, electrode update order, the range of frequencies spanned by the bandpass filters, and other parameters (Wilson *et al.*, 1995). Although predetermined values for some parameters may be appropriate for virtually all patients, the values of other parameters should be varied over certain ranges to optimize performance for individuals. An objective of current research in several laboratories is to identify values that can be fixed and values that must be varied to approximate optimal performance within and across patients. The results of such research may inform the development of improved and highly efficient fitting procedures. In the interim, it is important to understand that optimal fittings of speech processors cannot be accomplished without parametric manipulations and that control measures are necessary to gauge the effects of the manipulations. Such parametric studies take time, usually much more time than is typically allocated for the fitting of implant systems in clinical settings.

Importance of Strategy Implementations

The performance of a given strategy also can be affected by the quality of its implementation in speech processor hardware and software. As mentioned before, large increases in speech reception scores were produced in the study of Dowell *et al.* (1991) when the MSP implementation of the F0/F1/F2 strategy was substituted for the WSP III implementation of that strategy. In another two studies, Battmer *et al.* (1997a) and Kessler (1997) found significant improvements in speech reception scores when the Clarion version 1.2 implementation of a CIS strategy was substituted for the version 1.1 implementation of that strategy. Seemingly subtle changes in hardware and the programming of that hardware can produce large changes in performance. This fact complicates comparisons of processing strategies, in that one

or both of the strategies under test may not be implemented in the best possible way. For example, an apparent superiority of one of the strategies may be an artifact of a high-quality implementation of that strategy and a less than optimal implementation of the other strategy. This is a particular problem in comparisons involving CIS or CIS-like strategies, because those strategies have been implemented in different ways in a variety of commercial devices (including the Philips LAURA device, the Advanced Bionics Clarion device, the Med-El Combi 40 and Combi 40+ devices, and the Cochlear Ltd. CI24M device) and in a variety of custom processors for laboratory studies.

The details of the implementation are important. Examples of ways in which the implementation can go awry include use of microphones with poor frequency response or high levels of noise, use of amplifier and AGC circuits with low dynamic ranges or high levels of noise, use of digital filters with a reduced number of elements compared with conventional and well-behaved digital filters (a reduced number of elements have been used in devices with small memories or slow digital–signal–processing chips), use of current sources that are especially noisy, use of current sources that saturate or begin to saturate in the dynamic ranges of the electrodes for some or all patients (current sources saturate when the commanded current requires a voltage at the electrodes that approaches or is greater than the voltage limit of the device), and an excessive amount of digital or switching noise at the electrodes. Any one of these can degrade or destroy the performance of an otherwise good strategy.

Importance of the Patient Variable

Data indicating the importance of the patient variable are presented in Fig. 7.18. This figure shows a scatter plot of NU-6 word scores from the within-subject comparisons of CA and CIS processors described previously (scores are from Fig.

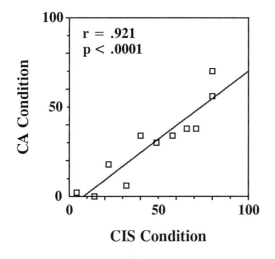

FIG. 7.18. Scatter plot of Northwestern University Auditory Test 6 scores for compressed analog (CA) and continuous interleaved sampling (CIS) processors. Each point represents scores for one subject, and the Pearson correlation coefficient, level of significance, and regression line are shown. (Adapted from Wilson *et al.*, 1993, with permission.)

7.15). These scores were obtained with careful and complete fittings of the two strategies and with high-quality implementations for both. Notice that relatively low scores for one strategy are associated with relatively low scores for the other strategy and vice versa. The data points in Fig. 7.18 are highly correlated ($r = 0.92$), indicating that 85% of the variance in the data is explained by the subject variable ($r^2 = 0.85$). Correlations for other tests not obviously distorted by ceiling effects also are quite high for these subjects and processors, in a range between 0.87 and 0.92 (Wilson *et al.*, 1993).

Although outcomes can be improved with a change in processing strategy, the patient variable can have an even greater effect. A patient who enjoys a high ranking among patients with one processor is likely to retain that ranking with another well-implemented and well-fit processor, and a patient who has a low ranking with one processor also is likely to retain that low ranking with another processor. Identification of the factor or factors that underlie the effects of the patient variable may lead to the development of reliable prognostic tests for prospective patients. Knowledge of the factor or factors also may help in the design of better implant systems, that take the factor or factors into account and minimize or eliminate their deleterious effects for

patients who otherwise would have relatively poor outcomes.

TRENDS AND CHALLENGES

One of the most striking findings from research on cochlear implants is that the range of performance across patients is large, even with the new processing strategies and current implant systems. Some patients score at or near 100% correct on standard audiologic tests of sentence and word recognition, whereas other patients obtain low scores using an identical speech processor and electrode array. Perhaps the greatest single challenge in improving implants is to identify the mechanisms underlying this variability in outcomes and to use that knowledge in developing new ways to help patients at the low end of the performance spectrum.

Another challenge is to provide more help for all implant users in listening to speech in competition with other speakers or background noise. Speech reception scores even for the best patients are markedly reduced in such situations.

Fortunately, multiple possibilities for improvements in implant systems are under investigation, including new electrode designs for placing electrode contacts close to the inner wall of the scala tympani and thereby reducing thresholds, increasing dynamic range, and increasing the spatial selectivity of stimulation; new ways of representing temporal variations within channels, such as use of very high carrier rates or high-rate conditioner pulses; and coordinated stimulation of bilateral implants, designed to restore sound lateralization abilities and the signal-to-noise advantages that accompany such abilities. These and other possibilities are described in detail in several recent articles (Clark, 1995; Klinke and Hartmann, 1997; Lenarz, 1997; Wilson, 1997 and 1999).

Research is in progress at several centers to identify the mechanisms underlying the wide variation in outcomes with current implant systems. Application of the results may lead to better performance through a reduction in the variation with improved devices. Implants of the near future are likely to be much better than those of today.

REFERENCES

Aubert L, Nicolai J, Staller S, Shaw S. Results of a pre-market evaluation of advanced speech encoders in the Nucleus 24 cochlear implant system [Abstract 68]. Presented at the *Fourth European Symposium on Paediatric Cochlear Implantation*; s'Hertogenbosch, The Netherlands, 1998.

Battmer RD, Feldmeier I, Kohlenberg A, Lenarz T. Performance of the new Clarion speech processor 1.2 in quiet and in noise. *Am J Otol* 1997a;18:S144–S146.

Battmer RD, Haake P, Lenarz T. Comparison study of the continuous interleaved sampling (CIS) and compressed analog (CA) strategies, using the CLARION cochlear implant system [Abstract 120]. Presented at the *Vth International Cochlear Implant Conference*; New York, NY, 1997b.

Blamey PJ, Dowell RC, Clark GM, Seligman PM. Acoustic parameters measured by a formant-estimating speech processor for a multiple-channel cochlear implant. *J Acoust Soc Am* 1987;82:38–47.

Böex C, Pelizzone M, Montandon P. Improvements in speech recognition with the CIS strategy for the Ineraid multichannel intracochlear implant. In: Hochmair IJ, Hochmair ES, eds. *Advances in cochlear implants.* Vienna: Manz, 1994:136–140.

Böex C, Pelizzone M, Montandon P. Speech recognition with a CIS strategy for the Ineraid multichannel cochlear implant. *Am J Otol* 1996;17:61–68.

Busby PA, Tong YC, Clark GM. The perception of temporal modulations by cochlear implant patients. *J Acoust Soc Am* 1993;94:124–131.

Clark GM. The University of Melbourne–Nucleus multi-electrode cochlear implant. *Adv Otorhinolaryngol* 1987;38:1–189.

Clark GM. Cochlear implants: future research direc-tions. *Ann Otol Rhinol Laryngol* 1995;104[Suppl 166]:22–27.

Clark GM, Tong YC, Patrick JF. *Cochlear prostheses.* Edinburgh: Churchill Livingstone, 1990.

Cohen NL, Waltzman SB, Fisher SG, et al. A prospective, randomized study of cochlear implants. *N Engl J Med* 1993;328:233–237.

Crosby PA, Daly CN, Money DK, Patrick JF, Seligman PM, Kuzma JA. Cochlear implant system for an auditory prosthesis. US patent 4532930, 1985.

Dorman MF. Speech perception by adults. In: Tyler RS, ed. *Cochlear implants: audiological foundations.* San Diego: Singular Publishing Group, 1993:145–190.

Dorman MF, Hannley MT, Dankowski K, Smith L, McCandless G. Word recognition by 50 patients fitted with the Symbion multichannel cochlear implant. *Ear Hear* 1989;10:44–49.

Dorman MF, Loizou PC. Changes in speech intelligibility as a function of time and signal processing strategy for an Ineraid patient fitted with continuous interleaved sampling (CIS) processors. *Ear Hear* 1997a;18:147–155.

Dorman MF, Loizou PC. Mechanisms of vowel recognition for Ineraid patients fit with continuous interleaved sampling processors. *J Acoust Soc Am* 1997b;102:581–587.

Dorman MF, Smith L, Parkin JL. Loudness balance between acoustic and electric stimulation by a patient with a multichannel cochlear implant. *Ear Hear* 1993;14:290–292.

Dowell RC, Dawson PW, Dettman SJ, et al. Multichannel cochlear implantation in children: a summary of current work at the University of Melbourne. *Am J Otol* 1991;12[Suppl 1]:137–143.

Dowell RC, Mecklenberg DJ, Clark GM. Speech recognition for 40 patients receiving multichannel cochlear implants. *Arch Otolaryngol Head Neck Surg* 1986;112:1054–1059.

Dowell RC, Seligman PM, Blamey PJ, Clark GM. Speech perception using a two-formant 22-electrode cochlear prosthesis in quiet and in noise. *Acta Otolaryngol* 1987a;104:439–446.

Dowell RC, Seligman PM, Blamey PJ, Clark GM. Evaluation of a two-formant speech-processing strategy for a multichannel cochlear prosthesis. *Ann Otol Rhinol Laryngol* 1987b;96[Suppl 128]:132–134.

Eddington DK. Speech discrimination in deaf subjects with cochlear implants. *J Acoust Soc Am* 1980;68:885–891.

Eddington DK, Dobelle WH, Brackman DE, Mladejovsky MG, Parkin JL. Auditory prosthesis research with multiple channel intracochlear stimulation in man. *Ann Otol Rhinol Laryngol* 1978;87[Suppl 53]:1–39.

Favre E, Pelizzone M. Channel interactions in patients using the Ineraid multichannel cochlear implant. *Hear Res* 1993;58:79–90.

Fishman K, Shannon RV, Slattery WH. Speech recognition as a function of the number of electrodes used in the SPEAK cochlear implant speech processor. *J Speech Hear Res* 1997;40:1201–1215.

Flanagan JL. *Speech analysis, synthesis and perception,* 2nd ed. Berlin: Springer-Verlag, 1972.

Gantz BJ. Cochlear implants: an overview. *Adv Otolaryngol Head Neck Surg* 1987;1:171–200.

Gantz BJ, McCabe BF, Tyler RS, Preece JP. Evaluation

of four cochlear implant designs. *Ann Otol Rhinol Laryngol* 1987;96[Suppl 128]:145–147.

Gantz BJ, Tyler RS, Knutson JF, *et al.* Evaluation of five different cochlear implant designs: audiologic assessment and predictors of performance. *Laryngoscope* 1988;98:1100–1106.

Hess W. *Pitch determination of speech signals*. Berlin: Springer-Verlag, 1983.

Hinojosa R, Marion M. Histopathology of profound sensorineural deafness. *Ann NY Acad Sci* 1983; 405:459–484.

Kessler DK. Clinical investigation of the CLARION Multi-Strategy—adult patient performance with Clarion version 1.2 [Abstract 118]. Presented at the *Vth International Cochlear Implant Conference*; New York, NY, 1997.

Kessler DK. New directions in speech processing II: The electrode connection [Abstract 159]. Presented at the *Fourth European Symposium on Paediatric Cochlear Implantation*; s'Hertogenbosch, The Netherlands, 1998.

Kiefer J, Müller J, Pfennigdorff T, *et al.* Speech understanding in quiet and in noise with the CIS speech coding strategy (Med-El Combi-40) compared to the multipeak and spectral peak strategies (Nucleus). *ORL J Otorhinolaryngol Relat Spec* 1996;58:127–135.

Klinke R, Hartmann R. Basic neurophysiology of cochlear implants. *Am J Otol* 1997;18:S7–S10.

Lawson DT, Wilson BS, Finley CC. New processing strategies for multichannel cochlear prostheses. *Prog Brain Res* 1993;97:313–321.

Lawson DT, Wilson BS, Zerbi M, Finley CC. Speech processors for auditory prostheses. First Quarterly Progress Report, NIH project N01-DC-5-2103. Bethesda: Neural Prosthesis Program, National Institutes of Health, 1995.

Lawson DT, Wilson BS, Zerbi M, Finley CC. Speech processors for auditory prostheses. Third Quarterly Progress Report, NIH project N01-DC-5-2103. Bethesda: Neural Prosthesis Program, National Institutes of Health, 1996.

Lenarz T. Cochlear implants—What can be achieved? *Am J Otol* 1997;18:S2–S3.

Loeb GE, Byers CL, Rebscher SJ, *et al.* Design and fabrication of an experimental cochlear prosthesis. *Med Biol Eng Comput* 1983;21:241–254.

Loizou PC. Mimicking the human ear: an overview of signal processing strategies for cochlear prostheses. *IEEE Sig Proc Mag* 1998;15:101–130.

Loizou P, Graham S, Dickens J, Dorman M, Poroy O. Comparing the performance of the SPEAK strategy (Spectra 22) and the CIS strategy (Med-El) in quiet and in noise [Poster abstract 64]. Presented at the *1997 Conference on Implantable Auditory Prostheses*; Pacific Grove, CA, 1997.

McDermott HJ, McKay CM, Vandali AE. A new portable sound processor for the University of Melbourne/ Nucleus Limited multielectrode cochlear implant. *J Acoust Soc Am* 1992;91:3367–3391.

McDermott HJ, Vandali AE. Spectral maxima sound processor. US patent 5597380, 1997.

McKay CM, McDermott HJ, Clark GM. Pitch percepts associated with amplitude-modulated current pulse trains in cochlear implantees. *J Acoust Soc Am* 1994;96:2664–2673.

McKay C, McDermott H, Vandali A, Clark G. Preliminary results with a six spectral maxima sound processor for the University of Melbourne/Nucleus multiple-electrode cochlear implant. *J Otolaryngol Soc Aust* 1991;6:354–359.

McKay CM, McDermott HJ, Vandali AE, Clark GM. A comparison of speech perception of cochlear implantees using the Spectral Maxima sound Processor (SMSP) and the MSP (MULTIPEAK) processor. *Acta Otolaryngol* 1992;112:752–761.

Merzenich MM. UCSF cochlear implant device. In: Schindler RA, Merzenich MM, eds. *Cochlear implants*. New York: Raven Press, 1985:121–130.

Merzenich MM, Rebscher SJ, Loeb GE, Byers CL, Schindler RA. The UCSF cochlear implant project. *Adv Audiol* 1984;2:119–144.

Millar JB, Blamey PJ, Tong YC, Patrick JF, Clark GM. Speech perception. In: Clark GM, Tong YC, Patrick JF, eds. *Cochlear prostheses*. Edinburgh: Churchill Livingstone, 1990:41–67.

Millar JB, Tong YC, Clark GM. Speech processing for cochlear implant prostheses. *J Speech Hear Res* 1984;27:280–296.

Moore BCJ. Speech coding for cochlear implants. In: Gray RF, ed. *Cochlear implants*. San Diego: College-Hill Press, 1985:163–179.

Osberger MJ. New directions in speech processing. I: Patient performance with simultaneous analog stimulation (SAS) [Abstract 158]. Presented at the *Fourth European Symposium on Paediatric Cochlear Implantation*; s'Hertogenbosch, The Netherlands, 1998.

O'Shaughnessy D. *Speech communication: human and machine*. Reading, MA: Addison-Wesley, 1987.

Papamichalis PE. *Practical approaches to speech coding*. Englewood Cliffs, NJ: Prentice-Hall, 1987.

Parkins CW. Cochlear prostheses. In: Altschuler RA, Hoffman DW, Bobbin RP, eds. *Neurobiology of hearing: the cochlea*. New York: Raven Press, 1986:455–473.

Patrick JF. The evolution of speech coding strategies [Abstract 5]. Presented at the *Vth International Cochlear Implant Conference*; New York, NY, 1997.

Patrick JF, Clark GM. The Nucleus 22-channel cochlear implant system. *Ear Hear* 1991;12[Suppl 1]:3S–9S.

Patrick JF, Seligman PM, Clark GM. Engineering. In: Clark GM, Cowan RSC, Dowell RC, eds. *Cochlear implantation for infants and children: advances*. San Diego: Singular Publishing Group, 1997:125–145.

Patrick JF, Seligman PM, Money DK, Kuzma JA. Engineering. In: Clark GM, Tong YC, Patrick JF, eds. *Cochlear prostheses*. Edinburgh: Churchill Livingstone, 1990:99–124.

Pelizzone M, Böex-Spano C, Sigrist A, *et al.* First field trials with a portable CIS processor for the Ineraid multichannel cochlear implant. *Acta Otolaryngol* 1995;115:622–628.

Pfingst BE. Stimulation and encoding strategies for cochlear prostheses. *Otolaryngol Clin North Am* 1986;19:219–235.

Rabiner LR, Shafer RW. *Digital processing of speech signals*. Englewood Cliffs, NJ: Prentice-Hall, 1978: 129–130.

Shannon RV, Adams DD, Ferrel RL, Palumbo RL, Grandgenett M. A computer interface for psychophysical and speech research with the Nucleus cochlear implant. *J Acoust Soc Am* 1990;87:905–907.

Skinner MW, Clark GM, Whitford LA, *et al.* Evaluation of a new spectral peak (SPEAK) coding strategy for the Nucleus 22 channel cochlear implant system. *Am J Otol* 1994;15[Suppl 2]:15–27.

Skinner MW, Holden LK, Holden TA, *et al.* Performance of postlinguistically deaf adults with the Wearable Speech Processor (WSP III) and Mini Speech Processor (MSP) of the Nucleus multi-electrode cochlear implant. *Ear Hear* 1991;12:3–22.

Tye-Murray N, Lowder M, Tyler RS. Comparison of the F0F2 and F0F1F2 processing strategies for the Cochlear Corporation cochlear implant. *Ear Hear* 1990;11:195–200.

Tye-Murray N, Tyler RS. Auditory consonant and word recognition skills of cochlear implant users. *Ear Hear* 1989;10:292–298.

Tyler RS, Lowder MW, Parkinson AJ, Woodworth GG, Gantz BJ. Performance of adult Ineraid and Nucleus cochlear implant patients after 3.5 years of use. *Audiology* 1995;34:135–144.

Tyler RS, Moore BCJ. Consonant recognition by some of the better cochlear-implant patients. *J Acoust Soc Am* 1992;92:3068–3077.

Tyler RS, Preece JP, Lansing CR, Otto SR, Gantz BJ. Previous experience as a confounding factor in comparing cochlear-implant processing schemes. *J Speech Hear Res* 1986;29:282–287.

Tyler RS, Tye-Murray N. Cochlear implant signal-processing strategies and patient perception of speech and environmental sounds. In: Cooper H, ed. *Cochlear implants: a practical guide.* San Diego: Singular Publishing Group, 1991:58–83.

White MW. Compression systems for hearing aids and cochlear prostheses. *J Rehab Res Dev* 1986;23:25–39.

White MW, Merzenich MM, Gardi JN. Multichannel cochlear implants: channel interactions and processor design. *Arch Otolaryngol* 1984;110:493–501.

Wilson BS. Signal processing. In: Tyler RS, ed. *Cochlear implants: audiological foundations.* San Diego: Singular Publishing Group, 1993:35–85.

Wilson BS. The future of cochlear implants. *Br J Audiol* 1997;31:205–225.

Wilson BS. New directions in implant design. In: Waltzman SB, Cohen N, eds. *Cochlear implants.* New York: Thieme Medical and Scientific Publishers, 1999:43–56.

Wilson BS, Finley CC, Farmer JC Jr, *et al.* Comparative studies of speech processing strategies for cochlear implants. *Laryngoscope* 1988a;98:1069–1077.

Wilson BS, Finley CC, Lawson DT. Speech processors for auditory prostheses. Seventh Quarterly Progress Report, NIH project N01-NS-3-2356. Bethesda: Neural Prosthesis Program, National Institutes of Health, 1985.

Wilson BS, Finley CC, Lawson DT, Wolford RD. Speech processors for cochlear prostheses. *Proc IEEE* 1988b;76:1143–1154.

Wilson BS, Finley CC, Lawson DT, Wolford RD, Eddington DK, Rabinowitz WM. Better speech recognition with cochlear implants. *Nature* 1991a;352:236–238.

Wilson BS, Lawson DT, Finley CC, Wolford RD. Coding strategies for multichannel cochlear prostheses. *Am J Otol* 1991b;12[Suppl 1]:56–61.

Wilson BS, Lawson DT, Finley CC, Wolford RD. Importance of patient and processor variables in determining outcomes with cochlear implants. *J Speech Hear Res* 1993;36:373–379.

Wilson BS, Lawson DT, Zerbi M. Advances in coding strategies for cochlear implants. *Adv Otolaryngol Head Neck Surg* 1995;9:105–129.

Zeng F-G, Shannon RV. Loudness balance between acoustic and electric stimulation. *Hear Res* 1992;60:231–235.

Cochlear Implants: Principles & Practices, edited by John K. Niparko, Karen Iler Kirk, Nancy K. Mellon, Amy McConkey Robbins, Debara L. Tucci, and Blake S. Wilson. Lippincott Williams & Wilkins, Philadelphia © 2000.

Assessment of Cochlear Implant Candidacy

8

Assessment of Cochlear Implant Candidacy

John K. Niparko

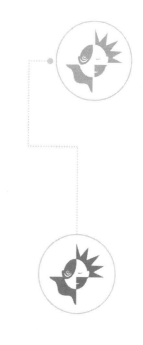

Assessing an individual's suitability for cochlear implantation requires consideration of a range of factors that affect performance and ultimately affect an individual's level of satisfaction with an implant. The importance of comprehensive assessment is underscored by several ideas:

- The cochlear implant is a communication tool and is not a curative intervention for hair cell dysfunction.
- Preoperative expectations largely shape postoperative satisfaction with any form of auditory rehabilitation (Ross and Levitt, 1997).
- The multifaceted nature of communication disorders often necessitates more than one rehabilitative strategy, particularly in children in whom deficits in auditory processing, speech production, cognitive ability, and attention may need to be addressed.
- Candidates should have the motivation (or motivated support system) and psychologic

makeup to learn to use and maintain the device to optimize performance.

For these reasons, it is advised that candidacy assessment and surgery be performed at a center that has a close working relationship with the clinicians who will provide the immediate postimplantation rehabilitation.

HEARING ASSESSMENT

Originally, candidacy for cochlear implantation required total or near-total sensorineural hearing losses as characterized by pure tone averages (PTAs at 0.5, 1, and 2 kHz) of 100 dB or greater, amplified thresholds that failed to reach 60 dB, and an absence of open-set speech recognition despite the use of powerful, best-fit hearing aids. Because clinical experience has indicated that mean speech reception scores with implants generally exceed those aided results of individuals with lesser impairments, the audiologic criteria have been relaxed to include those with PTAs higher than 90 dB or word understanding of up to 30% (for selected devices) on open-set sentence testing. Although thresholds as reflected by the PTA can provide a convenient indicator of impairment level, more important to implant candidacy is the individual's experience with

J. K. Niparko: Department of Otolaryngology—Head & Neck Surgery, The Listening Center at Johns Hopkins, The Johns Hopkins University, Baltimore, Maryland 21205-1809.

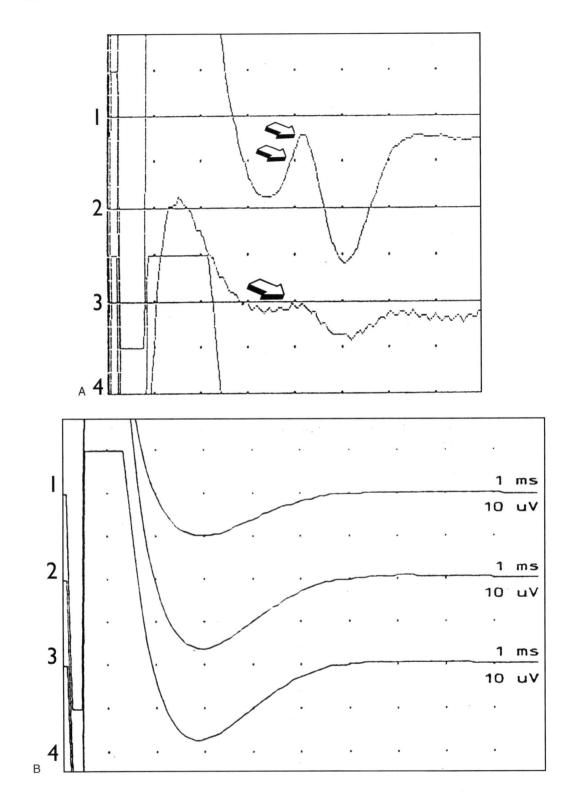

amplification. U.S. Food and Drug Administration (FDA) guidelines hold that candidates usually should have at least 6 months' experience with high-powered binaural amplification and undergo aided speech audiometry.

A standardized approach to audiologic assessment of implant candidacy is important for comparability across clinical trials. If the patient can detect speech in the best-aided condition, a series of speech tests are conducted with amplification in place and in a sound field of 55-dB sound pressure level.

Although audiologic criteria to be met for a particular device depend on FDA-approved labeling, candidacy for current devices requires that word discrimination scores do not exceed 30% in best-aided conditions (Lenarz, 1998). Mean speech recognition scores after implantation exceed these levels, and individuals with some preserved speech recognition ability preoperatively often score substantially higher than in their preoperative condition (Tyler *et al.*, 1989; Waltzman *et al.*, 1995).

Audiologic criteria for childhood candidacy follow similar guidelines. Children should demonstrate PTAs of 90 dB (HL) or greater to be considered for implantation. Acquiescence in hearing aid use can be an important indicator of the patient's preparation for wearing the external portion of an implant system. The development of aided communication abilities as reflected in the child's ability to acquire speech and language over a period of observation constitutes the critical criterion for determining candidacy in young children (Mecklenburg, 1990). For very young children who cannot be assessed with behavioral techniques, candidacy determination increasingly depends on threshold determination; extreme elevations in thresholds (consistent with profound deafness and lack of potential for speech understanding with amplification) can provide an indication for early implantation.

Assessment of the responsiveness of the auditory nerve to electrical activation before cochlear implantation is an adjunctive procedure for candidacy evaluation. The integrity of the auditory nerve may be verified with transtympanic stimulation with behavioral responses in adults or averaged, far-field auditory potentials in children (Kileny *et al.*, 1994). A monopolar needle electrode is placed through the posteroinferior quadrant of the drum adjacent to the annulus to approach the round window niche to deliver low-frequency sinusoids. Skin surface electrodes serve as a ground. Although the strict prognostic value of preoperative promontory testing is probably limited (Kileny *et al.*, 1991), the test is useful when asymmetries in the appearance of the cochlea are found on computed tomography (CT) scanning and in patients who are reticent about implantation because of concerns about the responsiveness of their ear to a novel stimulus (Fig. 8.1).

Otologic and Medical Assessment

Candidates for implantation often wonder whether the cause of their deafness can predict success or failure. Linkages between the cause and the degree of survival of neural elements (Nadol, 1984) in profound deafness have demonstrated prognostic value for only select pathologies (see Chapter 4). Nonetheless, establishing the precise origin of deaf-

---

FIG. 8.1. Brain stem evoked responses to electrical stimulation of the cochleas in a 4-year-old child with postmeningitis deafness. Recordings were obtained between electrodes placed in the midline scalp and opposite ear. Tracings represent the average responses to 11.1 stimulations per second, 0.1 milliseconds in duration, for 300 stimulations/trace. **A:** Robust responses are obtained with 0.8-mA *(arrow)* and 1.2-mA *(double arrows)* stimulation of the right cochlea. When present, the brain stem evoked response provides an indication of auditory nerve integrity. **B:** Lack of responsiveness is seen with stimulation of the left cochlea at levels similar to those used to evoke the responses observed in **A**.

ness can provide useful information in guiding the implantation process. For example, cochlear implants are often beneficial in cases of slowly progressive losses in which adaptive abilities such as lip-reading have developed and speech intelligibility is retained. Cochlear otosclerosis and temporal bone fractures may be more likely to manifest adventitial facial nerve stimulation with activation of the implant (Niparko *et al.*, 1991), thereby necessitating modifications of the processing program.

Cause alone is rarely a contraindication to implantation. Prior meningitis with associated cochlear ossification and chronic ear disease may necessitate adaptation of the implantation procedure. Profound sensorineu-

ral hearing loss associated with congenital absence of neural foramina (Jackler *et al.*, 1987) and profound loss from acoustic tumors are rare disorders in which the cause often obviates the option for cochlear implantation on the basis of inadequate auditory innervation. For patients with bilateral acoustic tumors (neurofibromatosis type II) producing profound sensorineural hearing loss, auditory brain stem implants offer a viable option to restore auditory access (Briggs *et al.*, 1994).

Preoperative high-resolution CT or MRI scans of the temporal bones provide the best means of determining cochlear patency. Although the radiographic appearance is not always predictive of scalar patency, results

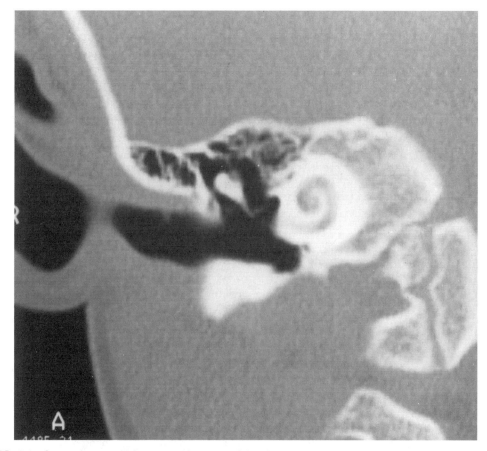

FIG. 8.2. Coronal computed tomography scan of the right temporal bone illustrates normal cochlear anatomy in a 6-year-old boy. Haziness of the cochlea represents averaging of tissue densities on the image, and the cochlea was found at surgery to be fully patent.

that are falsely negative or falsely positive are relatively uncommon (Jackler *et al.*, 1987; Wiet *et al.*, 1990). The radiographic appearance of the cochlea (Fig. 8.2) should be considered in light of clinical information, particularly when there is a history of meningitis or otosclerosis, cochlear dysgenesis is suspected, and particularly when considering the likelihood of complete insertion of the electrode array with the patient preoperatively.

General Health Assessment

Poor general health status is rarely a contraindication to cochlear implantation. Candidacy for implantation should include assessment of the patient's fitness for general anesthesia, the necessary mastoid surgery, and the effort required for device programming and postimplantation rehabilitation. Although implantation under local anesthesia has been described, this approach restricts the drilling and tissue dissection of the retrosigmoid tissues to effectively position and stabilize the internal device. Except for rare cases, there is little to recommend this approach.

Psychologic Assessment

The process of communication change can have far-reaching psychologic implications. A cochlear implant can most benefit individuals who possess sufficient motivation and support to complete a program of postimplantation device activation and rehabilitation. Motivations and expectations should be discussed in detail with the candidate. For pediatric candidates, parental expectations and attitudes should be carefully determined. The very best efforts of an implant team can be thwarted by patient or family frustrations based in unrealistic expectations. Although it is reasonable that a candidate or family would expect improved hearing, practical hearing gains usually require a period of training, and limitations always exist. Personality traits that may make program completion unlikely should be identified. Moreover, psychologic assessment should screen for other conditions that can hinder the implantation process such as psychopathology and organic brain disease.

REFERENCES

Briggs R, Brackmann D, Baser M, Hitselberger W. Comprehensive management of bilateral acoustic neuromas. *Arch Otolaryngol Head Neck Surg* 1994;120:1307–1314.

Jackler R, Luxford W, Schindler R, McKerrow W. Cochlear patency problems in cochlear implantation. *Laryngoscope* 1987;97:801–805.

Kileny P, Zimmerman-Phillips S, Kemink J, Schmaltz S. Effects of preoperative electrical stimulability and historical factors on performance with multichannel cochlear implants. *Ann Otol Rhinol Laryngol* 1991;100:563–568.

Kileny P, Young K, Niparko J. Acoustic and electrical assessment of the auditory pathway. In: Jackler R, Brackmann D, eds. *Neurotology.* St. Louis: Mosby, 1994:261–282.

Lenarz T. Cochlear implants: selection criteria and shifting borders. *Acta Otorhinology Belg* 1998;52:183–199.

Mecklenburg D. Cochlear implants and rehabilitative practices. In: Sandlin R, ed. *Handbook of hearing aid amplification,* vol II. Boston: College Hill Press, 1990:179–188.

Nadol J. Histological considerations in implant patients. Arch Otolaryngol 1984;110:160–163.

Niparko J, Oviatt D, Coker N, Sutton L, Waltzman S, Cohen N. Facial nerve stimulation with cochlear implants. *Otolaryngol Head Neck Surg* 1991; 104:826–830.

Ross M, Levitt H. Consumer satisfaction is not enough: hearing aids are still about hearing. *Semin Hear* 1997;18:1, 7–11.

Tyler R, Moore B, Kuk F. Performance of some of the better cochlear-implant patients. *J Speech Hear Res* 1989;32:887–911.

Waltzman S, Fisher S, Niparko J, Cohen N. Predictors of postoperative performance with cochlear implants. *Ann Otol Rhinol Laryngol* 1995;104[Supp 165]:15–18.

Wiet R, Pyle G, O'connor C, Russell E, Schramm D. Computed tomography: how accurate a predictor for cochlear implantation? *Laryngoscope* 1990;100: 687–692.

Appendix 8A

Professional Roles in Multidisciplinary Assessment of Candidacy

Betty Schopmeyer

Each candidate for cochlear implantation presents with a unique set of capabilities and needs. Although the factor of severely compromised hearing is common to this group, the population differs in virtually every other descriptor. Age; onset, origin, and progression of deafness; cognitive and educational level; attention; language competence; family and environment; sensory and motor skills; and personal motivation all influence the candidacy decision and the outcome of implantation. Although medical and audiologic criteria are typically decisive factors, other characteristics are likely to influence the benefit derived from use of the implant. A team approach to candidacy assessment ensures that as much information as possible is obtained about each candidate.

A multidisciplinary team brings together professionals offering different perspectives on a candidate's needs and capabilities. A typical progression through the candidacy process begins with audiologic and medical evaluations, and it may stop there if findings contraindicate implantation. Figure 8A.1 illustrates the probable tiers of professional assessment in the candidacy process.

CANDIDACY ASSESSMENTS

Audiology

Audiologists are typically the first contact made by potential cochlear implant users or

B. Schopmeyer: Cochlear Implant Rehabilitation, The Listening Center at Johns Hopkins, The Johns Hopkins University, Baltimore, Maryland 21287.

their families. The audiologist must determine the nature and severity of the individual's hearing loss. The audiology assessment includes diagnostic hearing tests, hearing aid evaluation and fitting, evaluation of speech perception skills, and neurodiagnostic testing if indicated. In addition to assessing the degree of aided benefit, the audiologist should provide critical details regarding implant candidacy.

Otology

Medical examination yields essential information about the health status of the candidate, identifying potential health concerns and determining suitability for a general anesthetic. A careful otologic evaluation includes history and physical examination and is essential to identifying structural changes in the temporal bone that may require a modified surgical approach. Clinical evaluation of the vestibular system may help to predict whether implantation will result in vestibular symptoms. Radiologic assessment typically includes a CT scan or magnetic resonance imaging to determine the status of the inner ear and temporal bone. If no audiologic or medical contraindications are identified, the cochlear implant candidate progresses to the next level of evaluations.

Auditory Skills Assessment

The auditory skills assessment evaluates the child's ability to attend to and integrate sound using conventional amplification. A child may demonstrate residual hearing on

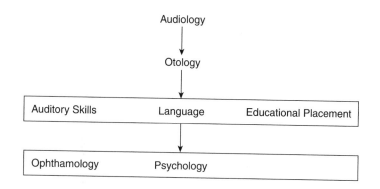

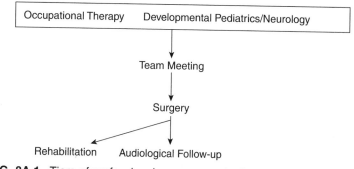

Audiology

Otology

| Auditory Skills | Language | Educational Placement |

| Ophthamology | Psychology |

Pre-Implant Training

| Occupational Therapy | Developmental Pediatrics/Neurology |

Team Meeting

Surgery

Rehabilitation   Audiological Follow-up

FIG. 8A.1. Tiers of professional assessment in the candidacy process.

an audiologic evaluation but not have the necessary skills to make use of that hearing. The auditory skills assessment determines the child's ability to use residual hearing to attend to speech and environmental sounds of various frequencies, integrate auditory perception with speech production as demonstrated by the ability to imitate what is heard, make meaningful associations with sound ranging from single words to conversational contexts, and integrate hearing in the context of communication.

The development of a child's residual hearing before implantation can provide a significant foundation for listening through the cochlear implant. This is accomplished through preimplantation training and ongoing evaluation.

Language Assessment

Assessing language in a child seeking a cochlear implant often requires evaluation of the very area that is most deficient in that child. In many cases, the child has no real language in the signed or spoken modality. Observation is the first tool employed by the speech-language pathologist to attempt to answer some questions. How does the child attempt to communicate with other people? What is the level of communicative intent, and what prelinguistic and linguistic strategies does the child use to support this intent?

Prelinguistic communication behaviors assessed include eye contact and eye gaze, gesture, pointing, vocalization, object and physical manipulation, turn-taking, imitation, and willingness to maintain engagement. The evaluation of linguistic communication examines receptive and expressive vocabulary in sign or speech; beginning syntax; use of grammatical markers; narration and conversation. The quantity and the variety of the child's vocabulary are important to language development.

Pragmatic development refers to the social use of language skills and applies to linguistic and prelinguistic behaviors. Pragmatic skills include communicating for a variety of purposes, such as to request, comment, gain attention or information, protest, choose, and demonstrate social conventions such as greetings. A child who displays appropriate social use of nonlinguistic and linguistic behaviors before implantation brings a degree of social engagement, communicative intent, and mastery motivation to the postimplantation rehabilitation process that can assist him in the task of attaching audition to his skills.

Psychologic Assessment

The candidate's skills in nonverbal problem solving, attention, and memory influence the postimplantation rehabilitation process and provide some predictive information concerning use and benefit. The psychologic assessment includes measurement of verbal and nonverbal intelligence, visual-motor integration, attention, motor development, child behavior, and parental stress. The evaluation also includes parent counseling regarding expectations.

Educational Placement Evaluation

A key factor in optimizing benefit from the implant is appropriate educational placement and opportunity for flexibility within that placement as the auditory skills of the child evolve and the supports required change. An appropriate school environment provides stimulation of audition, maximum attention to development of language, and a variety of communication opportunities. Encouragement for the use of spoken language, opportunities to interact verbally with adults and peers, appropriate support services, and school personnel who are supportive of cochlear implantation and willing to participate in a team approach are essential features of an appropriate school placement. A school visit by an implant team rehabilitation therapist initiates the collaboration with the child's teachers and therapists.

Ophthalmologic Evaluation

Vision plays a critical role in the deaf child's development. Even after implantation, the child may rely on vision to begin to associate meaning with auditory inputs. The ophthalmologic evaluation can identify visual abnormalities associated with congenital sensorineural deafness, including refractive errors, strabismus, adnexal anomalies, and cataracts (Siatkowski *et al.*, 1994). In some cases of unknown origin, rubella retinopathy, Usher's syndrome, and Waardenburg's syndrome have been diagnosed as a result of ocular examinations.

Occupational Therapy

Children with cochlear implants need to integrate their new sense of hearing with more developed sensory systems. Some children display subtle motor or sensory delays or differences that may impede the smooth acceptance and integration of new auditory stimulation. An evaluation by an occupational therapist may identify subtle vestibular, tactile, or proprioceptive deficits that may affect the child's ability to integrate auditory information, use language in a social context, engage with others, and gain volitional control over the movements of his body, especially those of his articulators.

Developmental Pediatric and Neurologic Assessments

Some deaf children present with clear global developmental issues that may be best evaluated by a developmental pediatrician or a neurologist. Such an assessment can screen for anomalies involving sensory and motor systems outside those routinely associated with communication deficits. For example, appropriate treatment of attention disorders may be required to ensure that the child can benefit from audiologic and rehabilitative services.

REFERENCE

Siatkowski R, Flynn J, Hodges A, Balkany T. Opthalmologic abnormalities in the pediatric cochlear implant population. *Am J Opthalmol* 1994;188:70–76.

Appendix 8B

Parental Response to the Diagnosis of Hearing Loss

Nancy K. Mellon

A crisis is a situation in which life events overwhelm an individual's ability to cope (Spink, 1976). For hearing parents, a diagnosis of deafness in a child often represents a crisis. The psychological reaction to diagnosis typically includes feelings of grief, helplessness, guilt, anger, and a sense of isolation (Kampfe, 1989). Parents' reactions to the diagnosis depends on factors such as the suddenness of the loss, the quality of their preparation for it, and the significance it holds for them.

Parents contemplating the birth of a child share a hope that their child will be normal. Because hearing loss is not a visible handicap, hearing parents who give birth to a deaf child are often unaware of the child's hearing loss. Though a child's hearing loss is not typically diagnosed until between 18 months and 3 years after birth (Mindel and Vernon, 1972; Marschark, 1997), the diagnosis often confirms the parent's growing suspicions. Parents have frequently experienced a long series of evaluations in attempting to discern the reasons for their child's lack of speech and come to the diagnosis with feelings of frustration, fear, and worry (Mindel and Vernon, 1972).

By the time deafness is diagnosed, parents have often established a series of expectations for their child based on the assumption that their child can hear. Diagnosis overturns these aspirations (Spink, 1976). Just as many deaf parents hope to have children who are deaf with whom they can share their experiences and culture (Lane and Bahan, 1998), hearing parents expect to share their language and culture with their children. They often expect, rather than hope, to have hearing children, because congenital deafness commonly occurs spontaneously in families where there is no history of hearing loss.

Parents adjusting to a child's hearing loss commonly experience a series of emotional stages. Luterman (1979) identifies these stages as shock, recognition, denial, acknowledgment, and constructive action. Successful resolution of anger and grief at diagnosis is important to the child's future, because these feelings otherwise may be manifested as depression (Luterman, 1979). Depression may negatively affect the child's outcome, because depressed mothers have been found to be less sensitive to their child's needs and therefore are less effective at nurturing language and socioemotional development in their children (Koester and Meadow-Orlans, 1990).

A child who cannot hear is not considered normal in a hearing society, because normality by definition presumes capabilities within

N. K. Mellon: The Listening Center at Johns Hopkins, The Johns Hopkins University, Baltimore, Maryland 21287.

the average range (Hetu, 1996). Acknowledgment of hearing loss in a child involves a loss of the parents hopes and dreams for a normal child (Luterman, 1979). Communication through hearing and speech are so basic to our sense of self that we take it for granted. A deaf child challenges the parents' sense of identity, causing them to reevaluate many of their most closely held beliefs and assumptions. Because hearing parents often have had little exposure to deaf people and culture, they are likely to share their culture's prejudices about hearing impairment. These perceptions may intensify feelings of grief and loss at diagnosis.

A period of mourning after diagnosis is expected. A failure to grieve is considered unhealthy, indicating that the parent has intellectually accepted the child's deafness but has not acknowledged the loss emotionally (Vernon and Wallrabenstein, 1984). Acceptance enables constructive actions such as seeking out and maintaining efforts at rehabilitation.

The child's hearing loss presents some daunting problems. Unlike visual problems that can be corrected by wearing glasses, the effects of profound sensorineural hearing loss often cannot be completely ameliorated by any hearing aid, even with intensive auditory and speech therapy (Vernon and Wallrabenstein, 1984). The deaf child may be educated in American sign language and find a sense of belonging in deaf culture but may never sound like a native speaker of any spoken language. The irreversible nature of profound hearing loss makes it particularly devastating to parents. Grief and depression are normal reactions to the sense of powerlessness and loss engendered by the parents inability to fix the child's deafness.

Reaction to a child's hearing loss is in part related to the parent's priorities and values (Kampfe, 1989). For example, parents who particularly value literacy and educational achievement may experience greater concern about the potential educational attainment of their child than parents less concerned with these values. The child's

rehabilitation requires an extra investment of time and energy from the parents. Quittner *et al.* (1991) examined patterns of stress and adjustment in parents of children with cochlear implants. Deafness poses a continuing challenge to families with regard to communication, discipline, and greater time demands. Difficulties in these areas are associated with higher levels of stress and depression in parents of hearing-impaired children.

After diagnosis, parents are encouraged to select a communication method for educating their child (Luterman, 1979). Selection of any option entails an investment of parental time and energy. For example, parents who select sign language as a communication strategy need to develop a proficiency in sign that continues to exceed their child's level of competence to keep the child's language developing optimally. Learning a second language is often difficult for adults (Marschark, 1997), and achieving linguistic competence in sign therefore represents a significant challenge for hearing parents. Parents selecting an oral method may be required to attend audiologic evaluations and auditory and speech therapy sessions for a period of years. In general, the daily frustrations associated with poor communication with their children may significantly increase parental stress and influence the perception of disability (Quittner *et al.*, 1991).

Access to support groups after diagnosis may play an important role in helping parents formulate realistic expectations regarding their child's disability (Kampfe, 1989). Constructive coping by parents is essential to providing appropriate intervention and depends on successful resolution of the parents feelings about the child's hearing loss (Vernon and Wallrabenstein, 1984). Adjustment to an exceptional child is an ongoing process marked by various degrees of grief, anger, and worry (Koester and Meadow-Orlans, 1990). Parents may re-experience these feelings periodically throughout the child's life. Acknowledgment of the hearing loss and its implications for the child's development must be understood and accepted as a first step to making informed decisions regarding the child's education.

REFERENCES

Hetu R. The stigma attached to hearing impairment. *Scandinavian Audiology* 1996;25[Suppl 43]:12–24.

Kampfe C. Parental reaction to a child's hearing impairment. *Am Ann Deaf* 1989;134:255–259.

Koester L, Meadow-Orlans K. Parenting a deaf child: stress, strength, and support. In: Moores D, Meadow-Orlans K, eds. *Educational and developmental aspects of deafness*. Washington, DC: Gaullaudet University Press, 1990:299–320.

Lane H, Bahan B. Ethics of cochlear implantation in young children: a review and reply from a deaf-world perspective. *Otolaryngol Head Neck Surg* 1998; 119:297–313.

Luterman D. *Counseling parents of hearing-impaired children*. Boston: Little, Brown, 1979.

Marschark M. *Raising and educating a deaf child*. New York: Oxford University Press, 1997.

Mindel E, Vernon M. *They grow in silence*. Silver Spring, MD: National Association of the Deaf, 1972:98–102.

Quittner A, Steck J, Rouiller R. Cochlear implants in children: a study of parental stress and adjustment. *Am J Otol* 1991;12[Suppl 1]:95–104.

Spink D. Crisis intervention for parents of the deaf child. *Health Social Work* 1976;1:140–160.

Vernon M, Wallrabenstein J. The diagnosis of deafness in a child. *J Commun Disord* 1984;17:1–8.

Appendix 8C

Maternal Attachment and Adjustment:
Impact on Child Outcomes

Nancy K. Mellon

Childhood hearing loss poses a significant challenge for parenting and family adjustment. The effects of chronic conditions such as deafness are likely to be pervasive, altering parent roles and expectations in multiple life domains (Quittner *et al.*, 1990). Parents of deaf children are faced with specific developmental stressors such as establishing daily routines, managing visits to therapists, and behavioral management. Parents also face chronic stressors, such as communication difficulty, and loss of expectations regarding optimal outcomes for the child (*e.g.*, educational achievement) and themselves (*e.g.*, deflated personal expectations).

Mothers typically assume more responsibility for caring for handicapped children (Wallander *et al.*, 1990; Brand and Coetzer, 1994) and exhibit more psychologic distress and lower levels of marital satisfaction than mothers of healthy children. Parenting a child with special needs requires an extra investment of parental time an emotional resources. Consequently, much of the psychosocial research on deaf children examines maternal adjustment and mother-infant interactions in relation to child psychosocial adjustment (Pratt, 1991). Accepting the assumption that deafness necessarily distorts attachment behavior, problems in deaf children have been attributed to poor parent-infant interaction and bonding (Schlesinger and Meadow, 1972). Behavioral and social problems in deaf children of hearing parents may result from a language system which is inadequate in speech or sign to enable socialization. Communication problems and an emotional overlay of distress may undermine appropriate development.

N. K. Mellon: The Listening Center at Johns Hopkins, The Johns Hopkins University, Baltimore, Maryland 21287.

Hearing parents may experience intense feelings of sadness and loss when deafness is diagnosed in their child. Hearing individuals generally regard communication as central to their sense of identity and may fear that communication problems will imperil their ability to know their deaf child (Koester and Meadow-Orlans, 1990). Unresolved grief feelings may interfere with establishment of mother-child attachment and may compromise the mother's ability to nurture the child across development. Consequently, the psychologic well-being of parents, particularly mothers, can be expected to influence child psychosocial adjustment.

In a metanalysis of 34 clinical studies of attachment, van Ijzendoorn *et al.* (1992) found that maternal problems such as psychopathology were more likely to lead to poor attachment than child problems such as deafness. These results suggest that the mother's psychological health plays a key role in shaping the quality of parent-child relationships. If the mother is able to adapt her responses to an infant's needs, normal attachment can develop (van Ijzendoorn *et al.*, 1992). It follows that parental depression at diagnosis may negatively impact the development of positive attachment if maternal distress results in less sensitive treatment of the deaf child (Sloman *et al.*, 1993; Koester and Meadow-Orlans, 1990).

Differences in mother-infant interaction have been found between hearing mothers and their deaf children and for deaf mother and deaf child dyads. Deaf mothers seem more attuned to infant facial expression and more adept at using nonverbal communication. Several studies have found more use of positive facial effect in deaf mothers of deaf children than in hearing mothers with deaf children and more neutral affect in the deaf children. These studies suggest that deaf children are attending to subtle shifts in facial expression in the parent and retain a neutral affect while concentrating on these cues (Hindley, 1997). Hearing mothers may need help understanding the neutral affect displayed by their deaf children as attention

rather than disinterest, but they can interact in a positive, reciprocal way with their infants without special training or support.

Lederberg and Mobley (1990) evaluated the quality of attachment and mother-toddler interaction in 41 hearing-impaired and 41 hearing children and their hearing mothers. Despite some communicative difficulties and delayed language development they found that hearing-impaired children were as likely to have warm, positive, secure, and reciprocal relationships with their mothers as hearing children. Despite the fact that hearing parents often do not know their children are deaf during infancy, parent-infant attachment generally proceeds normally (Koester and Meadow-Orlans, 1990). Lederberg and Mobley hypothesize that, even before the child is diagnosed, the infant is able to elicit the appropriate response from the mother by failing to be comforted by responses that are solely auditory. Hearing parents typically use visual, tactile, and kinesthetic cues when they interact with their infants regardless of the hearing status of the child (Koester and Meadow Orlans, 1990).

Studies of speech perception in infants suggest that hearing children perceive speech bimodally through vision and audition (Werker and Tees, 1992; Kuhl, 1994). Infants 18 to 20 weeks old can recognize auditory-visual correspondences for speech and look longer at a face producing a vowel matching a sound they have just heard than at a mismatched face (Kuhl, 1994). Deaf infants frequently are not diagnosed until 2 or 3 years of age, after the developmental stage in which they would normally learn to associate the auditory-visual correspondences of speech. This may explain the inability of most deaf individuals to read spoken language on the lips (Bench, 1992). The auditory experience has been found to be critical to the development of age-appropriate visual attention (Quittner *et al.*, 1994). This finding suggests that, even if a child is diagnosed early and given the appropriate language input through sign language, developmental differences may occur in the absence of auditory stimulation (Vaccari and Marschark, 1997).

Much of the literature on parent-child communication appears to implicate hearing parents in the poorer communicative competence displayed by their deaf children. Some research has characterized hearing mothers of deaf children as more intrusive, controlling, rigid, and disapproving than mothers of hearing children (Schlesinger and Meadow, 1972). Not surprisingly, their children have been found to be less happy, less creative, and less flexible than hearing children (Schlesinger and Meadow, 1972). Later research focused on the reciprocal nature of parent-child interactions and traces differences to poorly developed communication.

Deaf parents have an advantage in nurturing language development in their deaf children. They have in place a sophisticated language system to transmit to their children. Hearing parents must teach a language they themselves are unlikely to have mastered. Alternatively, they may try to teach spoken language to a child whose deafness is unlikely to be diagnosed during a critical developmental period and who in any case has imperfect access to the auditory information presented to them.

As a child matures, social interactions are increasingly based on language, and communication difficulties may begin to disturb mother-child interactions. Early in development, hearing and deaf children lack the strategies for controlling the flow of conversational interactions with their mothers. As the infant gains the ability to participate as a full communication partner, the mother begins to cede control and communication becomes bidirectional. Greater control exercised by hearing mothers in interactions with their deaf children may reflect the child's inability to fully participate in conversation rather than in differences in maternal personality traits (Vaccari and Marschark, 1997).

Viewed through this lens, some of the research on the communicative behaviors of hearing parents becomes more understand-able. For instance, Wood et al. (1986) found that during the preschool years hearing parents and teachers tend to be more directive, didactic, and demanding. They also observed that although adults typically engage children in conversation on various topics, they tend to question deaf children. Adults speaking with deaf children often demand short, factual answers, and they frequently correct the speech of the deaf child or request imitation. These tactics discourage dialogue and are not conducive to optimal development of the child's cognitive or psychosocial skills (Spencer and Gutfreund, 1990). These studies suggest that hearing parents need to value their child's communicative attempts and must refrain from constant corrections and demands to promote optimal language development. This balance may be difficult to maintain given the parent's responsibility for mentoring the child's language development.

Communication difficulties complicate parenting roles such as establishing daily routines and managing the child's behavior in public (Quittner et al., 1991). Ongoing stresses of these daily conflicts have been linked to maternal psychologic distress (Wallander et al., 1990). Quittner et al. (1990), associated chronic parenting stress with lower perceptions of emotional support, and greater symptoms of depression and anxiety. Surprisingly, support may act as a mediator for parental stress. Support for parents of deaf children is as likely to come from professional networks as from other parents. The investigators suggest that in chronic conditions such as deafness the advice and support of friends and relatives may be perceived as criticism by parents.

Children learn language through repeated exposure to it. They use language to learn behavioral and cognitive strategies and gain a knowledge of self and others (Vaccari and Marschark, 1997). Providing a rich language environment and improving access to ambient sound through cochlear implantation should improve child outcomes across multiple domains, including language, cognition, and socialization. Parents and children who are truly engaged in the process of learning language together are likely to find strategies to bridge the gaps posed by poor access to auditory input and consequent language delays. Nevertheless, hearing parents and their deaf children are faced with significant challenges in socializing with each other. Without an effective communication mode, parent-child asynchrony may develop during the preschool years and worsen thereafter (Greenberg, 1980; Pratt, 1991). Programs of deafness rehabilitation should strive to improve parent-child communication and can best promote such development through methodologic flexibility.

REFERENCES

Bench R. *Communication skills in hearing impaired children.* San Diego, California: Singular, 1992.

Brand H, Coestzer M. Parental response to their child's hearing impairment. *Psychol Rep* 1994;75:1363–1368.

Greenberg M. Social interaction between deaf preschoolers and their mothers: the effects of communication method and communicative competence. *Dev Psychol* 1980;16:465–474.

Hindley P. Psychiatric aspects of hearing impairments. *J Child Psychol Psychiatry* 1997;38:101–117.

Kuhl P. Learning and representation in speech and language. *Curr Opin Neurobiol* 1994;4:812–822.

Koester L, Measow-Orlans K. Parenting a deaf child: stress, strength and support. In: Moores DF, Meadow-Orlans KP, eds. *Educational and developmental aspects of deafness.* Washington, DC: Gallaudet University Press, 1990.

Lederberg A, Mobley C. The effect of hearing impairment on the quality of attachment and mother-toddler interaction. *Child Dev* 1990;61:1596–1604.

Pratt S. Nonverbal play interaction between hearing mothers and young deaf children. *Ear Hear* 1991;12:328–336.

Quittner A, Smith L, Osberger MJ, Mitchell T, Katz D. The impact of audition on the development of visual attention. *Psychol Sci* 1994;5:347–353.

Quittner A, Steck T, Rouiller J. Cochlear implants in children: a study of parental stress and adjustment. *Am J Otol* 1991;12:95–104.

Quittner A, Glueckauf R, Jackson D. Chronic parenting stress: moderating versus mediating effects of social support. *J Pers Soc Psychol* 1990;59:1266–1278.

Schlesinger HS, Meadow KP. *Sound and sign: childhood deafness and mental health.* Berkeley, CA: University of California Press, 1972.

Sloman L, Springer S, Vachon M. Disordered communication and grieving in deaf member families. *Fam Process* 1993;32:171–182.

Spencer PS, Gutfreund MK. Directiveness in mother-infant interactions. In: Moores DF, Meadow-Orlans KP, eds. *Educational and developmental aspects of deafness.* Washington, DC: Gallaudet University Press, 1991.

Vaccari C, Marschark M. Communication between parents and deaf children: implications of socio-emotional development. *J Child Psychol Psychiatry* 1997;38:793–801.

Van Ijzendoorn M, Goldberg S, Kroonenburg P, Frenkel O. The relative effects of maternal and child problems on the quality of attachment: a meta-analysis of attachment in clinical samples. *Child Dev* 1992;63:840–858.

Wallander J, Pitt L, Mellins C. Child functional independence and maternal psychosocial stress as risk factors threatening adaptation in mothers of physically or sensorially handicapped children. *J Consult Clin Psychol* 1990;58:818–824.

Werker J, Tees R. The organization and reorganization of human speech perception. *Annu Rev Neurosci* 1992;15:377–402.

Wood D, Wood H, Griffiths A, Howarth I. *Teaching and talking with deaf children.* Chichester, UK: John Wiley, 1986.

SECTION IV

Cochlear Implant Surgery

9

Medical and Surgical Aspects of Cochlear Implantation

Debara L. Tucci and John K. Niparko

Techniques for cochlear implantation have evolved over the past 25 years. This evolution has been driven by a number of factors, including changes in implant design and refinement of candidacy assessment and surgical technique, based on experience with implantation of more than 20,000 devices worldwide. The success of this technology in enhancing communication abilities in a large number of patients has encouraged the expansion of candidacy criteria to include patients for whom implants were deemed to be contraindicated in the early years of cochlear implantation. Children have been implanted in large numbers, and much work has focused on the special considerations required in caring for this population. In experienced hands, serious complications from cochlear implant surgery are rare; most ears can be safely implanted.

The beginning cochlear implant surgeon has access to a large body of literature to

gain expertise in this field. The competent surgeon possesses an armamentarium of techniques that may be applied in dealing with a variety of surgical findings, including anatomic variations and cochlear ossification, and the more predictable nuances required for implantation of the different devices available. Temporal bone dissection laboratory experience with the various devices to be used can be particularly valuable for the beginning implant surgeon.

PATIENT EVALUATION

General Medical and Otologic Assessment

Evaluation of candidacy for implantation should include an assessment of the patient's general health and ability to undergo a general anesthetic for the necessary mastoid surgery. Although implantation under a local anesthetic has been described, this approach constrains the soft tissue dissection behind the mastoid required for embedding the internal device and usually is not recommended.

Candidates and their families must also be aware that a period of rehabilitation is required for optimal use of the implant. Patients must be physically and psychologically capable of completing the course of recom-

D. L. Tucci: Division of Otolaryngology, Box 3805, Duke University Medical Center, Durham, North Carolina 27710.

J. K. Niparko: Department of Otolaryngology—Head & Neck Surgery, The Listening Center at Johns Hopkins, The Johns Hopkins University, Baltimore, Maryland 21205-1809.

mended programming and therapy. Personality traits that make program completion unlikely should be sought. Psychologic assessment may be indicated to screen for psychopathology and organic brain disease.

A complete medical history should be taken and appropriate laboratory studies obtained. An otologic history should focus on information that may provide insight into the cause and the time course of the hearing loss, including time of onset and pattern of progression of hearing loss. Cause alone is rarely a contraindication to implantation. Nonetheless, establishing a precise cause of deafness can provide useful information in guiding the implantation process. A history of amplification use should be obtained. Ear choice may depend on the chronology of deafness and previous use of amplification. A history of meningitis should prompt a discussion with the candidate of methods for implanting an ossified cochlea. Previous otologic operations should be documented.

Microscopic examination of the ear is performed to look for evidence of external or middle ear disease. Abnormalities such as tympanic membrane perforations should be treated before implant surgery. Patients with chronic suppurative otitis media that is resistant to medical and surgical treatment may be treated with obliteration of the mastoid cavity and external canal closure, followed by cochlear implantation at a second operation 3 to 6 months later (Gray and Irving, 1995). Patients with poor eustachian tube function and associated poorly pneumatized mastoid cavities or severe middle ear atelectasis may also be managed with mastoid obliteration and external canal closure (Parnes et al., 1993).

An increasing number of implant candidates are young children. Given the high prevalence of otitis media in this population, there is often concern about the advisability of implantation in a child who may be expected to have further episodes of otitis media after surgery. There has been speculation that bacteria may transgress the cochleostomy site into the inner ear, producing labyrinthitis or meningitis and associated reactive fibrosis and destruction of neural elements. In an effort to evaluate the risk of spread of infection from the middle ear into the implanted cochlea, Franz et al. (1987) inoculated the bullae of five bilaterally implanted cats with a suspension of group A streptococci. Despite a finding of inflammation in the round window niche in all ears, there was no evidence of inflammation in the cochlea of these animals. It was found that a protective seal had formed around the electrode as it entered the round window or the cochleostomy.

Luntz et al. (1996) reviewed their experience with 60 children implanted before 18 years of age. Whereas 74% of children had one or more episodes of acute otitis media before implantation, only 16% were diagnosed with acute otitis media after implantation. A decrease in the incidence of acute otitis media after implantation was also observed by House et al. (1985) and is thought to be caused by several factors, including a natural tendency for acute otitis media incidence to decrease with age, the use of intraoperative and perioperative antibiotics, and the beneficial effect of mastoidectomy. None of the children in these studies had inner ear or intracranial complications. Based on these studies and earlier reports, concerns about the potential for the development of intracochlear infections in children who have a history of otitis media appear not to be supported.

A related issue concerns the use of ventilation tubes in children undergoing cochlear implantation. Although it is best to remove a ventilation tube before implantation, implantation of an ear with a functioning ventilation tube has been reported (Luntz et al., 1996) and has not resulted in complications. Similarly, it is advisable to place a ventilation tube in an implanted child with frequent recurrent episodes of acute otitis media rather than risk complications associated with this disease process. Ventilation tube placement may also be indicated in individuals with severe middle ear atelectasis to prevent further tympanic membrane retraction and possible device extrusion (Parnes *et al.*, 1993).

Consideration should be given to conditions for which a patient may need future magnetic resonance imaging (MRI), because implantation of a magnet in the internal device is contraindicated in these patients. A nonmagnetic modification of one commercially available device can be used in patients who must be monitored with MRI (Heller *et al.*, 1996).

Etiologic Assessment

Determining the cause of hearing loss is important for two reasons. First, it can reveal information about the expected histopathology of the inner ear, particularly the spiral ganglion cell (SGC) population. Although many patient factors are deemed important in predicting success of speech recognition with the cochlear implant, survival of the first-order neurons is thought to be of particular importance. Second, the recognition of etiologic factors that are associated with cochlear abnormalities such as congenital malformations and ossification are critical for surgical planning and for patient and family counseling before implantation.

Nadol's (1997) studies of almost 100 temporal bones from patients with documented profound sensorineural hearing loss reveal patterns of SGC survival that are relatively consistent across diagnostic categories. Residual SGC counts were highest in individuals who were deafened by aminoglycoside ototoxicity or sudden idiopathic sensorineural hearing loss and least in those deafened by postnatal viral labyrinthitis or congenital causes. Counts for the two other largest etiologic categories in their sample—temporal bone neoplasms and bacterial labyrinthitis— fell in between. Age at time of death and duration of deafness were less predictive of SGC survival than was the cause of hearing loss. Survival was significantly greater for the apical than the basal half of the cochlea.

Labyrinthitis ossificans, or new bone formation in the inner ear, is a common finding

in the temporal bones of patients who are deafened by bacterial meningitis. Quantitative assessment of 11 temporal bones of these patients by Nadol (1997) revealed a significant negative correlation between SGC survival and the presence of bony occlusion. The correlation was weakest in the base of the cochlea (0 to 6 mm). However, even in segments with severe bony occlusion, significant numbers of SGCs remained. In a study of temporal bones from previously implanted patients, Linthicum *et al.* (1991) found that useful auditory sensations are reported by individuals whose temporal bones were found to have as few as 10% of the normal complement of cells. Although the presence of ossification is not considered a contraindication to implantation, the degree of ossification as demonstrated on imaging studies preoperatively should correlate with SGC survival and help to guide the implant team in selection of an ear for implantation.

Radiologic Assessment

Radiologic imaging is an essential part of the evaluation of the cochlear implant candidate. High-resolution computerized tomography (HRCT) scans of the temporal bone help to define the surgical anatomy and provide information about cochlear abnormalities that can aid the surgeon in surgical planning and patient counseling. Temporal bone CT scans should be obtained and reviewed for evaluation of temporal bone anatomy with attention to the degree of mastoid pneumatization, position of vascular structures, middle ear anatomy, and position of the facial nerve (Woolley *et al.*, 1997). Scans are also examined for evidence of cochlear malformation, cochlear ossification, enlarged vestibular aqueduct, and other inner ear and skull base anomalies.

Although HRCT is the gold standard for evaluation of most aspects of temporal bone anatomy, it does have limitations, particularly in the assessment of cochlear patency. Although some investigators report good correlation between CT findings and surgical findings of cochlear patency (Seicshnaydre et al., 1992; Langman and Quigley, 1996), others have reported significant discrepancies (Jackler et al., 1987c; Wiet et al., 1990; Bath et al., 1993; Frau et al., 1994; Seidman et al., 1994). False-negative results, or an underestimation of the degree of obstruction, occurred in 5% to 45% of patients in these series. Accuracy of detection of cochlear ossification is best when CT scans are interpreted by an experienced radiologist using specific criteria for assessment of cochlear patency (Frau et al., 1994). One classification scheme described by Balkany and Dreisbach (1987) describes four categories of cochlear patency: C0, normal cochlea; C1, indistinctness of the endosteum of the basal turn; C2, definite narrowing of the basal turn; and C3, bony obliteration of at least a portion of the basal or middle turn or the entire cochlea. Volume-averaging artifacts may be responsible for many of the reported discrepancies between CT and surgical findings (Seidman et al., 1994).

MRI may be a useful adjunct to HRCT for assessment of candidates for cochlear implantation (Harnsberger et al., 1987; Lasig et al., 1988; Tien et al., 1992; Casselman et al., 1993; Arriaga and Carrier, 1996). Although HRCT is the procedure of choice for detail-

ing bony anatomy, MRI is the ideal imaging technique for soft tissue structures such as the membranous labyrinth and neural structures. Using appropriate MRI techniques, it is possible to identify the presence or absence of fluid within the cochlear turns and the size of the cochlear and vestibular nerves within the internal auditory canals (Figs. 9.1 and 9.2). An extensive gadolinium-enhanced MR scan of the brain and temporal bone is probably not necessary to address the specific questions pertinent to a cochlear implant evaluation. Tien et al. (1992) first reported the use of fast spin-echo (FSE) MR techniques to image the inner ear. FSE imaging has an advantage over conventional spin-echo T1-weighted images, which lack tissue contrast between fluid, neural tissue, otic capsule septa, and surrounding temporal bone, and conventional T2-weighted images, which require considerably longer scanner times. The speed advantage of FSE allows the radiologist to obtain thin-section (2 mm) high-resolution T2-weighted images with excellent contrast in a fraction of the time needed for conventional spin-echo techniques. Images obtained with this technique can delineate the fluid-filled otic capsule and internal auditory canal.

Arriaga and Carrier (1996) report the use

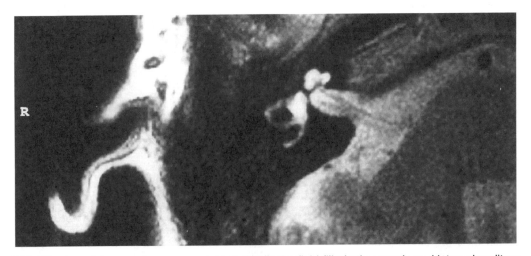

FIG. 9.1. An axial magnetic resonance scan details the fluid-filled otic capsule and internal auditory canal *(right)* in a normal ear.

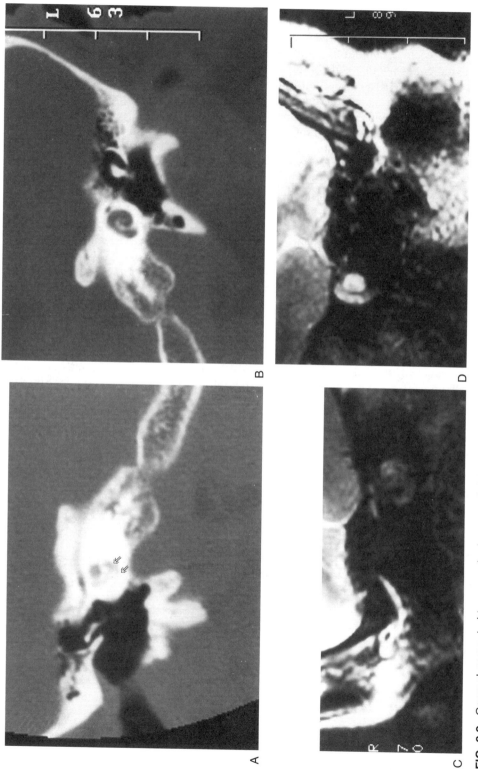

FIG. 9.2. Coronal computed tomography images of right (**A**) and left (**B**) cochleas show ossification, with more on the right (*arrows*) than the left. Coronal magnetic resonance images of right (**C**) and left (**D**) cochleas confirm greater cochlear patency on the left.

of a targeted MRI evaluation with a single fast spin echo T2-weighted sequence for evaluation of cochlear implant candidates. For 4 of 13 patients evaluated with this protocol and HRCT, the MRI provided information not provided by CT alone. Findings were helpful in making decisions regarding candidacy for surgery, side selection for surgery, and surgical technique for implantation. Nadol (1997) reports a strong positive correlation between the diameter of the cochlear and vestibular nerves and the total SGC count and suggests that modern imaging techniques such as MRI may be used to predict neuron survival in cochlear implant candidates.

SURGICAL ISSUES

Technique for Cochlear Implantation

Cochlear implant surgery is performed in the conventional otologic position using routine aseptic techniques (Luxford, 1994; Niparko, 1998). All implant systems in the United States use the transmastoid, facial recess approach to the round window and scala tympani. The mastoid is exposed using a pedicled flap. Several designs of scalp flaps are available for exposing the mastoid for cochlear implantation. All are designed to provide adequate exposure for implantation and preserve the blood supply to the auricle and periauricular soft tissue, ensuring long-term tissue coverage of the implant (Figs. 9.3 and 9.4). An anteriorly based C-shaped flap has the advantage of providing complete coverage of the internal receiver/stimulator and the electrode lead as it enters the mastoid cavity. One disadvantage of this flap design is that it does not allow gravity-based venous drainage, and flap edema may occur. This flap should cover the internal device with margins of at least 2 cm in all directions. Inverted U- and J-shaped flaps take advantage of the posterior arterial supply. Because these flaps have the disadvantage of crossing the electrode lead as it enters the mastoid cavity, it is necessary to create an anteriorly based musculofacial flap (*i.e.*, Palva flap) under the scalp flap to ensure electrode coverage. Other incisions include an extended endaural incision and an incision described by Miyamoto *et al.* (1992).

Intraoperative flap design and plans for device positioning are aided by use of a mock implant and mock behind-the-ear processor.

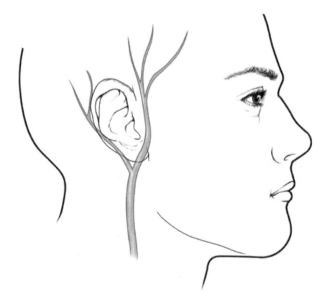

FIG. 9.3. Distribution of branches of the superficial temporal artery. Tissue flaps are designed to preserve this blood supply.

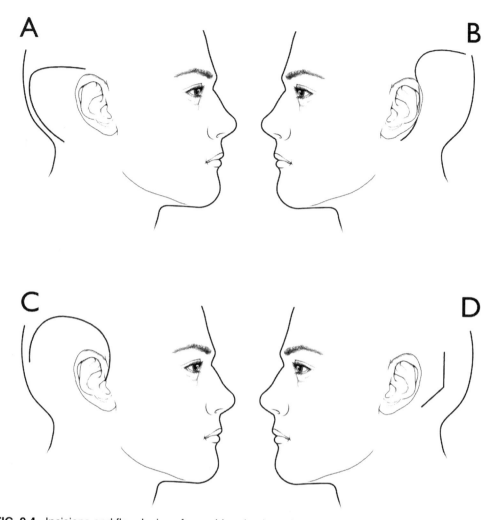

FIG. 9.4. Incisions and flap designs for cochlear implantation. **A:** Anteriorly based or C-shaped flap. **B:** Posteriorly based or inverted J flap. **C:** Inferiorly based flap or extended endaural incision. **D:** Superiorly and anteriorly based flap.

The planned position for the receiver/stimulator can be marked through skin to bone using methylene blue in a medium-bore needle. The flap is elevated to expose landmarks of the mastoid cortex—the spine of Henle, linea temporalis, and the mastoid tip—and at least 3 cm of bone above and beyond the mastoid.

A simple mastoidectomy is performed (Figs. 9.5 and 9.6), avoiding saucerization of the superior and posterior bony margins. The bone at the margins of the cavity can provide protection for connecting leads and a platform for stabilizing the receiver/stimulator. The facial recess is approached using strategies that maximize visualization: adequate thinning of the posterior canal wall and systematic exposure of the horizontal semicircular canal, fossa incudis, and chorda-facial angle. The facial recess is opened to visualize the incudostapedial joint and cochlear windows. It is usually possible to preserve the chorda tympani nerve in the course of facial recess exposure. If the facial recess is small

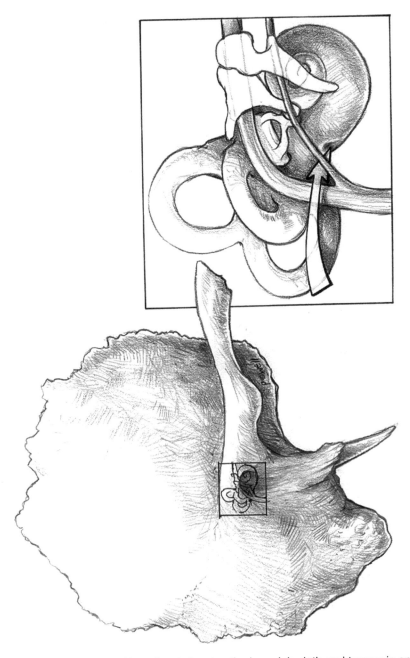

FIG. 9.5. Right temporal bone, with an inset showing the bony labyrinth and tympanic and mastoid segments of the facial nerve. The arrow points through the facial recess to the round window.

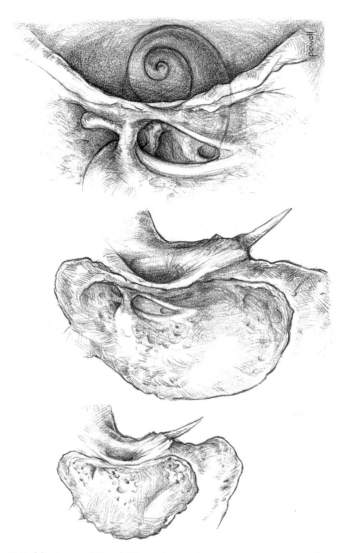

FIG. 9.6. Simple mastoidectomy of the right ear for cochlear implantation is achieved by transfacial recess exposure of the cochlear oval and round windows. The facial recess is opened by a successive drill-out of the chorda tympani–facial angle.

or the particular device implanted requires a generous facial recess exposure (Lalwani *et al.*, 1998), the nerve may be sacrificed. In this case, care should be taken not to damage the tympanic membrane as the chorda enters the middle ear at the level of the annulus. Bone on the anterior aspect of the vertical portion of the facial nerve should be removed to maximize visualization of the round window niche. If the anatomy of the round window is obscure, the surgeon should remember that the round window is never more than 2 mm from the inferior margin of the oval window and usually directly inferior in orientation (Proctor *et al.*, 1986; Takahashi and Sando, 1990; Takahashi *et al.*, 1995). Misinterpretation of the anatomy may lead the surgeon to insert the electrode into a hypotympanic air cell. If there is any concern that insertion may be suboptimal, a skull radiograph should be obtained before leaving the operating room to confirm the electrode's position.

The scala tympani may be opened in one of two ways: directly through the round window membrane or indirectly through the promontory. The preferred approach is to enter the scala tympani through a cochleostomy. This is created anterior and inferior to the round window, avoiding the "hook" region of the cochlea to allow direct insertion of the electrode array. A small diamond burr is used to create a fenestra slightly larger than the electrode to be implanted (Fig. 9.7).

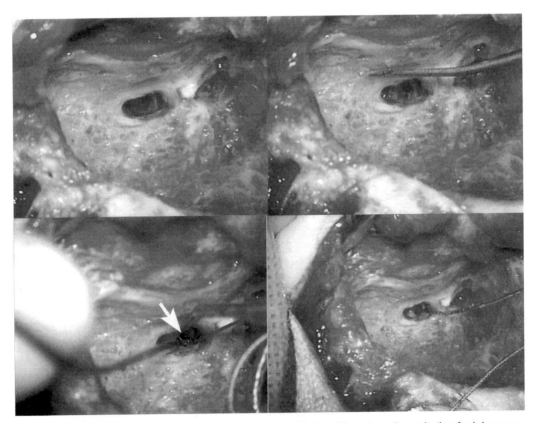

FIG. 9.7. Surgical views of a left ear cochlear implantation. The view through the facial recess reveals the round window *(upper panels)*, cochleostomy *(lower left panel, arrow)*, and inserted electrode array *(lower right panel)*.

Care should be taken in drilling the cochleostomy not to rest drill components or instruments on a potentially exposed facial nerve in the floor of the facial recess. The electrode array is inserted into the scala under direct visualization, using methods designed to minimize trauma to the membranous components of the cochlea (Cohen, 1997). If resistance to insertion is encountered, the electrode can be withdrawn slightly, rotated medially (counterclockwise for the right cochlea and clockwise for the left), and carefully advanced (Clark, 1977; Shepherd et al., 1983; Kennedy, 1987). Because buckling of the implant can produce spiral ligament, basilar membrane, and localized neural injury, aggressive insertion attempts should be avoided. Full insertion of the array within the basal turn of the cochlea represents an insertion depth of 25 to 30 mm, depending on array length. Those electrodes placed deepest (most apical) in the cochlea approach SGCs serving the lower frequencies, and those electrodes in the more proximal, or basal region, stimulate neurons serving the higher frequencies of hearing. Modification of conventional electrode designs promote greater proximity of the electrode to the modiolus and the SGC population and deeper insertion into the second cochlear turn (Fig. 9.8).

After the array is inserted, the cochleostomy is sealed around the electrode with fibrous tissue. The array can be stabilized in a variety of ways. The electrode lead is positioned within the mastoid cavity such that the natural spring of the electrode lead does not pull the electrode out of the cochleostomy. Fibrous tissue packing should not be relied on to retain an otherwise tenuous insertion. The lead can be tucked medial to the short process of the incus after removal of the medial portion of the "incus bridge" at the superior aspect of the facial recess (Balkany and Telischi, 1995). Other techniques described include the use of Dacron mesh ties to secure the proximal electrode to the edge of the mastoid cavity and a titanium clip to fix the electrode to the incus bridge (Cohen and Kuzma, 1995).

Before insertion of the electrode array, a depression is created in the bone behind the mastoid to accommodate the receiver/stimulator portion of the internal device (Fig. 9.9). The goals of receiver/stimulator placement are to minimize protrusion, thereby reducing vulnerability to external trauma, and to restrict device movement that can shear connecting leads. Creation of a deep well for embedding the stimulator and stabilization with permanent suture to the bony cortex are strongly advised. Overlying scalp should be thinned to less than 1 cm thick to enable stable, magnetic retention of the headset. The incision is closed in layers beginning with the periosteum for complete coverage of electrode leads extending from the receiver/stimulator into the mastoid cavity. Incisions may be closed over a drain, particularly if the larger C-shaped flap is used.

Minor modifications of the implant procedure as performed in conjunction with a labyrinthectomy for vertigo have been described (Zwolan et al., 1993). Revision implant surgery, including conversion from a single-channel to multichannel device, is feasible (Miyamoto et al., 1994; Rubenstein et al., 1998).

Intraoperative facial nerve monitoring may be helpful, particularly in cases of cochlear malformation that may be associated with an anomalous facial nerve and in cases of ossification that may require more extensive dissection for implantation. Perioperative antibiotics should be used and continued for 7 to 10 days after the operation. The monopolar cautery should not be used after the implant is in place and cannot be used in the head and neck region for any future surgery. Bipolar cautery can be safely used in these patients. Surgery usually is completed in 1.5 to 3 hours. Patients are typically discharged from the hospital either that day or the following day and seen for postoperative follow-up in 7 to 14 days. Activation of the implant takes place 4 to 6 weeks after

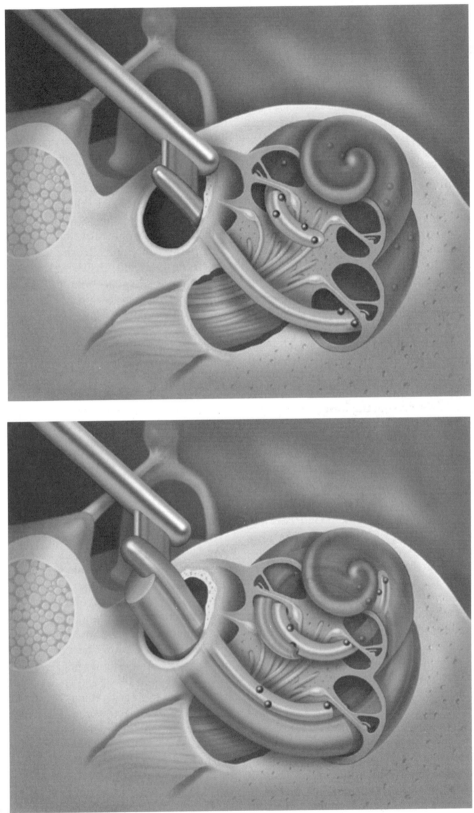

A

B

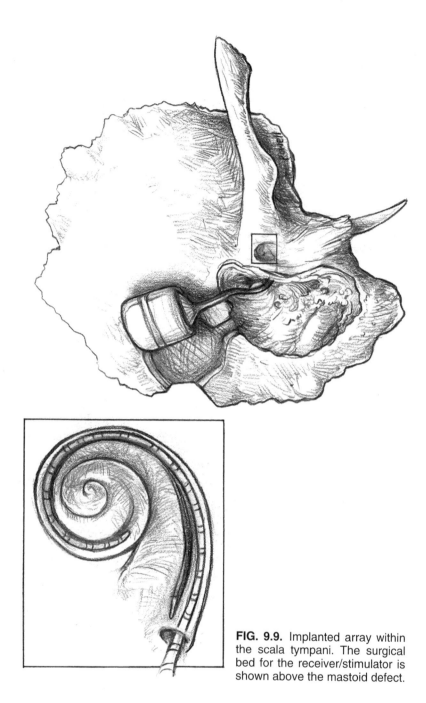

FIG. 9.9. Implanted array within the scala tympani. The surgical bed for the receiver/stimulator is shown above the mastoid defect.

FIG. 9.8. Modification of electrode insertion technique using a positioning device. **A:** Insertion of an electrode array into the scala tympani. **B:** Use of the positioner holds the electrodes closer to the modiolus and the spiral ganglion cell population and creates a deeper electrode insertion.

surgery, allowing ample time for the flap to heal and any edema to subside.

A postoperative radiograph usually is recommended to confirm that the array is intracochlear and to serve as a comparison for future studies in case extrusion of the device be suspected. Radiographs may be obtained intraoperatively, especially if there is a question that the electrode may be malpositioned or kinked. Particularly for the straight electrode arrays, a transorbital anterior-posterior plain skull radiograph should show position of the electrode in adequate detail. If a spiral electrode is used, it may be necessary to obtain a CT study for assessment of the three-dimensional anatomy, especially if a problem is suspected.

Cochlear Implantation in Children

Implantation of children, including those as young as 16 to 18 months, can be achieved safely and with no greater risk of complication than that observed for adults (Hoffman, 1997; Parisier et al., 1997; Waltzman and Cohen, 1998). Experience with implantation of young children has been reported by several centers, and initial results are encouraging (Gantz et al., 1993; Lenarz et al., 1997; Waltzman and Cohen, 1998). As our skills in identification and assessment of hearing loss in children improve, it is likely, based on the assertion that early intervention gives the best chance for optimal rehabilitation (see Chapter 1), that the trend toward implantation of younger children will continue.

Implant centers are challenged more by the difficulties involved in the audiologic assessment of very young children than by surgical difficulties related to the developing anatomy of the temporal bone. Nevertheless, implantation of the young child requires specific knowledge of the unique anatomy of the temporal bone in this age group and of the impact of skull growth on the implanted device. Although temporal bone growth has been shown to continue through adolescence, anatomy of the facial recess is fully

developed at birth (Bielamowicz et al., 1988; Eby, 1996). The most significant developmental changes are in the size and configuration of the mastoid cavity, which has been shown to expand in width, length, and depth from birth until at least the teenage years. Growth of the mastoid during this time parallels the growth patterns of the skull, with two periods of rapid development: one starts at birth and continues through early childhood, and another occurs at puberty. From 1 year of age to adulthood, the average mastoid can be expected to grow 2.6 cm in length, 1.7 cm in width, and 0.9 cm in depth for males and 2.0 cm in length, 1.7 cm in width, and 0.8 cm in depth for females. Based on these measurements, it has been recommended that 2.5 cm of electrode lead redundancy in the mastoid is necessary to accommodate for head growth and avoid electrode extrusion (Eby and Nadol, 1986). Investigation in the young primate has demonstrated that cochlear implantation had no adverse effects on skull growth (Burton et al., 1994).

The incision and flap are similar to those for an adult. As for all otologic surgery in children, the surgeon should remember that the lack of development of the mastoid tip, narrow tympanic ring, and lack of subcutaneous tissue in the young child place the main trunk of the facial nerve just below the skin, where it is easily injured by an incorrectly placed incision. Design of the postauricular skin flap is particularly important. In younger children, who have a thin scalp, elevation of the postauricular tissue in continuity with the skin flap may protect the flap from necrosis secondary to magnet pressure (Wang et al., 1990). The mastoidectomy, facial recess opening, and cochleostomy are similar to procedures followed for the adult. In older children, the lateral skull is usually thick enough to permit the creation of an adequate well for the receiver/stimulator. In younger children, in whom the skull is much thinner, the bone may be carefully taken down to the dura, or a mobile island of thin bone can be created over the dura in the center of the well for protection. Retention sutures around the well may be placed between the bone and dura. Electrode insertion and closure are similar to the procedures in the adult.

Implantation of Special Populations

Cochlear Ossification

Labyrinthitis ossificans results from severe inflammation of the inner ear and can be associated with a variety of pathology, including viral or bacterial labyrinthitis, advanced otosclerosis, trauma, autoimmune in-

ner ear disease, occlusion of the labyrinthine artery, and leukemia or other tumors of the temporal bone (Green *et al.*, 1991). This condition results in the formation of fibrous tissue or new bone growth within the fluid-filled spaces of the inner ear. Scala tympani especially in the basal turn (Fig. 9.10), is the most common site of fibrous tissue and new bone growth, regardless of the cause. Green *et al.* (1991) demonstrated that ossification due to meningogenic labyrinthitis (Fig. 9.11) extended further into the cochlea than ossification due to other causes (Fig. 9.12).

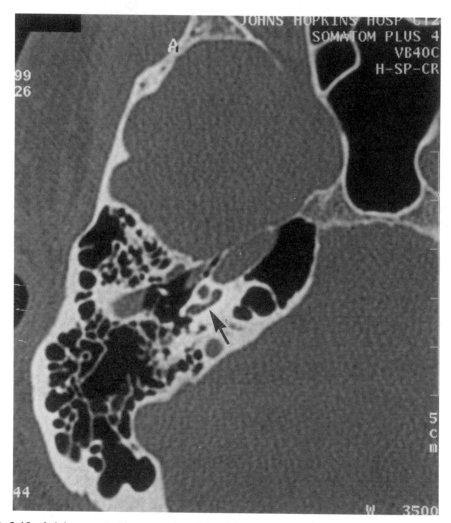

FIG. 9.10. Axial computed tomography of the right ear shows a patent scala tympani *(arrow)*.

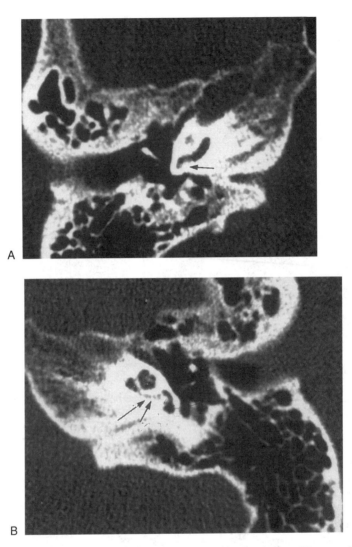

FIG. 9.11. Axial computed tomography through the temporal bones from a 52-year-old man with a history of meningitis occurring at 3 years of age. **A:** Scant ossification *(arrow)* is seen in the proximal basal turn on the right. **B:** Beadlike distribution of ossification *(arrows)* is seen in the proximal basal turn on the left.

Labyrinthitis ossificans was at one time considered a contraindication to implantation of a multi-electrode implant (Balkany et al., 1988; Balkany et al., 1996) for several reasons. First, it was considered difficult to achieve safe electrode insertion in an ossified cochlea. Second, it was unclear whether surviving neural elements could be adequately stimulated in the presence of bony obliteration. Third, histopathologic reports have shown a strong negative correlation between the degree of bony occlusion and the number of surviving SGCs (Nadol 1997), and it was unknown whether the population of surviving neurons would be adequate in most cases to support speech perception with the implant.

In most cases, ossification involves only

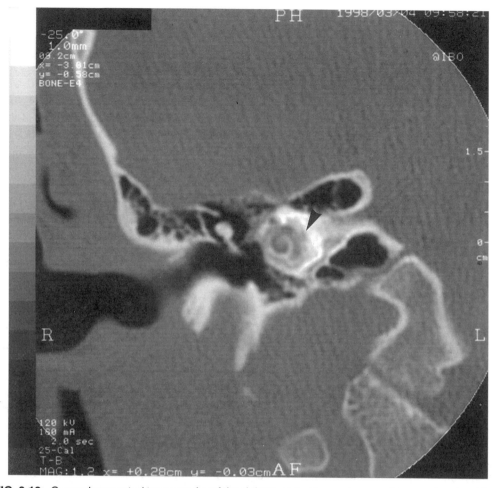

FIG. 9.12. Coronal computed tomography of the right temporal bone shows evidence of pericochlear osteolysis caused by extensive cochlear otosclerosis.

the most basal portion of the cochlea; total ossification of the cochlea is unusual [reported in 2 of 24 specimens by Green *et al.* (1991)]. In one series (Balkany *et al.*, 1988), 14% of patients were found to have cochlear ossification at the time of implant surgery. However, because the bony growth was typically confined to the most basal portion of the cochlea, electrode insertion was complete in all but 1 of the 15 patients in this series. Cohen and Waltzman (1993) reported that insertion of a multichannel cochlear implant was incomplete because of ossification in 8 (7%) of 110 patients in their series; the number of intracochlear electrodes implanted ranged from 10 to 18. The total number of patients with ossification was not reported. A study of implantation of 20 patients with otosclerosis (Fayad *et al.*, 1990) demonstrated some ossification of scala tympani that required drilling in 30%, but the extent of ossification did not exceed 5mm in any case. Performance with the implant was found to be similar to patients without ossification.

Survival of SGCs is poor in patients with labyrinthitis ossificans, particularly if caused by bacterial meningitis. In general, the greater the degree of ossification, the lower are the SGC counts. However, even in cases with severe bony occlusion, significant numbers of neurons remain (Nadol, 1997). Because patients with as few as 10% of the normal complement of SGCs are known to demonstrate at least average performance with the implant (Linthicum *et al.*, 1991), implantation is not contraindicated, even in patients with extensive ossification.

Several investigators have assessed cochlear implant performance in patients with ossification. Because many of these individuals function with partially inserted electrode arrays, performance may potentially suffer either because of smaller numbers of available channels for stimulation or because of poorer spine ganglion cell survival. However, studies of implant performance in patients with ossified cochleas have shown performance to be similar to patients with nonossified cochleas (Balkany *et al.*, 1988; Kemink *et al.*, 1992; Cohen and Waltzman, 1993). Implant performance after a radical mastoidectomy and cochlear drill-out (Gantz *et al.*, 1988) has not been assessed in a large number of patients. Reports by Gantz *et al.* (1988), Lambert *et al.* (1991), and Telian *et al.* (1996) indicate that performance in a limited number of patients is similar to that observed in patients with nonossified cochleas. However, no performance data are available to guide the surgeon in the choice of a more extensive drill-out procedure that may allow complete electrode insertion and a more limited, less invasive procedure that is likely to allow only partial insertion of the electrode array.

Surgical Procedure and Electrode or Device Choice

The implant surgeon should expect that ossification may be present and have an armamentarium of techniques available to deal with potentially unexpected findings. Balkany *et al.* (1996) describe a systematic approach to electrode insertion into the ossified cochlea. These investigators categorize intra-

cochlear bone growth according to the degree of obstruction:

1. Obliteration of the round window niche
2. Obstruction limited to the inferior, or straight, segment of the basal turn
3. Obstruction of the cochlea past the inferior segment (*i.e.*, into the ascending turn and beyond).

Surgical management of the ossified cochlea is best determined by the level of obstruction. The round window niche and membrane may be replaced with new bone growth and may not be readily identifiable. In these cases, it is important to keep in mind the expected position of the round window— 2 mm inferior to the inferior border of the oval window, and create a cochleostomy based on these measurements. A patent lumen is often encountered after drilling the cochleostomy. Inferior segment obstruction—less than 8 to 10 mm from the round window membrane and not obstructing the ascending turn—can be approached by removing the bony tissue obstructing the lumen or drilling through it. New bone growth is often softer and lighter in color than the bone of the otic capsule, and in many cases, a pick may be used to pull tissue out of the lumen. When the lumen is filled with hard bone and no space can be visualized, drilling is performed in an anteromedial direction, roughly parallel to the plane of the posterior canal wall, until a patent lumen is entered. In these cases, complete electrode insertion is possible.

In cases of obstruction of the ascending segment of the basal turn and beyond, three options are available to the surgeon. First, it is possible to drill a tunnel into the inferior segment and insert a portion of the electrode array into the scala tympani. The surgeon should monitor the depth of the drilled well, extending it no deeper than 8 to 10 mm, or until the carotid artery is visualized. In these cases, a straight electrode array is likely to be the most stable over time.

Second, Gantz *et al.* (1988) described a more aggressive approach that optimizes electrode insertion by creating a circumodiolar trough for the electrode using an extended transtympanic approach. A slight modification of this technique is described by Telian *et al.* (1996). The ear canal is divided and closed, and the ear canal skin, tympanic membrane, malleus, and incus are removed. The bony canal wall may be retained or taken down, but the prominence of the anterior bony external canal usually must be reduced to allow adequate visualization of the cochlear promontory. The carotid artery lies in proximity to the anterior basal turn of the cochlea and should be positively identified. A cochleostomy is created, and a bridge of bone at the round window niche is preserved to help secure the electrode. Osteogenic bone is then followed anteriorly, and the contour of the basal turn is developed with respect to the carotid artery. Care should be taken to remove only the outermost bone in an attempt to preserve neural tissue. Eventually a patent lumen may be encountered. If not, additional access may be gained by removing the tensor tympani muscle. The electrode array is then inserted beneath the bony bridge at the cochleostomy and into the lumen. Fibrous tissue is used to secure the electrode within the lumen. The facial nerve is at risk of injury during this procedure, and the use of facial nerve monitoring is recommended. At greatest risk of injury is the labyrinthine portion of the facial nerve, which is immediately superior to the superior portion of the descending segment of the basal turn of the cochlea.

Scala tympani is the preferred location for electrode insertion because of its size and proximity to the spiral ganglion. However, in cases of postmeningitic deafness, infection spreads initially into scala tympani, resulting in severe inflammation and subsequent osteogenesis in this location. The scala vestibuli is typically unaffected or less affected by bone growth (Green *et al.*, 1991). A third option for cochlear implantation of an ossified cochlea—implantation of scala vestibuli—has been described by Steenerson *et al.* (1990). Scala vestibuli implantation was

performed in two cases by extending the cochleostomy 1 to 2 mm superiorly; results in these cases were reportedly similar to those achieved after conventional implantation. If the scala vestibuli is ossified, a more extensive drill-out procedure is required to achieve full electrode insertion.

When ossification is suspected before the operation, the surgeon may take this information into account when the decision regarding device selection is made. Some manufacturers may recommend that a modification of their conventional electrode be used in cases of ossification. Two examples of modifications are the compressed array, which includes the same number of electrode contacts in a shorter length than the conventional array, and the "split" electrode, which offers the same number of electrode contacts on two carriers so that one can be inserted through the conventional cochleostomy and another through a more apical cochleostomy that may be created past the obstruction (Bredberg *et al.*, 1997; Lenarz *et al.*, 1997). Comparative studies have not been performed to confirm the benefit of these designs, and they may hold no advantage over conventional arrays.

A monopolar stimulation mode may be more advantageous than the bipolar modes for these patients, because it permits the use of an increased number of active channels and lower current for stimulation.

Cochlear Malformation

As in the case of cochlear ossification, identification of a bony cochlear malformation was once considered a contraindication to implantation. Concerns about the safety of the surgical procedure and postimplantation performance have been raised. Bony malformations of the cochlea have been associated with absence of the round and oval windows and with an aberrant course of the facial nerve. A thin cribriform area between the modiolus and a widened internal auditory canal is often observed; this is believed to be the route of cerebrospinal fluid (CSF) leak when it occurs during surgery or spontaneously, as in the case of microscopic occult leak and recurrent meningitis (Ohlms *et al.*, 1990; Tucci *et al.*, 1995). An anomalous internal auditory canal may suggest absence of the auditory nerve, a contraindication to implantation (Jackler *et al.*, 1987b; Shelton *et al.*, 1989) (Fig. 9.13). MRI may be used to delineate the intracanalicular neural anatomy in detail, and promontory stimulation testing may be performed to confirm the presence or absence of auditory nerve re-

sponse to electrical stimulation. Histopathologic studies of temporal bones with cochlear malformations have revealed substantially diminished and, in one case, bilaterally absent SGC populations (Otte *et al.*, 1978; Johnsson *et al.*, 1984; Monsell *et al.*, 1987).

Reports of experience with implantation of children and adults with cochlear malformations have demonstrated that implantation can be achieved without surgical complications and results in levels of performance not unlike patients with normal bony co-

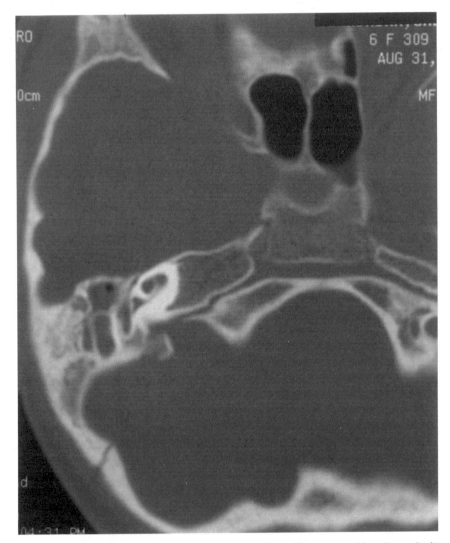

FIG. 9.13. Axial computed tomography demonstrates mild, right-sided cochlear hypoplasia with an absent internal auditory canal.

chlear anatomy (Tucci *et al.*, 1995; Slattery and Luxford, 1995; Luntz *et al.*, 1997). Modifications of conventional surgical implantation techniques are suggested and depend on a knowledge of the different types of malformations (Fig. 9.14). A classification of malformations based on embryogenesis is described by Jackler *et al.* (1987a):

1. *Cochlear aplasia:* no cochlear development; not candidates for implantation
2. *Common cavity deformity:* combined cochlea and vestibule with no internal structure
3. *Cochlear hypoplasia:* small cochlear bud
4. *Incomplete partition:* classic Mondini malformation, with loss of interscalar septum between the middle and apical turns; cochlea are often smaller than normal

Full or near-full electrode insertion can be achieved using routine implantation techniques in patients with incomplete partition (Mondini) deformity (Tucci *et al.*, 1995; Slattery and Luxford, 1995) (Fig. 9.15). A common cavity malformation is also likely to accommodate a multichannel electrode array, whereas the small size of the hypoplastic cochlea restricts the number of electrodes that can be positioned within the inner ear. Even so, the two patients with cochlear hypoplasia in one series were able to use 10 electrodes each (Tucci *et al.*, 1995) (Fig. 9.16). Because the electrodes may not be confined by scalar anatomy, electrode migration may occur, and individuals with cochlear malformations may require frequent reprogramming of the electrodes. Electrodes that are not intracochlear or that elicit facial nerve stimulation can be eliminated from the "map" (Tucci *et al.*, 1995), as can electrodes that elicit facial nerve stimulation in implanted normal cochleas (Niparko *et al.*, 1991).

Abnormalities of the round window and facial nerve anatomy should be expected, and the use of facial nerve monitoring is recommended. If the round window is absent, a cochleostomy should be placed according to the measurements described previously.

The round window may be found in a position more posterior and superior than usual, consistent with the deformity of the cochlea. Malposition of the facial nerve may necessitate a modification of usual implantation techniques, and implantation through a vestibulotomy has been described (Molter *et al.*, 1993).

CSF leak is common and is usually easily controlled with soft tissue packing at the cochleostomy. In cases of persistent CSF leak, a lumbar spinal drain can be placed at the time of surgery and left in place for 3 to 4 days to allow the fibrous tissue packing in the cochleostomy to seal, preventing further leakage. Control of a CSF leak may also be accomplished by more extensive soft tissue packing of the middle ear space and eustachian tube, with or without radical mastoidectomy and closure of the ear canal. No cases of meningitis have been reported after cochlear implantation in patients with cochlear malformations. CSF leak has also been reported in patients with enlarged vestibular aqueducts (Fig. 9.17) (Aschendorff *et al.*, 1997); these have been easily controlled with soft tissue packing.

Patients Requiring Magnetic Resonance Imaging for Follow-up

Some patients who are candidates for implantation require repeat MRI for monitoring of central nervous system disease. MRI is contraindicated in patients with conventional cochlear implants or with other types of implants that contain ferromagnetic materials because of the risk of implant movement. A nonmagnetic version of a multichannel cochlear implant is available for use in these patients (Heller *et al.*, 1996). In this modified device, the receiver/stimulator internal magnet, which is normally used to hold the external transmitter coil in place, is replaced with a silicone rubber plug. The external transmitter coil is held in place by magnetic attraction to a retainer disk that contains a steel plate and is held to the scalp with pressure-sensitive adhesive. If imaging

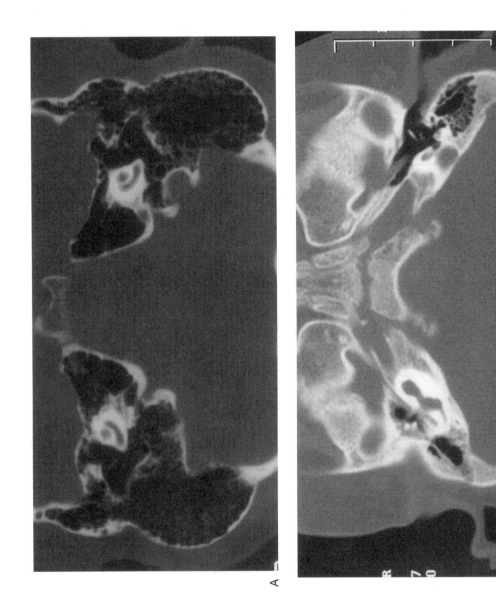

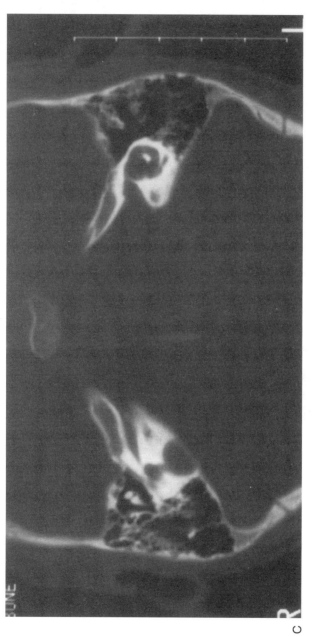

FIG. 9.14. Axial computed tomography shows a normal cochlea **(A)** and two types of cochlear malformations, including cochlear hypoplasia of the right ear **(B)** and common cavity of the left ear **(C)**.

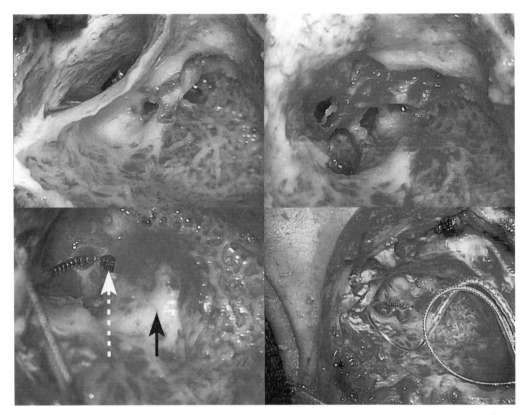

FIG. 9.15. Surgical views of left cochlear implantation performed in an ear with severe hypoplasia. The canal wall *(top left)* was taken down *(top right)* to better visualize the labyrinth. The vestibular labyrinth cochleostomy *(lower left)* is shown by a dotted arrow. An electrode *(lower right)* is inserted to approximately 19 mm.

is no longer required in the future, the device can be converted to a magnetic configuration during a relatively minor surgical procedure. Similar principles have been used to develop the auditory brain stem implant (ABI) for use in patients with bilateral acoustic neuromas who require follow-up MRI.

Neurofibromatosis type 2 (NF-2) patients with bilateral acoustic neuromas and resultant profound hearing loss are candidates for implantation. If the auditory nerve can be preserved in at least one ear, most likely after a failed attempt at hearing preservation surgery for resection of a relatively small tumor, cochlear implantation may be performed (Hoffman *et al.*, 1992). Similarly, patients with failed hearing preservation surgery for

a unilateral acoustic neuroma and contralateral deafness of another cause may be candidates for implantation in the ear with the resected tumor if the auditory nerve is intact (Lambert *et al.*, 1992). In cases of a small tumor with a profound hearing loss, use of a translabyrinthine approach with associated labyrinthectomy does not exclude the possibility of cochlear implantation (Levine, 1989; Zwolan *et al.*, 1993).

Auditory Brain Stem Implants

NF-2 patients who meet certain eligibility criteria may be candidates for the ABI, which is being implanted in several centers as part of a multicenter clinical trial. Eligibility

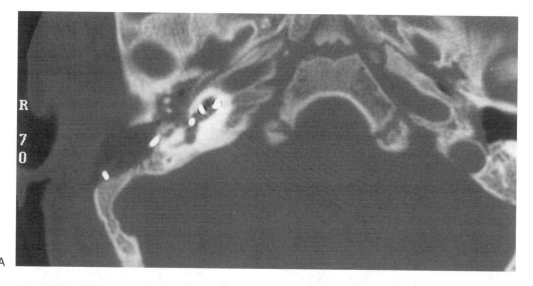

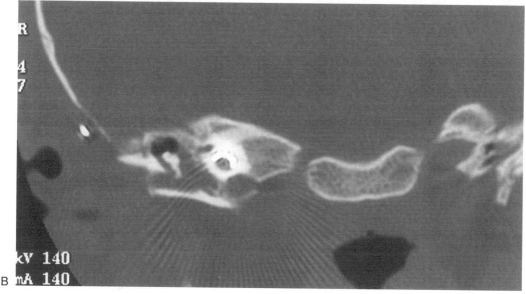

FIG. 9.16. Axial **(A)** and coronal **(B)** computed tomography scans show implantation of a hypoplastic cochlea (shown before implantation in Fig. 9.14B) with a labyrinthotomy approach. The electrode extends through the anterior limb of the horizontal semicircular canal into the vestibule and cochlea. The cochlear cavity measured 9 mm, and a compact or short electrode array was fully inserted.

criteria include evidence of bilateral eighth nerve tumors, competency in the English language, age of 15 years or older, psychologic suitability, and willingness to comply with the research protocol. Suitable candidates are patients undergoing translabyrinthine tumor removal who have nonaidable hearing, an only-hearing ear with a symptomatic tumor, or serviceable hearing in the contralateral ear but a contralateral tumor of sufficient size to indicate that hearing will likely be lost in a short period. This device may be

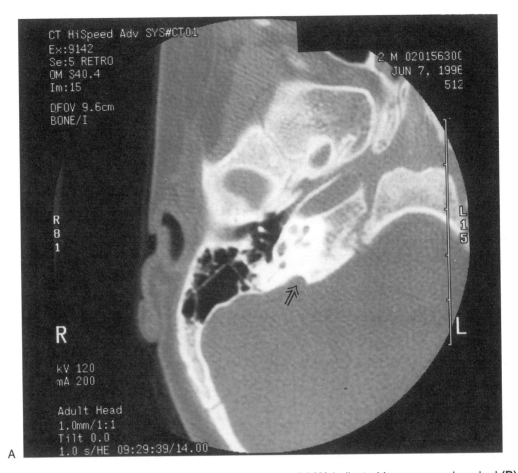

FIG. 9.17. Axial computed tomography images show mild **(A)** indicated by arrow, and marked **(B)** enlargement of the vestibular aqueduct.

implanted only at the time of tumor resection and not as a separate procedure (Briggs *et al.*, 1994).

RESULTS OF COCHLEAR IMPLANTATION

Complications after Cochlear Implantation in Adult Patients

The surgical portion of the cochlear implant procedure entails risks associated with mastoid surgery and the implanted device. Cohen *et al.* (1988) established a classification of implant-related complications as "major" if they require additional surgery or hospital-

ization for treatment or correction and "minor" if they resolve with minimal or no treatment. Facial nerve palsy or paralysis is considered a major complication even if no further surgery or inpatient treatment is required. An initial survey of 2,751 implants performed at multiple centers in the United States revealed the rate of major and minor complications to be 8% and 4.3%, respectively. A follow-up survey in 459 patients, published in 1991, revealed a complication rate of 5% and 7%, perhaps showing a decrease in the rate of major complications over time for a similar group of surgeons using a single device (Cohen and Hoffman, 1991).

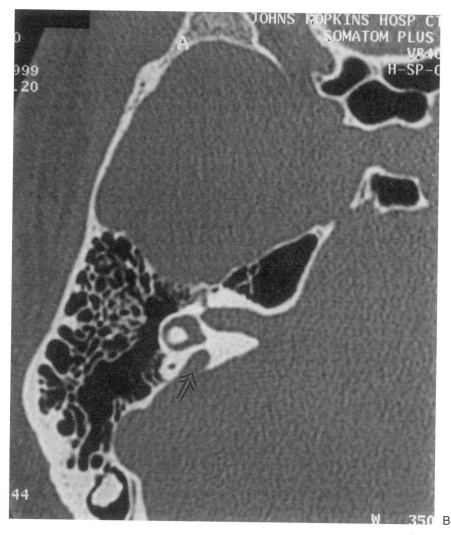

FIG. 9.17. *Continued.*

Several studies have shown that the most frequently reported major and minor complications are related to the incision and postauricular flap design. Problems range in severity from minor wound dehiscences or infections to major loss of tissue requiring removal of the device. In a report of surgical complications from a large series of patients implanted in Hannover and Melbourne, wound breakdown was the most common significant complication after cochlear implantation, requiring device removal in two cases (0.8%) of a total of 253 (Webb *et al.*, 1991). Many implant surgeons have emphasized the importance of good flap design and technical skill to avoid these complications. The flap must have adequate blood supply and venous drainage, allow adequate exposure of the operative site with adequate coverage of the device, and be carefully closed in layers without tension. The C-shaped incision is contraindicated when there is a previous postauricular incision (Harris and Cueva, 1987). Extrusion of the device can result from local flap necrosis, which can be managed by rotation of the device under an extended flap, usually to a more superior location where intact skin covers the device (Wang *et al.*, 1990; Haberkamp and Schwaber, 1992).

Facial nerve injury is a serious potential complication of cochlear implantation and has been reported to occur rarely. Only rare cases of transient weakness were reported in the series published by Cohen and Hoffman (1991) and Webb *et al.* (1991). House and Luxford (1993) described eight cases of facial paralysis or paresis that occurred after cochlear implantation. The most frequent mode of injury was the heat of the burr shaft rotating over the facial nerve in the facial recess. The investigators emphasize the importance of using copious irrigation during drilling, maintaining a thin sheet of bone over the facial nerve in this location, and maintaining an angle of drilling that keeps the burr shaft lateral and away from the floor of the facial recess. In some cases of paresis, steroid treatment has been employed. Notable instances of severe facial nerve injury include one child with a cochlear malformation and malposition of the facial nerve, and one patient who had undergone a radical mastoidectomy as a child and required reimplantation for a failed device implanted as a young adult.

Aside from wound breakdown, the incidence of major complications is low. Malpositioned hypotympanic or compressed or kinked electrode arrays can necessitate reoperation for repositioning, as can extrusion of the device. Potentially life-threatening complications are rare; two cases of meningitis in adults after cochlear implantation have been reported (Cohen and Hoffman, 1991; Daspit, 1991).

Although some patients may complain of tinnitus after implant surgery, the tinnitus may be suppressed or abolished by use of the implant in as many as 77% of implant users (Ito and Sakakihara, 1994). Patients in the older age group (60 to 80 years) are not at increased risk of surgical complications (Kelsall *et al.*, 1995). However, older individuals (>60 years) are more likely to have balance complaints postoperatively than are younger implant recipients (Brey *et al.*, 1995).

Approximately 70% of profoundly hearing-impaired individuals exhibit reduced vestibular function as indicated by tests of the vestibulocular reflex (Huygen *et al.*, 1994). For an ear with residual vestibular function, implantation ablates vestibular function in about 50%, yielding the possibility of postimplantation disequilibrium and vertigo. During the first week after surgery, patients often experience some degree of disequilibrium and unsteadiness. True vertigo that persists in the postoperative phase is rare (Dobie *et al.*, 1995). Extended periods of disequilibrium are also rare but, when present, are treatable with exercise regimens designed to elicit central compensatory mechanisms.

Complications in the Pediatric Population

Although it has been assumed that young children may be at greater risk of complication from cochlear implantation than adult patients, the published data on this issue reveal no increased risk of adverse effects in the pediatric population. Cohen and Hoffman (1991) cite as potential risk factors: small skull size, lack of mastoid development, potential for electrode movement or extrusion secondary to skull growth, and possibility of otitis media with associated complications. In a series of 309 children who were implanted with the Nucleus device by 25 surgeons in North America before 1991, the total complication rate (major and minor) was 7%, which compares favorably with the adult rate of 12%. The incidence of complications was lower in children older than 7 years of age. The lower rate of operative complications in the pediatric population as reported in this study may reflect the greater experience of surgeons who perform pediatric cochlear implants. The incidence of otitis media was lower after implantation, and the literature contains no reports of adverse sequelae.

Two additional studies report low complication rates for children. Miyamoto *et al.*

(1996) reviewed 100 consecutive pediatric cochlear implant surgeries performed by Miyamoto. Complications were limited to two cases: one case of transient facial paresis and one case of a CSF gusher in a patient with severe cochlear dysplasia. A number of children in this study were found to have otitis media, and two had delayed mastoiditis that required drainage. In no case, however, did a child contract meningitis or sequelae that required removal of the implant. Luetje and Jackson (1997) reviewed their experience with 55 children and found no surgical complications. The most important complication found in this study was device failure, which occurred in 5 children (9%). This failure rate is similar to that reported for children by Parisier et al. (1996).

Children are thought to be at increased risk for device failure, in part because of their high level of activity with the potential for traumatic injury to the internal receiver/stimulator. The connecting lead between the receiver/stimulator and the electrode array is vulnerable to shearing, particularly if the device is not properly secured. Accordingly, use of a well drilled in bone for embedding the device and fixation with permanent suture material is strongly advised. Manufacturer changes in implant design over the past few years have resulted in a decrease in device failure rates. Nevertheless, implant centers must be particularly vigilant in monitoring children who may be at higher risk for this problem.

Reimplantation Surgery

Reimplantation of an ear may be indicated for several reasons, including device failure, extrusion, or the desire to convert from an single-channel or experimental device (Tucci et al., 2000) to a conventional multi-electrode array. Although technically feasible, reimplantation requires considerable attention to surgical detail. The skin over the implant is often atrophic and must be handled carefully. The skin incision is through the original scar, and the flap is raised, exposing the receiver/stimulator. Bony or fibrous tissue probably surround the length of the electrode lead. New bone growth, thought to result from insertion trauma, is frequently found at the cochleostomy and may extend a few millimeters into the scala. The previously placed implant may be gently removed and any new bone growth removed with a pick or drill as for a primary procedure.

Audiologic results after conversion of a single channel to a multichannel device demonstrate a significant improvement in performance (Miyamoto et al., 1994; Rubenstein et al., 1998). Evaluations of patient performance after reinsertion of multi-electrode implants show that, although results are acceptable (Gantz et al., 1989; Parisier et al., 1991), there is a statistically significant decrease in insertion depth and channel activation compared with that achieved after initial implantation (Miyamoto et al., 1997). A multicenter review of 28 patients reimplanted after multi-electrode device failure reports that approximately one-fourth of these patients demonstrated poorer performance after reimplantation (Henson et al., 1998).

Histopathologic Study of Implanted Temporal Bones

The histologic results of cochlear implantation have been well studied (Kennedy, 1987; Fayad et al., 1991; Zappia et al., 1991; Nadol, 1994). Potential histopathologic findings can be divided into surgical and device-related injuries. Surgical trauma may include fractures of the osseous spiral lamina, perforation of the basilar membrane, and tears of the spiral ligament. Cochlear fibrosis and neossification are common findings in these studies. In general, traumatic changes appear to be limited to the most basal portions of the cochlea and are unlikely to exert significant negative effects on implant performance. Reactions to extended electrical stimulation (e.g., electrochemical tissue damage, neural degeneration) by current implants appear to be modest. Foreign body reactions and infection that extend along the implant array to involve membranous elements of the cochlea are likely to induce sensorineural degeneration. However, well-documented cases of such occurrences are lacking.

Findings of localized cochlear trauma after cochlear implantation have led to concerns that these traumatic injuries might result in associated SGC degeneration. Although two studies of temporal bone histopathology in individual patients with a unilateral cochlear implant reported a decrease in the normal SGC population ipsilateral to the implant (Zappia et al., 1991; Marsh et al., 1991), other studies in chronically implanted animals (Sutton and Miller, 1983; Shepherd et al., 1983) and humans (Clark et al., 1988; Linthicum et al., 1991; Nadol, 1994) showed no differences in SGC populations between the implanted and unimplanted ears. It is likely that many factors influence neuron survival, as evidenced by histopathologic studies, including previous pathology (which may vary between the two ears) and the amount of time between implantation (with possible end organ damage) and the time of death. Because the temporal association between SGC degeneration and end organ damage has not been clearly established for humans, histopathologic findings from implanted temporal bones are not always clearly interpretable. Although the duration of implant stimulation in the Linthicum study ranged from 1 to 14 years, Nadol's report was limited to the study of one set of temporal bones from a patient implanted 10 months before death. Animal studies have shown that the reintroduction of electrical activity through a cochlear implant may prevent degenerative changes in the central auditory system (Lousteau, 1987; Hartshorn et al., 1991; Tucci and Rubel, 1994) (see Chapter 1).

REFERENCES

Arriaga MA, Carrier D. MRI and clinical decisions in cochlear implantation. Am J Otol 1996;17:547–553.

Aschendorff A, Marangos N, Laszig R. Large vestibular aqueduct syndrome and its implication for cochlear implant surgery. Am J Otol 1997;18[Suppl 6]:S57.

Balkany T, Dreisbach J. Workshop: surgical anatomy and radiographic imaging of cochlear implant surgery. Am J Otol 1987;8:195–200.

Balkany T, Gantz B, Nadol JB. Multichannel cochlear implants in obstructed and obliterated cochleas. Otolaryngol Head Neck Surg 1988;98:72–81.

Balkany T, Gantz BJ, Steenerson RL, Cohen NL. Systematic approach to electrode insertion in the ossified cochlea. Otolaryngol Head Neck Surg 1996;114:4–11.

Balkany T, Telischi FF. Fixation of the electrode cable during cochlear implantation: the split bridge technique. Laryngoscope 1995;105:217–218.

Bath AP, O'Donoghue GM, Holland IM, Gibbin KP. Paediatric cochlear implantation: how reliable is computed tomography in assessing cochlear patency? Clin Otolaryngol 1993;18:475–479.

Bielamowiez SA, Coker NJ, Jenkins HA, Igarashi M. Surgical dimensions of the facial recess in adults and children. Arch Otolaryngol Head Neck Surg 1988; 114:534–537.

Bredberg G, Lindstrom B, Lopponen BH, Skarzynski H, Hyodo M, Sato H. Electrodes for ossified cochleas. Am J Otol 1997;18[Suppl 6]:S42–S43.

Brey RH, Facer GW, Trine MB, Lynn SG, Paterson AM, Suman VJ. Vestibular effects associated with implantation of a multiple channel cochlear prosthesis. Am J Otol 1995;16:424–430.

Briggs RJ, Brackmann DE, Baser ME, Hitselberger WE. Comprehensive management of bilateral acoustic neuromas. Arch Otolaryngol Head Neck Surg 1994;120:1307–1314.

Burton MJ, Shepherd RK, Xu SA, Franz BK-HG, Clark GM. Cochlear implantation in young children: histological studies on head growth, leadwire, design, electrode fixation in the monkey model. Laryngology 1994;104:167–175.

Casselman JW, Kuhweide R, Deimling M, Ampe W, Dehaene I, Meeus L. Constructive interference in steady state-3DFT MR imaging of the inner ear and cerebellopontine angle. AJNR Am J Neuroradiol 1993;14:47–57.

Clark FM, Shepherd RK, Franz BK-H. The histopathology of the human temporal bone and auditory central nervous system following cochlear implantation in a patient. Acta Otolaryngol (Stockh) Suppl 1988;448:6–65.

Clark GM. An evaluation of per-scalar cochlear electrode implantation techniques: a histopathological study in cats. J Laryngol Otol 1977;91:185–199.

Cohen NL. Cochlear implant soft surgery: fact or fantasy? Otolaryngol Head Neck Surg 1997;117:214–216.

Cohen NL, Hoffman RA. Complications of cochlear implant surgery in adults and children. Ann Otol Rhinol Laryngol 1991;100:708–711.

Cohen NL, Hoffman RA. Complications of cochlear implant surgery. In: Eisele D, ed. Complications in head and neck surgery. St. Louis: CV Mosby, 1993:722–729.

Cohen NL, Kuzman J. Titanium clip for cochlear implant electrode fixation. Ann Otol Rhinol Laryngol 1995;104[Suppl 166]:402–403.

Cohen NL, Waltzman SB. Partial insertion of the Nucleus multichannel cochlear implant: technique and results. Am J Otol 1993;14:357–361.

Daspit CP. Meningitis as a result of cochlear implantation: case report. *Otolaryngol Head Neck Surg* 1991;105:115.

Dobie R, Jenkins H, Cohen N. Surgical results. *Ann Otol Rhinol Laryngol* 1995;104[Suppl 165]:6–8.

Eby TL. Development of the facial recess: implications for cochlear implantation. *Laryngoscope* 1996; 106[Suppl 80]:1–7.

Eby TL, Nadol JB. Postnatal growth of the human temporal bone: implications for cochlear implants in children. *Ann Otol Rhinol Laryngol* 1986;95:356–382.

Fayad J, Linthicum FH, Otto SR, Galey FR, House WF. Cochlear implants: histopathologic findings related to performance in 16 human temporal bones. *Ann Otol Rhinol Laryngol* 1991;100:807–811.

Fayad J, Moloy P, Linthicum FH. Cochlear otosclerosis: does bone formation affect cochlear implant surgery? *Am J Otol* 1990;11:196–200.

Franz BK, Clark GM, Bloom DM. Effect of experimentally induced otitis media on cochlear implants. *Ann Otol Rhinol Laryngol* 1987;96:174–177.

Frau CN, Luxford WM, Lo W, Berliner KI, Telischi FF. High-resolution computed tomography in evaluation of cochlear patency in implant candidates: a comparison with surgical findings. *J Laryngol Otol* 1994;108:743–748.

Gantz BJ, Lowder MW, McCabe BF. Audiologic results following reimplantation of cochlear implants. *Ann Otol Rhinol Laryngol Suppl* 1989;142:12–16.

Gantz BJ, McCabe BF, Tyler RS. Use of multichannel cochlear implants in obstructed and obliterated cochleas. *Otolaryngol Head Neck Surg* 1988;98:72–81.

Gantz BJ, Tyler RS, Tye-Murray N, Fryauf-Bertschy H. Long-term results of multichannel cochlear implants in congenitally deaf children. In: Hochmair-Desoyer IJ, Hochmair ES, eds. *Advances in cochlear implants.* Vienna: International Interscience Seminars, 1993:528–533.

Gray RF, Irving RM. Cochlear implants in chronic suppurative otitis media. *Am J Otol* 1995;16:682–686.

Green JD, Marion MS, Hinojosa R. Labyrinthitis ossificans: histopathologic consideration for cochlear implantation. *Otolaryngol Head Neck Surg* 1991; 104:320–326.

Haberkamp TJ, Schwaber MK. Management of flap necrosis in cochlear implantation. *Ann Otol Rhinol Laryngol* 1992;101:38–41.

Harnsberger HR, Dart DJ, Parkin JL, Smoker W, Osborn AG. Cochlear implant candidates: assessment with CT and MRI imaging. *Radiology* 1987;164:53–57.

Harris JP, Cueva RA. Flap design for cochlear implantation: avoidance of a potential complication. *Laryngoscope* 1987;97:755–757.

Hartshorn DO, Miller JM, Altschuler RA. Protective effect of electrical stimulation in the deafened guinea pig. *Otolaryngol Head Neck Surg* 1991;104:311–319.

Heller JW, Brackmann DE, Tucci DL, Nyenhuis JA, Chou CK. Evaluation of MRI compatibility of the modified Nucleus multichannel auditory brainstem and cochlear implants. *Am J Otol* 1996;17:724–729.

Henson AM, Slattery WH, Mills D. Comparison of audiologic performance following reimplantation: a multicenter overview. Presented at the American Otologic Society meeting; Palm Beach, FL, May 1998.

Hoffman FA, Kohan D, Cohen NL. Cochlear implants in the management of bilateral acoustic neuromas. *Am J Otol* 1992;13:525–529.

Hoffman RA. Cochlear implant in the child under two years of age: skull growth, otitis media, and selection. *Otolaryngol Head Neck Surg* 1997;117:217–219.

House JR, Luxford WM. Facial nerve injury in cochlear implantation. *Otolaryngol Head Neck Surg* 1993; 109:1078–1082.

House WF, Luxford WM, Courtney B. Otitis media in children following cochlear implant. *Ear Hear* 1985;6:24S–26S.

Huygen PL, van den Broek P, Spies TH, Mens LH, Admiraal RJ. Does intracochlear implantation jeopardize vestibular function? *Ann Otol Rhinol Laryngol* 1994;103:609–614.

Ito J, Sakakihara J. Tinnitus suppression by electrical stimulation of the cochlear wall and by cochlear implantation. *Laryngoscope* 1994;104:752–754.

Jackler RK, Luxford WM, House WF. Congenital malformations of the inner ear: a classification based on embryogenesis. *Laryngoscope* 1987a;97[Suppl 20]: 2–14.

Jackler RK, Luxford WM, House WF. Sound detection with the cochlear implant in five ears of four children with congenital malformations of the cochlea. *Laryngoscope* 1987b;97[Suppl 40]:15–17.

Jackler RK, Luxford WM, Schindler RA, McKerrow WS. Cochlear patency problems in cochlear implantation. *Laryngoscope* 1987c;97:801–805.

Johnsson LG, Hawkins JE, Rouse RC, Kingsley TC. Four variations of the Mondini inner ear malformations as seen in microdissections. *Am J Otol* 1984;5:242–257.

Kelsall DC, Shallop JK, Burnelli T. Cochlear implantation in the elderly. *Am J Otol* 1995;16:609–615.

Kemink JL, Zimmerman-Phillips S, Kileny PR, Firszt JB, Novak MA. Auditory performance of children with cochlear ossification and partial implant insertion. *Laryngoscope* 1992;102:1001–1005.

Kennedy DW. Multichannel intracochlear electrodes: mechanism of insertion trauma. *Laryngoscope* 1987;97:42–49.

Lalwani AK, Larky JB, Wareing MJ, Kwast K, Schindler RA. The Clarion multi-strategy cochlear implant surgical techniques, complications, and results: a single institutional experience. *Am J Otol* 1998;19:66–70.

Lambert PR, Ruth RA, Hodges AV. Multichannel cochlear implant and electrically evoked auditory brainstem responses in a child with labyrinthitis ossificans. *Laryngoscope* 1991;101:14–19.

Lambert PR, Ruth RA, Thomas JF. Promontory electrical stimulation in postoperative acoustic tumor patients. *Laryngoscope* 1992;102:814–819.

Langman AW, Quigley SM. Accuracy of high-resolution computed tomography in cochlear implantation. *Otolaryngol Head Neck Surg* 1996;114:38–43.

Laszing R, Terwey B, Battmer RD, Hesse G. Magnetic resonance imaging (MRI) and high resolution computed tomography (HRCT) in cochlear implant candidates. *Scand Audiol Suppl* 1988;30:197–200.

Lenarz T, Battmer R, Bertram B. Cochlear implantation in children under the age of two. In: *Abstracts of the Vth International Conference on Cochlear Implants.* New York: NYU Post-Graduate Medical School, 1997:45.

Lenarz T, Battmer RD, Lesinski A, Parker J. Nucleus double electrode array: a new approach for ossified cochleae. *Am J Otol* 1997;6[Suppl 18]:S39–S41.

Levine SC. A complex case of cochlear implant electrode placement. *Am J Otol* 1989;10:477–480.

Linthicum FH, Fayad J, Otto SR, Galey FR, House WF. Cochlear implant histopathology. *Am J Otol* 1991;12:422–311.

Louosteau RJ. Increased spiral ganglion cell survival in electrically stimulated, deafened guinea pig cochleae. *Laryngoscope* 1987;97:836–842.

Luetje CM, Jackson K. Cochlear implants in children: what constitutes a complication. *Otolaryngol Head Neck Surg* 1997;117:243–247.

Luntz M, Balkany T, Hodges AV, Telischi FF. Cochlear Implants in children with congenital inner ear malformations. *Arch Otolaryngol Neck Surg* 1997; 123:974–977.

Luntz M, Hodges AV, Balkany T, Dolan-Ash S, Schloffman J. Otitis media in children with cochlear implants. *Laryngoscope* 1996;106:1403–1405.

Luxford WM. Surgery for cochlear implantation. In: Brackmann D, Shelton C, Moises AA, eds. *Otologic surgery*. Philadelphia: WB Saunders, 1994:425–436.

Marsh MA, Coker NJ, Jenkins HA. Temporal bone histopathology of a patient with a Nucleus 22-channel cochlear implant. Presented at the 26th Annual Scientific Meeting of the American Neurotology Society; Waikoloa, HI, May 1991.

Miyamoto RT, Osberger MJ, Cunningham L, *et al.* Single-channel to multi-channel conversions in pediatric cochlear implant recipients. *Am J Otol* 1994;15:40–45.

Miyamoto RT, Robbins AM, Osberger MJ. Cochlear implants. In: Cummings CW, Harker LA, Schuller DE, eds. *Otolaryngology—head and neck surgery*, 2nd ed. St. Louis: CV Mosby, 1993:3124–3151.

Miyamoto RT, Svirsky MA, Myres WA, Kirk KI, Schulte J. Cochlear implant reimplantation. *Am J Otol* 1997;6[Suppl 18]:S60–S61.

Miyamoto RT, Young M, Myres WA, Kessler K, Wolfert K, Kirk KI. Complications of pediatric cochlear implantation. *Eur Arch Otorhinolaryngol* 1996;253:1–4.

Molter DW, Pate BR, McElveen JT. Cochlear implantation in the congenitally malformed ear. *Otolaryngol Head Neck Surg* 1993;108:174–177.

Monsell EM, Jackler RK, Motta G, Linthicum FH. Congenital malformations of the inner ear. *Laryngoscope* 1987;97[Suppl 40]:18–24.

Nadol JB. Patterns of neural degeneration in the human cochlea and auditory nerve: implications for cochlear implantation. *Otolaryngol Head Neck Surg* 1997; 117:220–228.

Nadol JB, Ketten DR, Burgess BJ. Otopathology in case of multichannel cochlear implantation. *Laryngoscope* 1994;104:299–303.

Niparko JK, Kirk KI, Mellon NK, Robbins AM, Tucci DL, Wilson BS, eds. *Cochlear implants: principles and practices.* New York: Lippincott Williams & Wilkins, 1999.

Niparko JK, Oviatt DL, Coker NJ, Sutton L, Waltzman SB, Cohen NL. Facial nerve stimulation with cochlear implantation. *Otolaryngol Head Neck Surg* 1991; 104:826–830.

Ohlms LA, Edwards MS, Mason EO, Igarashi M, Alford BR, Smith RJ. Recurrent meningitis and Mondini dysplasia. *Arch Otolaryngol Neck Surg* 1990; 116:608–612.

Otte G, Schuknecht HF, Kerr AG. Ganglion cell populations in normal and pathological human cochleae: implications for cochlear implantation. *Laryngoscope* 1978;88:1231–1246.

Parisier SC, Chute P, Weiss M, Hellman S, Wang RC. Results of cochlear implant reinsertion. *Laryngoscope* 1991;101:1013–1015.

Parisier SC, Chute PM, Popp AL. Cochlear implant mechanical failures. *Am J Otol* 1996;17:730–734.

Parisier SC, Chute PM, Popp AL, Hanson MB. Surgical techniques for cochlear implantation in the very young child. *Otolaryngol Head Neck Surg* 1997;117:248–254.

Parnes LS, Gagne JP, Hassan R. Cochlear implants and otitis media: considerations in two cleft palate patients. *J Otol* 1993;22:5:345–348.

Proctor B, Bollobass B, Niparko J. Anatomy of the round window niche. *Ann Otol Rhinol Laryngol* 1986;95:444–446.

Rubinstein JT, Parkinson WS, Lowder MW, Gantz BJ, Nadol JB, Tyler RS. Single-channel to multichannel conversions in adult cochlear implant subjects. *Am J Otol* 1998;19:461–466.

Seicshnaydre MA, Johnson MH, Hasenstab MS, Williams GH. Cochlear implants in children: reliability of computed tomography. *Otolaryngol Head Neck Surg* 1992;107:410–417.

Seidman DA, Chute PM, Parisier S. Temporal bone imaging for cochlear implantation. *Laryngoscope* 1994;104:562–565.

Shelton C, Luxford WM, Tonokawa LL, Lo WWH, House WF. The narrow internal auditory canal in children: a contraindication for cochlear implants. *Otolaryngol Head Neck Surg* 1989;100:227–231.

Shepherd RK, Clark GM, Black RC. Chronic electrical stimulation of the auditory nerve in cats. *Acta Otolaryngol (Stockh) Suppl* 1983;399:19–31.

Slattery WH, Luxford WM. Cochlear implantation in the congenital malformed cochlea. *Laryngoscope* 1995;105:1184–1187.

Steenerson RL, Gary LB, Wynens MS. Scala vestibuli cochlear implantation for labyrinthine ossification. *Am J Otol* 1990;11:360–363.

Sutton D, Miller JM. Cochlear implant effects on the spiral ganglion. *Ann Otol Rhinol Laryngol* 1983; 92:53–58.

Takahashi H, Honjo I, Sando I, Takagi A. Orientation for cochlear implant surgery in cases with round window obstruction: a computer reconstruction study. *Eur Arch Otorhinolaryngol* 1995;252:102–105.

Takahashi H, Sando I. Computer-aided 3-D temporal bone anatomy for cochlear implant surgery. *Laryngoscope* 1990;100:417–421.

Telian SA, Zimmerman-Phillips S, Kileny PR. Successful revision of failed cochlear implants in severe labyrinthitis ossificans. *Am J Otol* 1996;17:53–60.

Tien RD, Felsberg GJ, Macfall J. Fast spin-echo high-resolution MR imaging of the inner ear. *AJR Am J Radiol* 1992;159:395–398.

Tucci DL, Telian SA, Zimmerman-Phillips S, Zwolan TA, Kileny PR. Cochlear implantation inpatients with cochlear malformations. *Arch Otolaryngol Head Neck Surg* 1995;21:833–838.

Tucci DL, Rubel EW. Central auditory system development and disorders. In: Jackler R, Brackmann D, eds. *Neurotology*. St. Louis: CV Mosby, 1994:567–617.

Waltzman SB, Cohen NL. Cochlear implantation in children younger than 2 years old. *Am J Otol* 1998;19:158–162.

Wang RC, Parisier SC, Weiss MH, Chute PM, Hellman SA, Sauris E. Cochlear implant flap complications. *Ann Otol Rhinol Laryngol* 1990;99:791–795.

Webb RL, Lehnhardt E, Clark GM, Laszig R, Pyman BC, Franz BK. Surgical complications with the cochlear multichannel intracochlear implant: experience at Hannover and Melbourne. *Ann Otol Rhinol Laryngol* 1991;100:131–136.

Wiet RJ, Pyle GM, O'Connor CA, Russell E, Schramm DR. Computed tomography: how accurate a predictor for cochlear implantation? *Laryngoscope* 1990;100: 687–692.

Woolley AL, Oser AB, Lusk RP, Bahadori RS. Preoperative temporal bone computed tomography scan and its use in evaluating the pediatric cochlear implant candidate. *Laryngoscope* 1997;107:1100–1106.

Zippia JJ, Niparko JK, Oviatt DL, Kemink JL, Altschuler RA. Evaluation of the temporal bones of a multichannel cochlear implant patient. *Ann Otol Rhinol Laryngol* 1991;100:914–921.

Zwolan TA, Shepard NT, Niparko JK. Labyrinthectomy with cochlear implantation. *Am J Otol* 1993; 14:220–223.

Cochlear Implants: Principles & Practices, edited by John K. Niparko, Karen Iler Kirk, Nancy K. Mellon, Amy McConkey Robbins, Debara L. Tucci, and Blake S. Wilson. Lippincott Williams & Wilkins, Philadelphia © 2000.

Results and Outcomes of Cochlear Implantation

10

Challenges in the Clinical Investigation of Cochlear Implant Outcomes

Cochlear implantation has been an approved method of treatment for persons with profound deafness since the mid-1980s (House and Berliner, 1991). Since that time, clinicians and researchers have seen great changes in the field. Continued technologic developments in the design of cochlear implant systems have brought us from the first device approved by the U.S. Food and Drug Administration (FDA), the 3M/House single-channel cochlear implant (Fretz and Fravel, 1985), to the present, when there are several commercially available, multichannel cochlear implant devices.

The criteria for candidacy also have evolved. Only adults with postlingual, profound deafness were considered suitable candidates in the early days of cochlear implantation; prelingually deafened children as young as 18 months of age now may be cochlear implant recipients.

Evolving technology and changes in candidacy criteria have prompted concomitant developments in measures of postimplantation performance. In the face of these changes, one fact remains constant: the benefits of

cochlear implantation vary tremendously across individuals. The range of receptive communication is wide even among users of the same cochlear implant system with similar otologic histories. Among adults and children, some cochlear implant recipients demonstrate substantial open-set speech recognition, whereas others may not consistently discriminate certain speech features when they are presented in a limited, closed set. This variability raises a number of questions concerning the outcomes of cochlear implantation. How do we evaluate the benefits of cochlear implants in such a heterogeneous population? What constitutes success with a cochlear implant? What factors are key in making precise predictions of postimplantation benefits? This chapter considers some of the challenges inherent in the clinical investigation of cochlear implants and reviews the results of cochlear implantation in adults and children.

CHALLENGES IN THE CLINICAL INVESTIGATION OF COCHLEAR IMPLANTS

Determining the benefits of cochlear implant use by adults and children is essential to the clinical care of implant patients and to re-

K. I. Kirk: Department of Otolaryngology, Indiana University, Indianapolis, Indiana 46202.

searching new directions for deafness rehabilitation (Robbins and Kirk, 1996). For
adults and children with postlingual deafness, the evaluation of speech perception
abilities before and after implantation provides important clinical information about
progress over time and about the need for
adjusting the speech processor settings. A
more extensive battery of outcome measures
is needed to assess the potential benefits of
cochlear implant use in children with prelingual or early-acquired deafness. These children must use the auditory information from
a cochlear implant to aid in spoken word
recognition, to develop intelligible speech
production abilities and to acquire spoken
language. For such children, periodic assessments of their speech perception, speech
production, and language skills provide
clinical information that is needed for determining the goals of aural rehabilitation
and selecting appropriate educational programs.

The assessment of cochlear implant benefits has important research implications as
well. Empirical data concerning the benefits
of implantation are used to modify candidacy
criteria, to evaluate the effectiveness of different cochlear implant systems and speech
processing strategies, and to identify patient
and treatment characteristics that maximize
performance. Because improvements in
communication abilities emerge over time
after cochlear implant use, longitudinal studies are needed to determine the ultimate benefits of cochlear implants. This is especially
true when investigating the effects of cochlear implant use by children with prelingual deafness.

EVOLUTIONARY NATURE OF COCHLEAR IMPLANT RESEARCH

The evolution of cochlear implant technology and cochlear implant candidacy criteria
offers a particular set of challenges for clinical researchers. Longitudinal studies of an
intervention that is continually evolving can
put into competition the adequacy of re-

search design and the relevance of observations. Ideally, researchers would like to examine the effects of cochlear implant use in
a large group of individuals while holding all
other subject factors constant. New cochlear
implant systems or new speech processing
strategies for existing cochlear implant systems offer the possibility of improved patient
performance, but they also introduce additional sources of variability into a study design. Researchers sometimes must choose
between monitoring the progress of patients
who started implant use with older processing strategies and initiating new studies
with users of current implant technology. As
new studies are initiated, researchers may
have difficulty recruiting enough participants
to effectively evaluate performance differences between implant systems.

Criteria for cochlear implant candidacy
also have evolved. In the early days of cochlear implantation, clinicians and researchers were uncertain of the benefits that might
be obtained from the relatively simple single-
channel implant systems. Only adults with
postlingual, total deafness were considered
for implantation. These patients had nothing
to lose from placing an implant array within
the cochlea because they received no benefit
from conventional hearing aids. Initial subjects selected as candidates were postlingually deafened and could compare the
sound perceived through an implant to their
memory for speech. To determine the benefits of cochlear implantation in this population, researchers generally conducted within-
subject longitudinal studies wherein each
participant served as his or her own control.
Preimplantation speech perception abilities
were compared with performance on the
same tasks measured at periodic postimplantation intervals.

As clinicians and researchers learned more
about the benefits of cochlear implant use,
implantation was extended to children with
prelingual deafness and to listeners with severe to profound hearing losses who obtained some minimal benefit from their hearing aids. Current FDA guidelines permit the

implantation of children as young as 18 months of age, and many suitable cochlear implant recipients demonstrate some level of aided open-set word recognition (*i.e.*, 30% correct on tests of word [within sentence] recognition) before implantation.

The procedures for determining benefit and defining appropriate control groups have evolved along with candidacy criteria. In children, postimplantation improvements in communication abilities may result from implant use, from maturation, or from their combined effects. The use of a within-subject design to assess cochlear implant performance does not permit researchers to separate the effects of maturation and cochlear implant use. Osberger *et al.* were among the first to address this problem. They compared the communication abilities of children with cochlear implants to those of age-matched children with similar hearing thresholds who used other sensory aids, such as hearing aids or vibrotactile aids (Miyamoto *et al.*, 1996; Miyamoto *et al.*, 1989; Osberger *et al.*, 1991; Osberger *et al.*, 1996). This remains the preferred approach to determining cochlear implant benefit. However, the audiologic characteristics of the control groups have evolved as patients with more residual hearing have been implanted.

SELECTING APPROPRIATE OUTCOME MEASURES

The individual variability among cochlear implant recipients in terms of their demographic characteristics (*e.g.*, age, residual hearing) and their speech perception, production, and language skills presents challenges to researchers in the selection of appropriate outcome measures. The primary benefit of cochlear implant use for adults with profound, postlingual deafness is improved speech perception and spoken word recognition. In contrast, cochlear implantation in children may have a profound impact on all aspects of communication, and the assessment battery employed for children should be broad enough to reflect these

changes. Clinical researchers must have available a wide array of age-appropriate outcome measures that allows them to target different aspects of communication development.

Speech Perception Outcome Measures: Considerations

A speech perception test battery should permit the evaluation of a hierarchy of skills, ranging from discrimination of vowel and consonant speech features through the comprehension of connected speech. Several methodologic factors are likely to affect results. These include the method of stimulus presentation, the response format of the tests, the use of competing noise during stimulus presentation, and the sensory modality in which the speech signal is presented.

Recorded vs. Live-Voice Stimulus Presentations

The use of recordings as opposed to live voice administration of speech perception tests has been widely debated. Proponents of recorded materials point out that speakers differ, and therefore results obtained with live voice presentation are not comparable across clinics or research centers unless speaker equivalence can be demonstrated. Subtle changes in presentation may improve performance over the testing interval. Several clinicians and researchers have argued that consistency in presentation between listeners or over time can be maintained only through the use of recorded test stimuli (Carhart, 1965; Mendel and Danhauer, 1997). However, there may be as much difference between recordings as between two different talkers administering live-voice tests. Live-voice testing provides greater flexibility for the examiner. It often takes less time than using recorded versions. In general, the use of recorded tests is preferred for assessing performance in adults so that results can be compared across centers and testing intervals. Very young children frequently require flexible testing situations.

The need to customize the length and pace of testing often necessitates live-voice testing.

Open-Set vs. Closed-Set Test Formats

Most cochlear implant test batteries use open-set and closed-set test measures of speech understanding in auditory-only conditions. Open-set tests are those in which the listener theoretically has an unlimited number of response possibilities. On hearing the test item, no response alternatives are provided and the listener typically repeats what is heard. Closed-set tests are those that restrict the listener to one of a fixed number of possible responses (*e.g.*, a multiple-choice test).

Open-set tests are advantageous in that the demands simulate those encountered in natural listening situations. For example, performance on open-set tests of spoken word recognition is influenced by cognitive (top-down) processing, just as is real-world speech comprehension. Cognitive processing is facilitated by an individual's general knowledge (including vocabulary and linguistic knowledge), and by expectations based on the situational (*i.e.*, the who, what, where, and why) and linguistic context of the speech event.

Sometimes, researchers wish to evaluate an individual's sensory capabilities without the influence of cognitive factors (Tyler, 1993). For example, researchers may wish to determine which speech features are well conveyed by a particular cochlear implant system. Closed-set tests of word or nonsense syllable recognition assess speech feature perception in the absence of cognitive influences. The target speech signal is embedded among foils that are acoustically or phonetically similar. Such closed-set tests of speech feature perception also are useful in assessing implant performance in those with minimal open-set speech understanding through audition alone. These listeners may have fairly good speech understanding when certain speech features that are well conveyed by the cochlear implant (*e.g.*, manner of consonant articulation) are combined with lip-reading cues.

Use of Competing Noise

Administering tests of speech perception and spoken word recognition in quiet yields estimates of speech understanding under optimum listening situations. However, it may not accurately estimate performance in daily living where there are many sources of competing noise. Test administration in quiet may produce ceiling effects for cochlear implant recipients with excellent spoken word recognition. Conversely, for adults with poor speech understanding, testing only in noise can produce floor effects. Ceiling and floor effects can interfere with a clinician's decision regarding the best device settings. These effects can also reduce the accuracy with which researchers identify and weight factors that affect performance. Whenever possible, it is best to evaluate word recognition in quiet and in noise.

Multimodal Speech Perception

Information in the speech signal is conveyed through the auditory and visual modalities. Listeners with cochlear implants differ greatly in their ability to understand speech through listening alone and in their ability to integrate auditory and visual speech information. Perceptual performance can be assessed using auditory-only, visual-only, and auditory-plus-visual modalities. Results from independent-modality and multimodality testing provide information about how well speech is conveyed through an implant alone and about the speech perception enhancement obtained when auditory and visual cues are combined. Assessing performance in the auditory-plus-visual modality may better estimate real-world performance when modes of speech information are available.

Speech Perception Outcome Measures for Adults

Ideally, researchers and clinicians evaluating the benefits of cochlear implants should use the same assessment materials and procedures so that results can be compared across centers and devices. Early researchers found that traditional audiologic tests such as the Northwestern University Auditory Test 6 (Tillman and Carhart, 1966) were too difficult for many of the initial cohort of implant candidates and recipients, and other test batteries were developed.

One of the first was the Minimal Auditory Capabilities (MAC) Battery (Owens *et al.*, 1985; Owens *et al.*, 1981). The MAC consisted of a hierarchy of 14 subtests (13 auditory subtests and 1 audiovisual enhancement subtest) assessing skills ranging from environmental sound recognition and closed-set suprasegmental speech perception through open-set word and sentence recognition. The MAC was suitable for adults with widely varying skills, but it had several drawbacks. One was that the sound quality of the original version was poor. Second, administration of the MAC battery took approximately 2 to 3 hours, making it difficult to use clinically.

To address these problems, researchers at The University of Iowa developed their own battery of tests (Tyler *et al.*, 1983). Some of the subtests were the same as those in the MAC battery. However, the Iowa cochlear implant tests yielded additional information about patient performance. This speech perception test battery used laser videodisc technology so that many of the subtests could be administered in the auditory-only, visual-only, and auditory-plus-visual modalities, including tests of vowel and consonant recognition, and two tests of sentence recognition. Like the MAC battery, the Iowa speech perception battery required several hours to complete if all subtests were administered.

As speech perception performance by adults with cochlear implants improved through the late 1980s and early 1990s, many of the relatively simple tests of closed-set speech perception became obsolete. Most adult cochlear implant recipients could be tested with more standard open-set tests of word and sentence recognition.

There was a need for a relatively brief assessment battery that could be used in busy clinical settings.

A subcommittee of the American Academy of Otolaryngology—Head and Neck Surgery met with representatives of cochlear implant manufacturers and the FDA to select a minimum battery of speech perception tests for adults with cochlear implants. Their goal was to facilitate the comparison of results across centers and cochlear implant systems through the use of a standard test battery of speech perception. This battery consists of one monosyllabic word recognition test, the Consonant–Nucleus–Consonant (CNC) word lists (Lehiste and Peterson, 1959; Peterson and Lehiste, 1962), and one sentence test, The Hearing in Noise Test (HINT) (Nilsson *et al.*, 1994).

Clinicians may wish to use additional tests to evaluate performance when assessing adults with limited open-set word recognition through audition alone. For example, closed-set tests of speech feature or word recognition from the MAC or Iowa speech perception batteries and tests of audiovisual speech recognition such as the City University of New York (CUNY) Sentences (Boothroyd *et al.*, 1985) provide useful information about speech understanding and audiovisual speech enhancement. A detailed description of other test measures that are suitable for adults has been provided by Mendel and Danhauer (1997).

Outcome Measures for Children

Children with cochlear implants must use the sound they receive to acquire speech production and spoken language skills. Although measures of speech perception may be the most direct method of determining cochlear implant benefits (Tyler, 1993), they alone are not adequate. We must consider also the impact of cochlear implant use on the development of other communication abilities, and subsequently on the educational options available to children with cochlear implants. In this section we examine several approaches to assessing speech perception and speech production by children with cochlear implants. The development of language abilities is addressed in Chapters 12 and 13.

Speech Perception Test Batteries

Two general approaches have been followed in the development of a speech perception battery for children with profound deafness who use cochlear implants or other sensory aids. One approach, followed by Geers *et al.* (Geers and Moog, 1989) at the Central Institute for the Deaf (CID), assumes that children acquire speech perception abilities in a hierarchical fashion starting from simple detection through spoken word comprehension (Erber, 1982). Test administration follows this hierarchy, and children are required to reach criterion scores at each level before being administered more difficult measures. The outcome of this testing is used to categorize the children's speech perception abilities and determine auditory training goals.

Table 10.1 presents the CID speech perception categories and Table 10.2 lists the

tests in the CID battery. An advantage of the hierarchical approach is that less time is required to complete testing. This may be especially important for assessing young children with limited attention spans. The disadvantages of hierarchical testing and categorization of results are twofold. First, some skills may develop in parallel rather than hierarchically, and administering only part of a test battery might not reveal the development of more sophisticated listening skills. Second, categorizing children's responses often obscures individual differences in performance and makes it more difficult to identify factors that influence spoken word recognition (Tyler, 1993).

A second approach, described by Kirk *et al.* (1997), makes no *a priori* assumptions concerning the sequence of auditory skill development. Instead, children are administered a battery of tests that evaluate a range of speech perception abilities and are then assigned scores for each test in the battery. The speech perception batteries employed at Indiana University School of Medicine (IUSM) exemplify this latter approach and permit researchers to describe all aspects of a child's communication. There are two batteries, one for children younger than 6 years (Preschool Battery) and one for children 6 years or older (School-Age Battery). Tables 10.3 and 10.4 list the measures in the two IUSM speech perception batteries.

The CID and IUSM speech perception test batteries assess skills using closed-set and open-set test formats. Both also evaluate performance in the auditory-only, visual-only, and auditory-plus-visual modalities to measure speech perception enhancement. Because the speech perception tasks and materials must be appropriate for the age, developmental and linguistic levels of the children being tested, the CID and IUSM batteries have separate tasks for very young children and older, school-aged children. Table 10.2 lists the speech perception and lipreading measures for the CID battery; the IUSM speech perception batteries are presented in Tables 10.3 and 10.4. A more de-

TABLE 10.1 *Central Institute for the Deaf speech perception categories*

Category	Speech Perception Skills
0	No detection of speech (*e.g.*, aided speech detection threshold >65-dB HL)
1	Speech detection
2	Pattern perception (discrimination based on temporal or stress cues; *e.g.*, airplane versus baby)
3	Beginning word identification (closed-set word identification based on phoneme information; *e.g.*, airplane versus lunch box)
4	Word identification through vowel recognition (closed-set word identification based on vowel information; *e.g.*, boat versus bat)
5	Word identification through consonant recognition (closed-set word identification based on consonant information; *e.g.*, pear versus chair)
6	Open-set word recognition (word recognition without contextual cues through listening alone)

Adapted from Geers, 1994.

TABLE 10.2 *The Central Institute for the Deaf speech perception and lip-reading enhancement battery*

Test	Stimulus	Presentation	Response format	Perceptual skill
Speech detection threshold	Speech	Auditory only	Closed-set	Detection
ESP[a] Test	Patterns (1-, 2-, or 3-syllable words)	Auditory only	Closed-set	Word ID (stress and duration cues)
	Spondees	Auditory only	Closed-set	Word ID (spectral cues)
	Monosyllables	Auditory only	Closed-set	Word ID (vowel cues)
WIPI[b]	Monosyllables	Auditory only	Closed-set	Word ID (consonant cues)
Matrix test[c]	Phrases	Auditory only	Closed-set	Word ID in phrases
Phonetic task evaluation[d]	Syllables	Auditory only	Closed-set	Speech feature discrimination
PBK[e]	Monosyllables	Auditory only	Open-set	Word recognition
GAEL-P[f]	Words	Auditory; auditory + visual	Closed-set	Word ID
Craig Lip-reading Inventory[g]	Monosyllabic words	Auditory; auditory + visual	Closed-set	Word ID
	Sentences	Auditory; auditory + visual	Closed-set	Sentence ID
Monsen sentences[h]	Sentences	Auditory; auditory + visual	Open-set	Word recognition in simple sentences
CID sentences[i]	Sentences	Auditory; auditory + visual	Open-set	Word recognition in complex sentences
CUNY sentences[j]	Stories	Auditory; auditory + visual	Open-set	Connected discourse recognition

CID, Central Institute for the Deaf; CUNY, City University of New York; ESP, Early Speech Perception test; GAEL-P, Grammatical Analysis of Elicited Language—Presentence Level; ID, identification; PBK, Phonetically Balanced Kindergarten word list; WIPI, Word Intelligibility by Picture Identification.
[a]Moog and Geers, 1990.
[b]Ross and Lerman, 1979.
[c]Tyler and Holsted, 1978.
[d]Mecklenburg *et al.*, 1987.
[e]Haskins, 1949.
[f]Moog *et al.*, 1983.
[g]Craig, 1992.
[h]Monsen, 1978.
[i]Davis and Silverman, 1978.
[j]Boothroyd *et al.*, 1985.
Adapted from Geers, 1994.

tailed description of these test batteries is offered by Kirk *et al.* (1997).

Speech Production Test Batteries

A battery of tests often is used to assess a wide range of speech production skills in children with cochlear implants. One common approach is to evaluate vowel and consonant production in a variety of tasks ranging from imitation of nonsense syllables through elicited and spontaneous productions in words and sentences (Tobey *et al.*, 1994). As Tobey (1993) pointed out, imitation is an important task because the examiner knows the phonologic structure of the target and can compare the stimulus and the uttered response. Speech tasks that elicit productions (such as picture naming or object description) require

TABLE 10.3 *The Indiana University preschool speech perception battery*

Test	Stimulus	Presentation	Response format	Perceptual skill
SCIPS[a]	1-, 2-, or 3-syllable words	Auditory[b]	Closed-set	Pattern perception; word identification
GAEL-P[c]	1-, 2-, or 3-syllable words	Auditory[b]	Closed-set object selection	Word identification
Mr. Potato Head task[d]	Mr. Potato Head and his "Bucket of Parts" toy	Auditory[b]	Modified open-set	Key word identification; sentence comprehension
PSI[e]	Single words and sentences	Auditory only[b]; visual only; auditory[b] and visual	Closed-set	Word and sentence identification
MAIS[f]	10 probes	Structured interview	Parent report	Detection through comprehension in daily living situations

SCIPS, Screening Inventory of Perceptual Skills; GAEL-P, Grammatical Analysis of Elicited Language-Presentence Level; PSI, Pediatric Speech Intelligibility Test; MAIS, Meaningful Auditory Integration Scale.
[a]Osberger et al., 1991.
[b]Administered by means of live voice.
[c]Moog *et al.*, 1983.
[d]Robbins, 1994.
[e]Jerger *et al.*, 1980.
[f]Robbins *et al.*, 1991.

the child to produce target sounds in the absence of a model from the examiner. Spontaneous samples provide a representative sample of the child's usual speech. When assessing speech production skills, it is common for the examiner to score the child's responses on-line or to record the responses for later transcription by another clinician. This type of scoring may be influenced by the examiner's familiarity with the child or with the speech of other deaf talkers. An additional approach followed at IUSM is to record children's productions and play them later to listeners who are unfamiliar with the speech of children with profound deafness. These naive listeners are asked to record in

TABLE 10.4 *Indiana University school-age speech perception battery*

Test	Stimulus	Presentation	Response format	Perceptual skill
Minimal Pairs Test[a]	1-syllable words	Auditory[b]	Closed-set	Word discrimination based on vowel and consonant features
MLNT[c]	2-, 3-syllable words	Auditory	Open-set	Word identification
LNT[c]	1-syllable words	Auditory[d]	Open-set	Word identification
PB-K[e]	1-syllable words	Auditory*	Open-set	Word identification
Common phrases[e]	2- to 6-word phrases	Auditory only[b]; visual only; auditory[b] + visual	Open-set	Sentence identification

MLNT, Multisyllabic Lexical Neighborhood Test; LNT, Lexical Neighborhood Test; PBK, Phonetically Balanced Kindergarten word list.
[a]Robbins *et al.*, 1988.
[b]Administered by means of live voice.
[c]Kirk *et al.*, 1995.
[d]Recorded word lists.
[e]Haskins, 1949.
[f]Robbins *et al.*, 1995.

writing the children's utterances, and their written responses are scored as the percent of words correctly identified. Such scores may yield better estimates of the children's speech intelligibility to unfamiliar listeners. It is beneficial to have productions scored by familiar and unfamiliar listeners. Table 10.5 lists the speech production tasks included in the IUSM Speech Production Battery.

Accounting for Individual Variability in Performance

Results obtained from previous studies concerning cochlear implant benefits highlight one of the most important challenges facing clinical researchers: how to account for the individual variability in performance across adults with postlingual deafness (*e.g.*, Cohen *et al.*, 1993; Dorman *et al.*, 1989; Gantz *et al.*, 1988) and across children with prelingual deafness (*e.g.*, Miyamoto *et al.*, 1989; Osberger *et al.*, 1991; Staller *et al.*, 1991). This variability makes it difficult to compare the relative benefits of different cochlear implant

systems or to predict who might benefit most from cochlear implantation.

Previous investigations have attempted to account for variability among adult listeners by focusing on sensory and neural factors that can influence performance in the early stages of perceptual processing. For example, electrically evoked auditory brain stem responses have been used to investigate the effects of cochlear nerve survival in adults (Simmons *et al.*, 1984; Gantz *et al.*, 1988; Kileny *et al.*, 1991; Kileny *et al.*, 1994) and pyschophysical tests have been used to evaluate the relationship between temporal processing and word recognition in adults with cochlear implants (Hochmair-Desoyer *et al.*, 1985; Shannon, 1993). Previous clinical researchers have focused on the study of demographic variables (such as age at onset of hearing loss or length of profound deafness) in predicting or explaining individual variability (Gantz *et al.*, 1993; Miyamoto *et al.*, 1994). Peripheral processing and demographic variables play a role in successful implant use. However, these factors appear

TABLE 10.5 *Indiana University School of Medicine speech production battery*

Test	Targeted production	Production task	Transcribed	Production skill
Nonsense Imitative Test of Syllables[a]	CV syllables	Imitation of examiner's spoken model	Clinician	Vowel and consonant feature production
Minimal Pairs II[b]	CVC words	Elicited (picture naming)	Clinician	Production of vowel and consonant contrasts
Goldman Fristoe Test of Articulation[c]	Isolated words	Elicited (picture naming)	Clinician	Vowel and consonant production by word position
Beginner's Intelligibility Test[d] **or**	Sentences	Elicited (object description)	3 naive listeners	Word intelligibility
Monsen sentences[e]	Sentence	Elicited (written sentences)	3 naive listeners	Word intelligibility
Meaningful Use of Speech Scale[f]	This parent questionnaire uses a structured interview to evaluate the children's speech production skills in daily living situations			

CV, consonant-vowel; CVC, consonant-vowel-consonant.
[a]Robbins and Osberger, 1987.
[b]Robbins *et al.*, 1988.
[c]Goldman and Fristoe, 1972.
[d]Osbergeret *et al.*, 1994.
[e]Monsen, 1978.
[f]Robbins and Osberger, 1991.

to account for only some of the variability in speech perception achieved by adults or children with cochlear implants.

Investigators have begun to examine the role of more central speech processing capabilities (such as lexical access and perceptual normalization) or cognitive factors (such as attention or working memory capacity) that may underlie superior cochlear implant performance (Kirk *et al.*, 1995; Knutson *et al.*, 1991; Pisoni and Geers, 1998). Other investigators (Pisoni *et al.*, 1997) have attempted to identify the factors underlying superior implant performance in children by examining the relationship among spoken word recognition, speech intelligibility, and spoken language processing in children with superior spoken word recognition abilities. Through such studies, researchers hope to learn more about the underlying perceptual factors employed in spoken word recognition and how these processes contribute to individual differences in performance. The following sections review the audiologic results of cochlear implant use in adults and children and consider factors that contribute to superior speech understanding in listeners with cochlear implants.

RESULTS OF COCHLEAR IMPLANTATION IN ADULTS

Speech Perception Performance

Single-Channel Cochlear Implant Systems

Two single-channel cochlear implant systems were used in the United States, the 3M/House device (Fretz and Fravel, 1985) and the 3M/Vienna cochlear implant (Hochmair and Hochmair-Desoyer, 1983). Patients who had been totally deaf before implantation demonstrated a number of auditory skills with these devices. These patients could detect speech at well below conversational levels (Tyler *et al.*, 1985) and identify environmental sounds with a fair degree of accuracy (Gantz *et al.*, 1988). Subjects appeared to discriminate some vowels from a closed-set based primarily on fundamental frequency

(Gantz *et al.*, 1989) or first formant cues (Dorman, 1993; Tyler *et al.*, 1989) and discriminate some consonants from a closed-set based on duration and voicing distinctions (Gantz *et al.*, 1989). Few patients demonstrated open-set speech understanding with these single-channel devices (Gantz *et al.*, 1988; Tye-Murray and Tyler, 1989), but many obtained substantial improvements in speech recognition when the auditory signal received through an implant was combined with lip-reading cues (Gantz *et al.*, 1988; Tyler *et al.*, 1985).

Multichannel Cochlear Implant Systems

Multichannel, multi-electrode cochlear implant systems are designed to take advantage of the tonotopic organization of the cochlea to encode spectral (frequency) cues. The incoming speech signal is filtered into frequency bands, each corresponding to a given electrode in the electrode array. Multichannel cochlear implant systems use place coding to convey spectral information in the speech signal in addition to the durational and intensity cues provided by single channel systems. Three cochlear implant systems have received FDA approval and are commercially available in the United States. Each of these multichannel cochlear implant systems differs in electrode design and in the signal processing strategies that may be used.

Nucleus Cochlear Implant Systems

Two of the FDA-approved cochlear implants, the Nucleus 22-channel cochlear implant system (Clark *et al.*, 1981) and the Nucleus-24 channel cochlear implant system, are manufactured by Cochlear Corporation. The Nucleus 22-channel cochlear implant system was the first cochlear implant to receive FDA approval for use in adults and children. It has been used by more patients than any other cochlear implant system. More than 20,000 Nucleus cochlear implants have been implanted worldwide (Patty Arndt, personal communication). The Nucleus 24-channel cochlear implant received FDA approval for adults and children in June 1998. As of July 1998, 1,079 adults (18 years of age or older) have received this system (Fig. 10.1).

Several generations of speech processors were designed for use with the Nucleus 22-channel cochlear implant. The early speech processing strategies used a feature-extraction scheme that conveyed information about key speech features. The F0F2 strategy presented three acoustic features of speech: the amplitude of the waveform presented as the amount of current charge, fundamental frequency (F0) presented as the rate of pulsatile stimulation, and the spectral range of the second formant frequency presented by varying the site of stimulation along the electrode array (Hollow *et al.*, 1995). In the F0F1F2 strategy that followed, an additional stimulating electrode was added to present information about the spectral range of the first formant frequency. The performance of patients who used these processing strategies was superior to that demonstrated previously by patients with single-channel cochlear implants (Cohen *et al.*, 1993; Gantz *et al.*, 1988; Gantz *et al.*, 1989). Vowel recognition was generally superior to consonant recognition with these multichannel speech processing strategies. For example, Blamey *et al.* (1987) reported mean vowel recognition scores of 49% compared with 37% for consonant recognition. Blamey and Clark (1990) reported that vowel recognition by cochlear implant users with the F0F1F2 strategy could be accounted for in large part by the place coding of the first and second formant frequencies. Using information transmission analysis (Miller and Nicely, 1955) of patients' consonant confusions, Tye-Murray *et al.* (1992) found that the consonant features of envelope cues, nasality, frication and voicing were relatively well conveyed by the F0F1F2 processing strategy; place of articulation cues were not well conveyed. In contrast to patients with single channel cochlear implants, most patients with the F0F1F2 processing strategy demonstrated at least some open-set speech recognition (Dowell *et al.*, 1986; Gantz *et al.*, 1988; Hollow *et al.*, 1995; Tyler and Lowder, 1992). Hollow

et al. (1995) reported that the percent of words correctly identified in a sentence context by patients with the F0F1F2 processing strategy ranged from 2% to 98%, with a mean of 38.5% words correct.

The third-generation feature-extraction coding strategy was the Multipeak (MPEAK) strategy. Parkinson *et al.* (1996) referred to this as the F0F1F2B3B4B5 processing strategy because in addition to estimating fundamental frequency and the first and second formant frequencies, higher frequency information was encoded by stimulating two of three more basal, fixed electrodes. The goal of the MPEAK strategy was to provide additional information that would yield improved consonant recognition scores. Parkinson *et al.* (1996) reported that other vowel and consonant recognition scores did not differ significantly between the F0F1F2 and the MPEAK strategies. However, a number of studies demonstrated that open-set word and sentence recognition was significantly higher with the MPEAK than with the F0F1F2 processing strategy (Hollow *et al.*, 1995; Parkinson *et al.*, 1996; Skinner *et al.*, 1991). Skinner *et al.* (1991) reported that monosyllabic word recognition increased from 14% with the F0F1F2 strategy to 29% correct with the MPEAK strategy. Hollow *et al.* (1995) reported that patients with the MPEAK strategy correctly recognized from 1% to 100% of words presented in sentences, with a mean of 59.1% words correct. Dorman (1993) suggested that closed-set tests of phoneme recognition might not be sensitive enough to detect improvements in the perception of consonant features provided by the MPEAK strategy.

The latest speech processing strategy developed by Cochlear Corporation is the spectral peak (SPEAK) strategy. This strategy received FDA approval for use with the Nucleus 22-channel system in 1994 and is one strategy currently provided with the Nucleus 24 implant system. In contrast to the previous generations of Nucleus speech processors, the SPEAK strategy does not employ a feature extraction scheme. This strategy filters

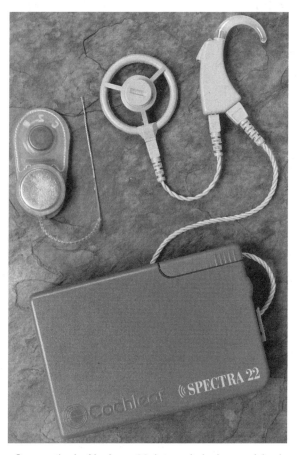

A

FIG. 10.1. A: Cochlear Corporation's Nucleus 22 internal device and body-worn processor. **B:** Cochlear Corporation's Nucleus 24 internal device ear-level (Esprit) processor. **C:** Cochlear Corporation's Nucleus 24 body-worn (SPRINT) process.

the incoming speech signal into 20 frequency bands. The filter bank is repetitively scanned at an adaptive rate, and the largest outputs of these filters are then presented to stimulating electrode pairs. On each stimulation cycle the number of electrodes stimulated may vary from 1 to 10, with an average of six electrodes stimulated. The rate of stimulation varies adaptively between 180 and 300 pulses per second.

A number of investigators have demonstrated that the performance of patients using the SPEAK strategy is superior to that obtained with the MPEAK processing strategies (Holden *et al.*, 1997; Hollow *et al.*, 1995; Keifer *et al.*, 1996; Skinner *et al.*, 1996; Staller

et al., 1997; Whitford *et al.*, 1995). According to Holden *et al.* (1997), average monosyllabic word recognition scores were 13% higher with the SPEAK strategy than with the MPEAK; mean word recognition in sentences improved by approximately 35% words correct. Whitford *et al.* (1995) reported that the largest improvements were seen for sentence recognition in noise. Staller *et al.* (1997) described the performance of 73 adults with postlingual deafness who were consecutively implanted with a Nucleus cochlear implant and tested while using the SPEAK processing strategy. These investigators reported that patients demonstrated a rapid acquisition of open-set speech recognition

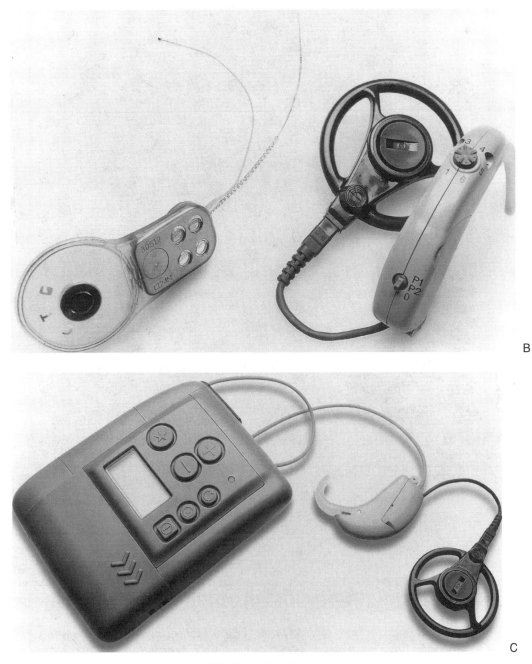

FIG. 10.1. (*Continued*)

skills in the initial postoperative period. After two weeks of implant use the mean sentence recognition score was 54% words correct. After six months of device experience, the adults correctly recognized an average of 36% of the monosyllabic words, and an average of 74% of the words presented in sentences.

Clarion Cochlear Implant System

The third commercially available device is the Clarion multichannel cochlear implant

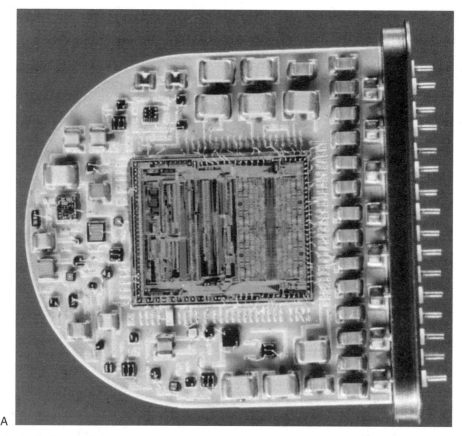

A

FIG. 10.2. A: Internal circuitry of the Advanced Bionics (Clarion) cochlear receiver/stimulator. **B:** Advanced Bionics (Clarion) implantable device and body-worn processor. **C:** Advanced Bionics (Clarion) ear-level processor.

system (Schindler and Kessler, 1987; Kessler and Schindler, 1994; Schindler and Kessler, 1993) manufactured by the Advanced Bionics Corporation (Fig. 10.2). This device has been approved by the FDA for use in adults (1996) and children (1997). Approximately 3,000 patients worldwide have received the Clarion cochlear implant. About 40% of these patients were implanted as adults (D. Kessler, personal communication).

The Clarion multichannel cochlear implant has an eight-channel electrode array that uses a radial bipolar configuration. Electrode pairs are positioned adjacent to the osseous spiral lamina in a 90-degree orientation (Schindler and Kessler, 1987). Theoretically, the radial bipolar orientation is more beneficial in achieving channel separation.

The Clarion multichannel cochlear implant system originally offered two types of processing strategies, both of which were designed to convey information about the speech waveform (Wilson, 1993). No specific features of speech are extracted and encoded by these processing strategies. The compressed analog (CA) strategy first compresses the analog signal into the restricted range for electrical hearing and then filters the signal into a maximum of eight channels for simultaneous presentation to the corresponding electrodes. Speech information is conveyed by the relative amplitudes of information in each channel and the temporal

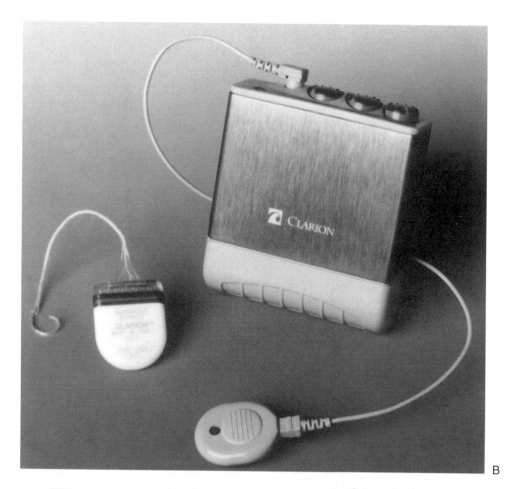

B

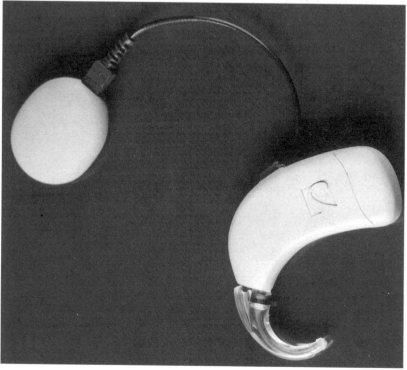

C

FIG. 10.2. (*Continued*)

details of the waveforms in each channel (Wilson et al., 1991). A new generation of the compressed analog system, the simultaneous analog strategy (SAS) has been introduced.

The other processing strategy available with the Clarion cochlear implant is the continuous interleaved sampling (CIS) strategy (Wilson et al., 1991). The CIS strategy filters the speech signal into eight bands, obtains the speech envelope, and then compresses the signal for each channel. On each cycle of stimulation, a series of interleaved digital pulses rapidly stimulates consecutive electrodes in the array. This sequential stimulation of the different electrodes in the array prevents channel interaction. The CIS strategy is designed to preserve fine temporal details in the speech signal by using high rate, pulsatile stimuli.

Most early Clarion cochlear implant users were fitted with the CIS processing strategy rather than the CA strategy (Battmer et al., 1995; Kessler et al., 1995; Tyler et al., 1996). According to Kessler et al. (1995), nearly 90% of the patients preferred the CIS speech processing strategy. Tyler et al. (1996) reported preliminary speech perception findings from 19 patients with the Clarion multichannel system who were implanted at the University of Iowa. Because of limitations in current output, only six patients could be fit successfully with the CA processing strategy. Average scores for these patients were approximately 60% correct for closed-set vowel and consonant recognition, 37% correct for open-set monosyllabic word recognition, and 61% words correct in open-set sentence contexts. Similar performance levels have been reported by other investigators. Doyle et al. (1995) examined closed-set consonant recognition by Clarion cochlear implant users who used the CA or the CIS processing strategy. On average, both groups correctly identified about 50% of the consonants presented in a closed-set format. Information transmission analysis revealed that duration was the best conveyed feature for the CA users (50%) with the features of place of articulation, manner of articulation, and nasality following (29%, 28%, and 27%, respectively). For users of the CIS strategy, the features of voicing, place of articulation and duration were among the best conveyed (41%, 40%, and 37%, respectively). Schindler et al. (1995) examined open-set word recognition performance in 40 adults with the Clarion implant. They reported mean word recognition scores of 30% correct for monosyllabic words and 60% words correct in sentences, scores that are similar to those from the Iowa study. Kessler (1998) reported that with the advent of Clarion electrode modifications (i.e., increasing the distance between contacts in bipolar pairs) more patients can be fit with the analog speech processing strategy, SAS. She reported that approximately 30% of the patients currently implanted with the Clarion system are choosing the SAS strategy rather than CIS. Osberger (1998) compared the word recognition performance of adults who preferred the SAS strategy (n = 11) with that of adults who preferred the CIS strategy (n = 16). She reported a trend toward improved performance for patients with the SAS strategy. Mean word recognition scores were 48% and 31% correct for users of the SAS and CIS strategies, respectively.

COMBI 40 Cochlear Implant System

Two additional cochlear implant systems, the COMBI 40H and COMBI 40+, manufactured by the Medical Electronics Corporation are currently undergoing FDA clinical trials in the United States. The COMBI 40H cochlear implant system has eight electrode pairs, whereas the COMBI 40+ has 12 electrode pairs and has the capability of deep electrode insertion into the apical regions of the cochlear (Gstöttner et al., 1997). Both devices use the CIS processing strategy and have the capacity to provide the most rapid stimulation rate of any of the cochlear implant systems currently available. More than 2,700 COMBI 40 cochlear implant systems are in use worldwide (D. Franz, personal communication). Of these about 1000 have been provided to children.

The Med-El cochlear implant systems have been used most widely in Europe. An extensive multicenter clinical study of patient performance with the 8-electrode system was conducted at 19 different centers; 16 of these centers were in German-speaking countries (Helms *et al.*, 1997). Participants in the study met the following inclusion criteria: 18 years of age or older, duration of deafness less than half the participant's lifetime, and preimplantation monosyllabic word recognition scores 10% or less correct. Sixty adults met these criteria and were included as participants (Fig. 10.3). Their speech recognition performance was assessed using closed-set vowel and consonant tests and using open-set tests of word and sentence recognition administered in each participant's native language (including German, English, Polish, and Hungarian). Participants were evaluated before implantation and then at 3, 6, and 12 months after implantation. Twenty-five participants had completed 12 months of device use at the time of the study. Results demonstrated that vowel and consonant recognition improved most during the first three months of cochlear implant use. In contrast, word and sentence recognition scores improved over the first year of device use. By 12 months after implantation, all participants scored near 30% correct for both vowel and consonant recognition. By 1 year after implantation, all subjects demonstrated some open-set speech understanding. Monosyllabic word recognition scores ranged from 5% to 85% correct, with a mean of 54%, and the percent of words correctly identified in a sentence context ranged from 30% to 100%, with a mean of 89%.

Factors Influencing Speech Perception by Adults

The results reported previously demonstrate that the current multichannel cochlear implant systems provide moderate open-set speech understanding, on average, to most adult users. However, there remains much variability in performance. The improvements gained with each new generation of the Nucleus processing strategy indicate that device characteristics do influence patient performance. However, within each device group, some adults are unable to understand any speech through listening alone, whereas others can communicate successfully on the telephone. As Wilson *et al.* (1993) pointed out, several within-subject factors also contribute to successful cochlear implant use.

Investigators have examined possible subject factors that may contribute to the observed variability in performance. Across these studies, the demographic factors of age at implantation and length of profound deafness are among the best predictors of performance. For example, Gantz *et al.* (1988) administered an extensive battery of tests covering audiologic thresholds, speech perception, cognition, electrophysiologic performance, psychophysics, psychologic measures of compliance, and demographic characteristics. There was a significant negative correlation between speech perception performance and age at implantation and duration of deafness. That is, the longer the period of profound deafness before implantation, the poorer the prognosis for achieving superior postimplantation speech perception abilities. The predictive power of these demographic factors has been demonstrated by other investigators as well (Battmer *et al.*, 1995; Blamey *et al.*, 1992; Cohen *et al.* 1993; Gantz *et al.*, 1993; Shipp and Nedzelski, 1995; Shipp *et al.*, 1997). However, these factors account for only part of the variance in cochlear implant patient performance. The findings regarding other predictive factors have been less conclusive. For example, Gantz *et al.* (1988) found that measures of cognitive ability were not associated with patient performance, whereas Cohen *et al.* (1993) reported that measures of IQ were significantly associated with good speech perception skills. Other factors that have been found to significantly correlate with adult outcomes include lip-reading ability (Cohen *et al.*, 1993; Gantz *et al.*, 1993), residual hearing before implantation (Gantz *et*

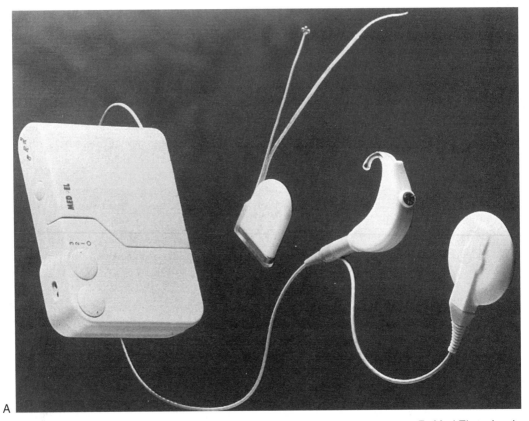

A

FIG. 10.3. A: Med El COMBI 40 implantable device and body-worn processors. **B:** Med El ear-level processor.

al., 1988; Gantz et al., 1993), gap detection abilities (Hochmair-Desoyer et al., 1985; Blamey et al., 1992), and greater dynamic ranges for intracochlear electrical stimulation (Blamey et al., 1992).

Auditory Brain Stem Implants

Conventional cochlear implants cannot be used by patients whose auditory nerve has been damaged during acoustic tumor removal (Dorman, 1993). An electrode array that can be placed on the cochlear nucleus has been designed for these patients. The first auditory brain stem implant was implanted by William House and William Hitselberger in 1979 (Edgerton et al., 1982). This first device was based on the 3M/House single-channel cochlear implant system and used the same speech processor. Patients

with this device had awareness of environmental sounds and obtained lip-reading enhancement. In 1992, a multichannel brain stem implant based on the Nucleus 22 channel cochlear implant was developed in a collaborative effort by the House Ear Institute, Cochlear Corporation and Huntington Medical Research Institute (Otto and Staller, 1995). This system combines the receiver/stimulator from the Nucleus multichannel cochlear implant system, an eight electrode surface array designed for the human cochlear nucleus and state of the art Nucleus speech processing strategies.

Clinical trials with the auditory brain stem implant were initiated in 1993. Original criteria for participation in the clinical trials included the following:

1. Diagnosis of Neurofibromatosis type 2

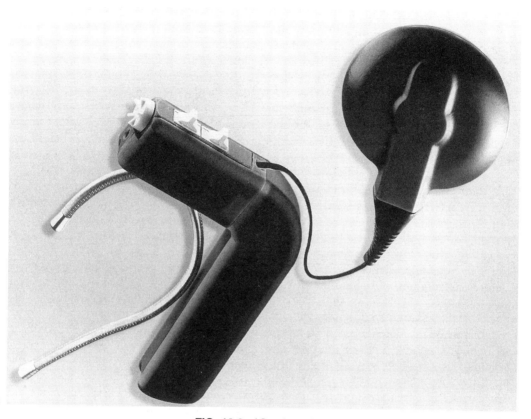

B

FIG. 10.3. (*Continued*)

2. Being in imminent need of removal of an eighth nerve tumor
3. Fifteen years of age or older
4. Competence in English
5. Reasonable expectations
6. Capable of complying with the investigational protocol

The criteria since have been modified to include patients 12 years of age and older. As of October 1998, 94 patients have been implanted in the United States, and approximately 40 more patients have been implanted in Europe (K. Evinger, personal communication). The performance of 20 patients who had used the mutichannel auditory brain stem implant for at least 3 months was summarized (Otto *et al.*, 1998). Three of these patients demonstrated sound-only sentence recognition (49% to 58% words cor-

rect). The most consistent benefits for the majority of recipients were environmental sound awareness, speech pattern perception, and enhanced lip-reading abilities. These benefits can yield substantial improvements in the quality of life experienced by users of the Nucleus auditory brain stem implant.

RESULTS OF COCHLEAR IMPLANTATION IN CHILDREN

Speech Perception Performance

Single-Channel Cochlear Implant Systems

In 1980, after extensive experience with the 3M/House single-channel cochlear implant system in adults, William House decided to expand his clinical cochlear implant program to include the implantation of children. The use of cochlear implants in children was quite controversial at that time. Many scientists believed that the limited auditory information provided by a single-channel cochlear implant was not sufficient for children to acquire speech perception and speech production abilities. However, Dr. House received approval to initiate FDA clinical trials for pediatric implantation and by 1984, 164 children were implanted. Most of these children were adventitiously deafened; their mean age at onset of hearing loss was 1.7 years, and their mean age at time of implantation was 8.4 years (Berliner and Eisenberg, 1985). Initial pediatric performance results were reported in 1985 by House, Berliner, and Eisenberg. Audiologic performance was similar to that of adults (Thielemeir et al., 1985). Before implantation, most children were unable to detect speech. With their cochlear implants, the children could recognize environmental sounds, detect speech at conversational levels, and perform auditory discriminations of different speech stress patterns (e.g., syllable number). Some children could discriminate among spondees presented in a closed-set, but most could not. Similarly, a few of the earlier-implanted children exhibited some open-set speech understanding, but most did not (Berliner et al., 1989). The FDA premarket approval process was never completed, and the 3M/House device never received approval for use in children.

Multichannel Cochlear Implant Systems

Nucleus Cochlear Implant Systems

Pediatric clinical trials with the Nucleus 22-channel cochlear implant began in 1986, and in 1990 the FDA approved this device for use in children. Children initially implanted with the Nucleus 22-channel system used the F0F1F2 feature extraction speech processing strategy. Children implanted after 1989 were provided with the MPEAK strategy, and the SPEAK strategy was approved in 1994. Pediatric clinical trials for the Nucleus 24-channel device with the SPEAK strategy were initiated in April, 1997 and FDA approval was

received in June, 1998. More than 1,700 children have been implanted with the Nucleus 24 channel system (P. Arndt, personal communication).

Early comparisons demonstrated that children with the Nucleus device obtained greater closed- and open-set speech perception abilities than children with the 3M/House device (Miyamoto et al. 1989; Miyamoto et al., 1992), but the number of participants in each group was relatively small. One of the first large-scale reports of pediatric performance with the Nucleus cochlear implant was presented by Staller et al. (1991). These investigators reported speech perception data from 80 children with the Nucleus 22-channel cochlear implant system who were tested as part of the FDA clinical trials. The mean age at onset of deafness was 2 years and 8 months, and the mean age at implantation was 9 years and 10 months for this group of children. The children's performance was classified by the highest category of speech perception achieved. Comparisons were made between their speech perception performance before implantation and again at 12 months after implantation. After 12 months of cochlear implant use, 63% of the children showed significant improvements in the closed-set speech perception tasks and 46% of the children demonstrated significant improvements on at least one open-set speech perception task. This improvement in open-set speech perception was encouraging, given that single channel implant systems yielded minimal open-set speech benefits. However, open-set speech abilities were still relatively modest. Children could correctly identify a mean of only 10% of the monosyllabic PB-K words.

Similar findings were reported by Osberger, Miyamoto et al. (1991) for 28 children who had used the Nucleus 22-channel implant for an average of 1.7 years. Most children (n = 23) used the F0F1F2 strategy and the remaining children used the MPEAK strategy. The children's speech perception abilities improved significantly after implantation; 17 of the children demonstrated open-set speech perception (at least one open-set score higher than 0%) through audition alone. The 28 children correctly identified an average of 71% of the sentences on the Common Phrases test presented in the auditory-plus-visual modality. Most children tested with the early Nucleus cochlear implant processing strategies demonstrated at least some open-set word recognition, and performance was generally good when auditory and visual cues were available.

The introduction of newer generation Nucleus processing strategies yielded greater speech perception benefits in children just as in adults. Osberger *et al.* (1996) compared the performance of six children who used the F0F1F2 processing strategy with that of six children who used the MPEAK strategy. The children in each group were matched by age at onset of deafness and age at implantation. After 1 year of implant use, the children with the MPEAK device were significantly better at discriminating vowel height and consonant place of articulation cues on the Minimal Pairs test. However, the two groups did not differ after 3 years of cochlear implant use. The investigators concluded that children show an accelerated rate of learning with improved speech processing strategies.

Similar improvements have been found for children who switch from the MPEAK to the SPEAK processing strategies. Cowan *et al.* (1995) and Cowan *et al.* (1997) compared the open-set recognition of words and sentences by children who converted from the MPEAK to the SPEAK strategy. Six subjects were tested in the first and 11 in the latter study. All subjects had more than 1 year of experience with MPEAK; only children who demonstrated some open-set word recognition in the auditory-only modality were included. In both studies, all but one participant recognized a significantly greater percent of words in noise with the SPEAK compared with the MPEAK processing strategy.

Sehgal *et al.* (1998) extended this investigation by comparing speech perception performance with a feature extraction strategy to that obtained with SPEAK in 11 children

who demonstrated a wide range of speech perception abilities with their earlier strategy. Before switching to the SPEAK strategy, three children used the F0F1F2 and eight children used the MPEAK strategy; they had used their original strategies for various periods (6 months to 6 years) before switching to the SPEAK strategy. The children demonstrated high levels of vowel and consonant feature discrimination on the Minimal Pairs Test (mean, 80% correct) with their original processing strategy but various amounts of open-set speech understanding. Figures 10.4 and 10.5 present the individual subjects open-set monosyllabic word and phoneme recognition, respectively, on the Lexical Neighborhood Test (LNT) before and after the signal processing conversion. Mean LNT word recognition scores improved significantly, from 28% words correct with the original strategy to 58% words correct with the SPEAK strategy. Nine of the 11 children showed significant improvements on at least one open-set speech perception test with the SPEAK processing strategy. Examination of data collected from the four most experienced users revealed distinct patterns of performance for children switching to SPEAK. Two of these children clearly benefited from using SPEAK, even one whose open-set skills with the MPEAK strategy had reached a plateau. In contrast, the child with minimal open-set skills showed no change in performance, and the last experienced a decrement in performance that did not return to MPEAK baseline levels until 2 years of SPEAK use. However, all children subjectively preferred the SPEAK strategy. Sehgal *et al.* (1998) concluded that one needs to consider a variety of factors, objective and subjective, when considering a change to a new speech perception strategy.

Clarion Cochlear Implant System

Pediatric clinical trials of the Clarion multichannel cochlear implant system began in 1995 and the device received FDA approval for use in children in 1997. Zimmerman-Phil-

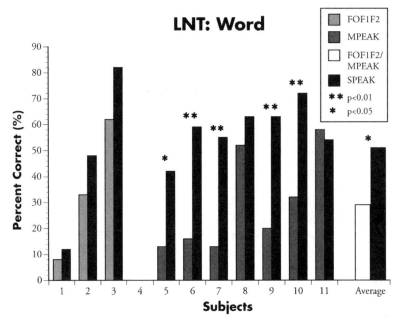

FIG. 10.4. Percentage of words correctly identified on the Lexical Neighborhood Test (LNT) with each processing strategy. Symbols above the bars for individual subjects represent a significant change in performance. (From Sehgal *et al.*, 1998, with permission.)

lips *et al.* (1997) summarized the initial results of the children's preoperative performance with hearing aids compared with their postoperative performance with the Clarion device. The mean age of the group of children implanted by 1996 was approximately 5 years ($n = 124$). Data were reported for children tested at 3 months after implantation ($n = 60$) and 6 months after implantation ($n = 23$). After only 3 months of device use, mean scores were higher than the preimplantation performance, and many of the children demonstrated some open-set speech recognition. By 6 months after implantation, mean word recognition scores were 23% for the PB-K and 38% for a test of word recognition in a sentence context, the Glendonald Auditory Screening Procedure (GASP) (Erber, 1982).

In a second study, Osberger *et al.* (1998) examined the performance of children implanted with the Clarion device after the age of 5 years who had at least six months of device experience ($n = 30$). The children were divided into two groups based on communication method. After 6 months of device use, children in the Oral group correctly identified an average of 27% of the words on the PB-K. The average PB-K word score for children in the Total Communication group was 8% correct.

COMBI 40 Cochlear Implant System

The pediatric FDA clinical trial for the COMBI 40 was initiated in 1998. As of Fall 1998, approximately 40 children in the United States have received this device. The clinical trial has not yet yielded sufficient data to draw conclusions regarding the benefits to be received by these children.

Speech Perception Performance in Children

In summary, children with multichannel cochlear implants demonstrate significant improvements in closed-set speech discrimination, enhanced lip-reading ability, and most

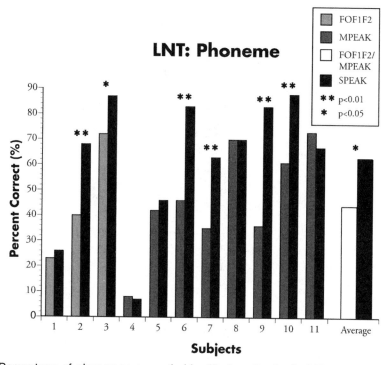

FIG. 10.5. Percentage of phonemes correctly identified on the Lexical Neighborhood Test (LNT) with each processing strategy. Symbols above the bars for individual subjects represent a significant change in performance. (From Sehgal *et al.*, 1998, with permission.)

obtain some open-set speech understanding with their devices. The rate of auditory skills development seems to be increasing as cochlear implant technology improves and children are implanted at a younger age. Early studies reported significant increases in the discrimination of nonsegmental speech cues after only six months of implant use. However, significant increases in the discrimination of vowels and consonant features were not evident until 1.5 years of cochlear implant experience and auditory-only open-set skills continued to improve long after this time period. Studies have shown that many children achieve open-set speech recognition within the first year of device use (Miyamoto, Kirk, Svirsky, and Sehgal, 1998; Osberger *et al.*, 1998), but these skills still continue to develop over time (Fryauf-Bertschy *et al.*, 1992; Fryauf-Bertschy *et al.*, 1997; Gantz *et al.*, 1994; Miyamoto *et al.*, 1994; Miyamoto *et al.*, 1996; Osberger *et al.*, 1996). Miyamoto *et al.* (1996) found continued improvements in spoken word recognition even after 5 years of multichannel cochlear implant use. These findings highlight the need to conduct longitudinal studies to determine the ultimate benefits of implant use in children.

Comparison of Sensory Aid Use in Children

Osberger *et al.* have conducted a number of studies at Indiana University School of Medicine to compare the the speech perception performance of pediatric cochlear implant users to that of their peers with mutichannel tactile aids or conventional hearing aids (Kirk *et al.*, 1995; Miyamoto *et al.*, 1994; Miyamoto *et al.*, 1995; Miyamoto *et al.*, 1996; Osberger *et al.*, 1991; Osberger *et al.*, 1996). A similar study was conducted by Geers and

Moog (1994) at the Central Institute for the Deaf in St. Louis. In contrast to children with multichannel cochlear implants, children who use vibrotactile aids achieve only modest speech perception improvements over time (Geers and Brenner, 1994; Kirk *et al.*, 1995; Miyamoto *et al.*, 1995). Most children with multichannel vibrotactile aid achieve the ability to recognize speech patterns with their device, but few acquire the ability to recognize words from even a closed-set using spectral information (*e.g.*, vowel and consonant cues) or to understand speech under sound-alone conditions.

The speech perception abilities of children with multichannel cochlear implants are often compared with those of children using conventional hearing aids. Such comparisons are valuable as these children can be matched for communication environment and lifestyle. At preimplantation intervals, the speech perception skills of the children with cochlear implants were similar to those of pediatric hearing aid users with unaided pure tone thresholds between 101 and 110 dB HL (the $PTA_{101-110}$ group), but poorer than those of hearing aid users with unaided pure tone thresholds between 90-100 dB HL (the PTA_{90-100} group). After 2 or more years of device use, the speech perception abilities of children with multichannel cochlear implants typically exceed those of children in the $PTA_{101-110}$ group and approach those of children in the PTA_{90-100} group.

Figure 10.6 illustrates the differences in speech perception performance among pediatric users of multichannel cochlear implants, multichannel tactile aids, or hearing aids. These data suggest that multichannel cochlear implants provide substantial information to children with profound hearing impairments who receive minimal benefit from conventional amplification. Many of the children in these studies used the older,

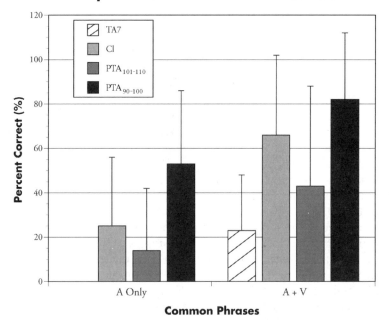

Open-Set Sentence Identification

FIG. 10.6. Average sentence recognition scores in the auditory-only *(A Only)* and auditory-plus-visual *(A + V)* modality for users of the Nucleus multichannel cochlear implant *(CI)*, the Tactaid 7 multichannel vibrotactile device *(TA7)*, and two groups of hearing aid users differing in their unaided pure tone threshold averages in the better-hearing ear. (From Kirk *et al.*, 1995, with permission.)

feature extraction speech processing strategies.

With advances in the design of speech processors, researchers have compared the performance of pediatric cochlear implant users to that of children with more residual hearing who use conventional hearing aids. Levi *et al.* (1998) conducted a preliminary study comparing the performance of one child with the Nucleus 22 channel implant and the SPEAK processing strategy to that of a child with bilateral hearing aids whose unaided pure tone average in the better-hearing ear was 70 dB HL. The children were matched by age, date of initial hearing aid fitting, communication mode, and educational setting. Their performance was similar on two tests of isolated word recognition, the LNT and the MLNT. However, the performance of the hearing aid user was superior on a more difficult task, recognizing words in sentences presented in background noise. Further research is needed to determine whether children with implants can achieve the same performance levels as their peers with severe hearing losses who use hearing aids.

Just as with adults, individual children vary greatly in their ability to perceive speech with a cochlear implant. In the next section, we consider some factors that contribute to individual differences in the outcomes of pediatric cochlear implantation.

Factors Influencing Speech Perception in Children with Cochlear Implants

Age at onset of hearing loss, age at time of implantation, length of cochlear implant use, communication mode and amount of residual hearing before implantation are all demographic factors that have been shown to influence performance results. Early results demonstrated that age at onset and duration of deafness significantly affected speech perception performance (Fryauf-Bertschy *et al.*, 1992; Osberger *et al.*, 1991; Staller *et al.*, 1991). That is, the children with a later onset of deafness and a shorter period of auditory deprivation before implantation had better

speech perception skills than children who were deafened earlier and had a longer duration of deafness before implantation. When only children with prelingual deafness (*i.e.*, less than 3 years) are considered, age at onset of hearing loss is no longer a significant factor. The speech perception performance of children with congenital deafness is similar to that of children with adventitious deafness acquired before age 3 years (Miyamoto *et al.*, 1993; Osberger *et al.*, 1991).

It is clear that earlier implantation yields superior cochlear implant performance. Fryauf-Bertschy *et al.* (1997) compared closed- and open-set word recognition in children implanted before and after 5 years of age. They found that closed-set performance did not differ between the two groups. However, children implanted before 5 years of age had significantly better open-set word recognition than did those implanted at a later age. Similarly, Miyamoto *et al.* (1997) found that children implanted before 5 years of age had significantly better multisyllabic word recognition on the MLNT did children implanted after that time (Fig. 10.7).

Waltzman *et al.* conducted several studies to examine the speech perception abilities of children implanted before the age of 5 years (between 2 and 5 years) (Waltzman and Cohen, 1998; Waltzman *et al.*, 1995; Waltzman *et al.*, 1997). Waltzman *et al.* (1995) reported the performance results of 14 children who were implanted before age 3 years and had used their device for at least 3 years. All children used the Nucleus cochlear implant with the MPEAK processing strategy and all used oral communication. After 1 year of implant use, seven of the children demonstrated consistent open-set speech perception abilities. After 2 years, this number increased to 13 children. The mean PB-K word recognition score at 3 years after implantation was 47% correct. Similar performance results also were reported for a group of 11 children implanted before the age of 2 years (Waltzman and Cohen, 1998).

One of the most consistent findings is that the speech perception abilities of children

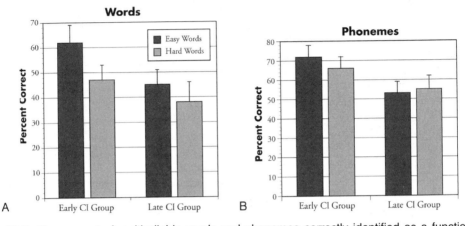

FIG. 10.7. The percent of multisyllabic words and phonemes correctly identified as a function of age at time of cochlear implantation (CI) and of lexical difficulty. Children in the Early-CI group were implanted before the age of 5 years; children in the Late-CI group were implanted after that time. Lexically easy words are those that occur often in the language and have few phonemically similar words with which they can be confused; lexically hard words have the opposite characteristics. (From Miyamoto *et al.*, 1997, with permission.)

with cochlear implants improve with increased device experience (*e.g.*, Fryauf-Bertschy *et al.*, 1997; Miyamoto *et al.*, 1994; Quittner and Steck, 1991). Miyamoto *et al.* (1994) used multiple regression analyses to examine the relationship between children's performance on closed- or open-set word recognition tests and a variety of demographic and device factors. The participants were 61 children (prelingually or postlingually deafened) who used a Nucleus cochlear implant. Age at onset of hearing loss, age at implantation, duration of deafness, length of cochlear implant use, processor type (F0F1F2 vs MPEAK), and communication mode accounted for about 40% of the variance in open-set word recognition. Among these factors, length of device use account for the most variance on all speech perception measures.

The variables of communication mode and unaided residual hearing also influence speech perception performance (Cowan *et al.*, 1997; Osberger and Fisher, 1998; Zwolan

et al., 1997). It is important to note that these factors may covary. Children with greater amounts of residual hearing before implantation are more likely to succeed in an Oral educational setting than those with very limited residual hearing. Osberger and Fisher (1998) examined preoperative variables that could predict open-set speech perception performance at 12 months after implantation. They found that preoperative communication mode and the presence of open-set speech recognition before implantation were significant and independent predictors of postoperative speech perception performance. The highest postoperative performance was obtained by children who used Oral communication and had at least minimal open-set speech perception before implantation (*i.e.*, > 1% on the GASP word test). The poorest performance was demonstrated by children who used Total Communication and had no preoperative open-set speech understanding.

Zwolan *et al.* (1997) compared the postoperative performance of 12 children who demonstrated some aided open-set speech recognition before implantation (the Borderline candidacy group) with that of 12 matched controls who had no preimplantation speech recognition (the Traditional candidacy group). Candidacy for study participation was based on preimplantation binaural aided speech testing and the children were subsequently implanted in their poorer hearing ear. The mean preoperative audiograms did not differ for the implanted ears in the two groups. By 1 year after implantation, children in the Borderline group had significantly higher scores than children in the Traditional group on all six speech perception measures employed. The investigators suggested that increased auditory experience before implantation facilitated the development of speech perception skills postimplant. Their results highlight the need to consider aided thresholds and speech perception abilities when determining candidacy for a cochlear implant. That is, children with some residual hearing should be considered for implantation if their speech perception performance is less than that obtained by the average pediatric cochlear implant recipient.

Speech Production Performance by Children

Most pediatric cochlear implant users are congenitally or prelingually deafened. These children must use the auditory input from their devices in learning to produce spoken language. Investigations concerning the effects of cochlear implant use on speech production in children began during the pediatric clinical trials of the 3M/House single-channel system (Kirk and Hill-Brown, 1985). The children's productions of prosodic speech features (*e.g.*, duration and rhythm), vowels, consonants, and consonant blends were assessed imitatively in nonsense syllables and in spontaneous speech using the Phonetic Level Speech Evaluation and the Phonologic Level Speech Evaluation, respectively (Ling, 1976). Kirk and Hill-Brown

developed a method of quantifying these evaluations to measure speech production changes over time. In their system, higher numeric scores reflected the production of more speech sounds, the production of those sounds in more difficult articulatory contexts, or increased consistency of production. After 1 year of single-channel implant experience, children in this study demonstrated significant improvements in the production of nonsegmental speech features, vowels, and consonants, but not in the production of consonant blends. Children implanted at an earlier age demonstrated greater speech production improvements than those implanted later. The children using Oral communication had better speech production skills than those children who used Total Communication.

Tobey *et al.* (Tobey, 1993; Tobey *et al.*, 1991; Tobey and Hasenstab, 1991; Tobey *et al.*, 1988) adapted some of the procedures developed by Kirk and Hill-Brown to evaluate the speech production abilities of children participating in the Nucleus 22-channel implant clinical trials (most of whom used the F0F1F2 speech processing strategy). They developed categories to describe the clinical significance of the speech production scores achieved on Ling's evaluations. Speech production changes over time were considered clinically significant if the child's postimplant score fell in a higher category than their preimplantation performance. Of 61 children in the study, 31% demonstrated clinically significant improvements in imitative nonsegmental speech production and 67% improved in imitative segmental speech production after 1 year of cochlear implant use (Tobey *et al.*, 1991). About one-half of the children showed significant clinical improvement in their spontaneous speech production abilities. More children implanted at a younger age achieved significant gains than children implanted at a later age.

Other investigators have examined more carefully the spontaneous production of nonsegmental and segmental aspects of speech. Tobey *et al.* (1991) analyzed the spontaneous speech samples of children implanted with the Nucleus 22-channel device. The speech samples were transcribed and the frequency of occurrence of phonemes was tabulated. Their results revealed that after 1 year of cochlear implant use, more children produced stop, fricative, glide and nasal consonants than before they were implanted.

Osberger *et al..* (1991) analyzed speech samples from three groups of children with sensory aids, 3M/House users, Nucleus users, and Tactaid II users (a two-channel vibrotactile aid). They classified the children's productions as nonspeech, speechlike, or speech. Nonspeech sounds were vocal noises such as a tongue trill or a raspberry. Speechlike sounds were vocalic segments or glottal fry segments. They then calculated the percent of vocalizations and the percent of phonetic approximations (speechlike or speech) produced. Samples were analyzed before and after 1 year of device use. The largest improvements occurred for users of the Nucleus multichannel implant; however, only 67% of their utterances were judged to be phonetic approximations. Before implantation, all children produced stop consonants with the greatest frequency, followed by nasal consonants. After 1 year of device use, the Nucleus children showed increases in the number of stops, fricatives and glides, and a reduction in nasal consonant production.

Additional studies have been conducted that compare speech production in children with multichannel cochlear implants to that of children with tactile aids or conventional hearing aids (Ertmer *et al.,* 1997; Kirk *et al.,* 1995; Osberger *et al.,* 1994; Sehgal *et al.,* 1998; Tobey *et al..,* 1994). Tobey *et al.* (1994) conducted one of the most carefully controlled comparisons. Over a 3-year period, they examined the speech production and speech intelligibility of 13 triads of sensory aids users matched by age, unaided thresholds, intelligence, family support and speech and language skills. All children had average pure tone thresholds of 100 dB HL or more in their better hearing ear. In each triad, one child used the Nucleus 22-channel cochlear

implant, one child used a hearing aid (the HA group), and one child used a vibrotactile aid (the Tactaid II or the Tactaid VII). After the initiation of the study, an additional group of 13 hearing aid users with pure tone average thresholds between 90-100 dB HL were added and tested one time (the HA+ group). After 3 years of device use, the Nucleus multichannel implant users showed significantly greater increases in imitative speech production (36%) than children in the Tactaid and HA groups (20% for both). Children in the HA+ group had significantly better imitative speech production skills that children in the Tactaid and HA groups. The nonsegmental speech production abilities of children in the HA+ group were significantly better than those of the Nucleus users, but the two groups did not differ in their abilities to imitate segmental aspects of speech. After 3 years of device use, the spontaneous speech production abilities of the Nucleus users exceeded those of the Tactaid and HA groups, but were similar to those of the HA+ group.

Speech Intelligibility of Children with Cochlear Implants

Measures of imitative speech production provide information that is important for diagnostic and therapeutic purposes. However, they are only weakly related to spontaneous speech production abilities (Tye-Murray and Kirk, 1993). It is therefore necessary to conduct additional measures to evaluate the effectiveness of cochlear implant use in promoting the development of intelligible speech.

Osberger was among the first investigators to compare the speech intelligibility of children with different sensory aids (Osberger *et al.,* 1994) using naive listeners who were unfamiliar with the speech of deaf talkers. Children's elicited productions of 10 sentences were recorded, digitized and then played to panels of three naive listeners who wrote down what they thought was said. Intelligibility was scored as the mean percent of words in the sentences that were correctly identified by the panel. Using this technique, the authors compared the speech intelligibility of children with the Nucleus cochlear implant to that of three groups of hearing aid users divided by their unaided pure tone thresholds: PTA_{90-100}, $PTA_{101-110}$, and $PTA_{>110}$ out through 5 years of device use.

Children in the $PTA_{>110}$ group were those who met the criteria for cochlear implantation. Children in the cochlear implant group were tested longitudinally whereas children in the hearing aid groups generally were tested one time only. After 2.5 years of implant use, the speech intelligibility of the Nucleus users exceeded that of children in the $PTA_{101-110}$ group. By 4 years after implantation, the mean intelligibility score for the Nucleus users was approximately 40%, nearly 20% higher than the mean for children in the $PTA_{101-110}$ group. The intelligibility of the Nucleus users never reached that of children in the $PTA_{101-110}$ group. Similar results were later reported by other investigators at IUSM (Miyamoto *et al.*, 1996; Miyamoto *et al.*, 1997).

Svirsky and others (Miyamoto *et al.*, 1997; Svirsky *et al.*, 1998) expanded on the work of Osberger by analyzing the speech intelligibility data obtained from each hearing aid group as a function of chronologic age. For each hearing aid group, they used regression analyses to estimate the rate of improvement expected per year in the absence of a cochlear implant (*i.e.*, through maturation alone). These estimates then served as a baseline for comparing preimplantation and postimplantation speech intelligibility performance. Any differences between the observed and predicted growth rates presumably should reflect the effects of cochlear implant use.

Svirsky *et al.* (1998) compared the speech intelligibility of 44 children with cochlear implants (the Nucleus with the SPEAK strategy or the Clarion with the CIS strategy) to that of children in the PTA_{90-100} group. Children with newer state-of-the-art processing strategies demonstrated substantial improvements in speech intelligibility over time. After 1.5 to 2.5 years of cochlear implant use, the speech intelligibility of the cochlear implant users was similar to that of the PTA_{90-100} group, a finding not previously demonstrated in pediatric cochlear implant users with older speech processing strategies.

NEW DIRECTIONS IN PEDIATRIC COCHLEAR IMPLANT RESEARCH: CORRELATES OF EXCEPTIONAL PERFORMANCE IN CHILDREN

Children with profound, prelingual deafness have demonstrated the ability to achieve substantial amounts of open-set spoken word recognition and high levels of speech intelligibility using cochlear implants with the latest processing strategies. These results are extremely encouraging, and support the notion of carefully considering all young children with profound hearing loss as potential cochlear implant candidates (Svirsky and Chin, in press; Zwolan *et al.*, 1997). This broadening of cochlear implant candidacy highlights again the primary challenge facing clinical cochlear implant researchers: how to account for variability in performance.

Prior research has concentrated on identifying the key demographic variables that play an important role in predicting postimplant speech perception and production abilities of children with prelingual deafness. Although these studies have been informative, much of the variability in performance remains unexplained. Pisoni *et al.* initiated a series of studies to examine the more perceptual, cognitive, or linguistic factors that contribute to the individual differences in communication abilities demonstrated by children with cochlear implants.

Pisoni *et al.* (1997) examined the performance of two groups of pediatric cochlear implant users with at least 2 years of device experience. Children were categorized as "Stars" if their 2-year postimplantation scores on the PB-K placed them in the top 20% of the children followed as part of the IUSM longitudinal study. Children were placed in the control group if their scores placed them in the bottom 20% of the participants in the longitudinal group. Scores from behavioral tests of speech perception, spoken word recognition, language development and speech intelligibility were compared between the two groups at the preimplantation interval and again at testing intervals of 1, 2, and 3 years after implantation. Scores on several psychologic tests administered before implantation were compared.

Stars did not score consistently better than children in the control group on all behavioral measures. Rather, the differences between the groups depended on the test administered and the specific task demands. The children with superior implant performance were consistently better on measures of speech perception (*i.e.*, vowel and consonant recognition), spoken word recognition, comprehension, language development and speech intelligibility than children in the control group. However, the two groups did not differ on measures of vocabulary knowledge, nonverbal intelligence, visual-motor integration or visual attention. The superior performance of the Stars on measures of spoken language processing and speech intelligibility was not due to some global difference in overall performance but to differences in the processing of auditory information provided by the cochlear implant.

Pisoni *et al.* (1997) also examined the relationship among performance on the various behavioral tests of communicative ability administered after 1 year of cochlear implant use. Strength-of-correlation analyses revealed a consistent pattern of very strong and highly significant associations between spoken word recognition, language development and speech intelligibility for the Stars but not for children in the control group. The investigators concluded that superior performance stemmed from the ability to process language and to develop phonologic and lexical representations for words. The strong relationship between spoken word recognition and speech intelligibility for the superior im-

plant performers suggests that there is a transfer of knowledge between perception and production and that perception and production share a common system of internal representation.

According to Pisoni *et al.*, the exceptional performance of the Stars appears to be because of their superior abilities to perceive, encode and retrieve information about spoken words from lexical memory. This information is used in a variety of processing tasks that require the manipulation and transformation of the phonologic representations of spoken words.

In a second study, Pisoni and Geers (1998) investigated the role of working memory in speech perception, speech intelligibility, language processing and reading in a group of 43 children with prelingual deafness who had used their cochlear implants for more than 4 years. The investigators examined the relationship between the children's ability to recall lists of digits presented in the auditory-only modality and their performance in each area listed earlier. Moderate to high correlations were found between auditory memory for digits and performance in each outcome area, suggest that working memory plays an important role in mediating performance across a range of different tasks. Pisoni and Geers (1998) concluded that the commonality among the perceptual processes employed in each task may be related to the ability to extract or encode speech sounds from the acoustic signal and to a process of rehearsal used to encode and retrieve the representations of spoken words from lexical memory.

According to Pisoni *et al.* (1997), future research concerning cochlear implant use by children should focus on informational processing operations such as perceptual learning, categorization, attention and working memory. Studies concerning the nature of linguistic interactions between children and their caregivers during the early periods of cochlear implant use should provide information about the nature and effects of the early input children receive through their sensory aid. Such studies currently are underway at Indiana University School of Medicine.

ACKNOWLEDGMENT

The author was supported in part by NIH-NIDCD grant K08 DC00126 while preparing this manuscript.

REFERENCES

Battmer RD, Gupta SP, Allum-Mecklenburg DJ, Lenarz T. Factors influencing cochlear implant perceptual performance in 132 adults. *Ann Otol Rhinol Laryngol* 1995;166[Suppl 166]:185–187.

Battmer RD, Lenarz T, Allum-Mecklenburg DJ, Strauss-Schier A, Gnadeberg D, Rost U. Postoperative results for adults and children implanted with the Clarion device. *Ann Otol Rhinol Laryngol* 1995;166[Suppl]:254–255.

Berliner KI, Eisenberg LS. Methods and issues in the cochlear implantation of children: an overview. *Ear Hear* 1985;6[Suppl]:6S–13S.

Berliner KI, Tonokawa LL, Dye LL, House WF. Open-set speech recognition in children with single-channel cochlear implants. *Ear Hear* 1989;10:237–242.

Blamey J, Clark GM. Place coding of vowel formants for cochlear implant patients. *J Acoust Soc Am* 1990;88:667–673.

Blamey PJ, Dowell RC, Brown AM, Clark GM, Seligman PM. Vowel and consonant recognition of cochlear implant patients using formant-estimating speech processors. *J Acoust Soc Am* 1987;82:48–57.

Blamey PJ, Pyman BC, Gordon G, et al. Factors predicting postoperative sentence scores in postlingually deafened cochlear implant patients. *Ann Otol Rhinol Laryngol* 1992;101:342–348.

Boothroyd A, Hanin L, Hnath T. *A sentence test of speech perception: reliability, set equivalence, and short term learning* (internal report RCI 10). New York: City University of New York, 1985.

Carhart R. Problems in the measurement of speech discrimination. *Arch Otolaryngol* 1965;82:253–260.

Clark G, Tong Y, Dowell R, et al. A multiple channel cochlear implant: an evaluation using nonsense syllables. *Ann Otol Rhinol Laryngol* 1981;90:227–230.

Cohen NL, Waltzman SB, Fisher SG, et al. A prospective, randomized study of cochlear implants. *N Engl J Med* 1993;328:233–237.

Cowan RSC, Brown C, Whitford LA, et al. Speech perception in children using the advanced SPEAK speech-processing strategy. *Ann Otol Rhinol Laryngol* 1995;104[Suppl 166]:318–321.

Cowan RSC, DelDot J, Barker EJ, et al. Speech perception results for children with implants with different levels of preoperative residual hearing. *Am J Otol* 1997;18, 125–126.

Cowan RSC, Galvin KL, Klieve S, et al. Contributing

factors to improved speech perception in children using the Nucleus 22-channel cochlear prosthesis. In: Honjo I, Takahashi H, eds. *Cochlear implant and related sciences update.* Basel: Karger, 1997:193–197. (*Advances in otorhinolaryngology, 52.*)

Craig WN. *Craig lip-reading inventory: word recognition.* Englewood, CO: Resource Point, 1992.

Davis H, Silverman S. *Hearing and deafness,* 4th ed. New York: Holt, Rinehart & Winston, 1978.

Dorman MF. Speech perception by adults. In Tyler RS, ed. *Cochlear implants: audiological foundations.* San Diego: Singular Publishing Group, 1993:145–190.

Dorman MF, Hannley M, Dankowski K, McCandless K, Smith L, McCandless G. Word recognition by 50 patients fitted with the Symbion multichannel cochlear implant. *Ear Hear* 1989;10:44–49.

Dowell RC, Mecklenburg DJ, Clark GM. Speech recognition for 40 patients receiving multichannel cochlear implants. *Acta Otolaryngol* 1986;112:1054–1059.

Doyle KJ, Mills D, Larky J, Kessler D, Luxford WM, Schindler RA. Consonant perception by users of Nucleus and Clarion multichannel cochlear implants. *Am J Otol* 1995;16:676–681.

Edgerton BJ, House WF, Hitselberger W. Hearing by cochlear nucleus stimulation in humans. *Ann Otol Rhinol Laryngol* 1982;91:117–124.

Erber NP. *Auditory training.* Washington, DC: Alexander Graham Bell Association for the Deaf, 1982.

Ertmer D, Kirk KI, Sehgal ST, Riley AI, Osberger MJ. A comparison of vowel production by children with multichannel cochlear implants or tactile aids: perceptual evidence. *Ear Hear* 1997;18:307–315.

Fretz RJ, Fravel RP. Design and function: a physical and electrical description of the 3M House cochlear implant system. *Ear Hear* 1985;6[Suppl]:14S–19S.

Fryauf-Bertschy H, Tyler RS, Kelsay DM, Gantz BJ. Performance over time of congenitally deaf and postlingually deafened children using a multichannel cochlear implant. *J Speech Hear Res* 1992;35:913–920.

Fryauf-Bertschy H, Tyler RS, Kelsay DMR, Gantz BJ, Woodworth GG. Cochlear implant use by prelingually deafened children: the influences of age at implant use and length of device use. *J Speech Hear Res* 1997;40:183–199.

Gantz BJ, Tye-Murray N, Tyler RS. Word recognition performance with single-channel and multichannel cochlear implants. *Am J Otol* 1989;10:91–94.

Gantz BJ, Tyler RS, Knutson JF, et al. Evaluation of five different cochlear implant designs: audiologic assessment and predictors of performance. *Laryngoscope* 1988;98:1100–1106.

Gantz BJ, Tyler RS, Woodworth G, Tye-Murray N, Fryauf-Bertschy H. Results of multichannel cochlear implant in congenital and acquired prelingual deafness in children: five-year follow-up. *Am J Otol* 1994;15[Suppl 2]:1–8.

Gantz BJ, Woodworth GG, Abbas PJ, Knutson JF, Tyler RS. Multivariate predictors of audiological success with multichannel cochlear implants. *Ann Otol Rhinol Laryngol* 1993;102:909–916.

Geers AE. Techniques for assessing auditory speech perception and lip-reading enhancement in young deaf children. *Volta Rev* 1994;96:85–96.

Geers AE, Brenner C. Speech perception results: audition and lip-reading enhancement. *Volta Rev* 1994;96:97–108.

Geers AE, Moog JS. Evaluating speech perception skills: tools for measuring benefits of cochlear implants, tactile aids, and hearing aids. In: Owens E, D Kessler, eds. *Cochlear implant in young deaf children.* Boston: College-Hill Press, 1989:227–256.

Goldman R, Fristoe M. *Goldman-Fristoe test of articulation.* Circle Pines, MN: American Guidance Service, 1972.

Gstöttner WK, Baumgartner WD, Franz P, Hamzavi J. Cochlear implant deep-insertion surgery. *Laryngoscope* 1997;107:544–546.

Haskins HA. *A phonetically balanced test of speech discrimination for children.* Master's thesis. Evanston, IL: Northwestern University, 1949.

Helms J, Muller J, Schon F, *et al.* Evaluation of performance with the COMBI 40 cochlear implant in adults: a multicentric clinical study. *ORL J Otorhinolaryngology Relat Spec* 1997;59:23–35.

Hochmair ES, Hochmair-Desoyer IJ. Percepts elicited by different speech-coding strategies. In: Parkins CW, Anderson SW, eds. *Cochlear prostheses: an international symposium.* New York: Raven Press, 1983:268–279.

Hochmair-Desoyer IJ, Hochmair ES, Stiglbrunner HK. Psychoacoustic temporal processing and speech understanding in cochlear implant patients. In: Shindler RA, Merzenich MM, eds. *Cochlear implants.* New York: Raven Press, 1985:291–304.

Holden LK, Skinner MW, Holden TA. Speech recognition with the MPEAK and SPEAK speech-coding strategies of the Nucleus cochlear implant. *Otolaryngol Head Neck Surg* 1997;116:163–167.

Hollow RD, Dowell RC, Cowan RSC Skok MC, Pyman BC, Clark GM. Continuing improvements in speech processing for adult cochlear implant patients. *Ann Otol Rhinol Laryngol* 1995;166[Suppl]:292–294.

House WF, Berliner KI. Cochlear implants: from idea to clinical practice. In: Cooper H, ed. *Cochlear implants: a practical guide.* San Diego: Singular Publishing Group, 1991:9–33.

House WF, Berliner KI, Eisenberg LS. The cochlear implant: an auditory prosthesis for the profoundly deaf child. *Ear Hear* 1985;6[Suppl]:1S–69S.

Jerger J, Lewis S, Hawkins J, Jerger J. Pediatric speech intelligibility test I: generation of test materials. *Int J Pediatr Otorhinolaryngol* 1980;2:101–118.

Kessler DK. New directions in speech processing II: the electrode connection. Paper presented at the 7th Symposium on Cochlear Implants in Children; Iowa City, IA, 1998.

Kessler DK, Loeb GE, Barker MJ. Distribution of speech recognition results with the Clarion cochlear prosthesis. *Ann Otol Rhinol Laryngol* 1995; 166[Suppl]:283–285.

Kessler DK, Schindler RA. Progress with a multistrategy cochlear system: the Clarion. In: Hochmair-Desoyer IJ, Hochmair ES, eds. *Advances in cochlear implants.* Wein: Manz, 1994:354–362.

Kiefer J, Muller J, Pfennigdorff T, *et al.* Speech understanding in quiet and in noise with the CIS speech coding strategy (Med-EL COMBI 40) compared to the multipeak and spectral peak strategies (nucleus). *J Otol Rhinol Laryngol* 1996;58:127–135.

Kileny P, Zimmerman-Phillips S, Kemink J, Schmaltz S. Effects of preoperative electrical stimulability and historical factors on performance with multichannel cochlear implants. *Ann Otol Rhinol Laryngol* 1991;100:563–568.

Kileny P, Young K, Niparko J. Acoustic and electrical assessment of the auditory pathway. In: Jackler R, Brackmann D, eds. *Neurotology.* St. Louis: CV Mosby, 1994:261–282.

Kirk KI, Diefendorf E, Riley A, Osberger MJ. Consonant production by children with multichannel cochlear implants or hearing aids. In: Uziel AS, Mondain M, eds. *Cochlear implants in children.* Basel: Karger, 1995:154–159. *(Advances in Otorhinolaryngology, 50.)*

Kirk KI, Diefendorf AO, Pisoni DB, Robbins AM. Assessing speech perception in children. In: Mendel LL, Danhauer JL, eds. *Audiologic evaluation and management and speech perception assessment.* San Diego: Singular Publishing Group, 1997:101–132.

Kirk KI, Hill-Brown C. Speech and language results in children with a cochlear implant. *Ear Hear* 1985;6[Suppl]:36S–47S.

Kirk KI, Osberger MJ, Robbins AM, Riley AI, Todd SL, Miyamoto RT. Performance of children with cochlear implants, tactile aids, and hearing aids. *Semin Hear* 1995;16:370–381.

Kirk KI, Pisoni DB, Osberger MJ. Lexical effects on spoken word recognition by pediatric cochlear implant users. *Ear Hear* 1995;16:470–481.

Knutson JF, Hinrich JV, Tyler RS, Gantz BJ, Schartz HA, Woodworth GG. Psychological predictors of audiological outcomes of multichannel cochlear implants: preliminary findings. *Ann Otol Rhinol Laryngol* 1991;100:817–822.

Lehiste I, Peterson GE. Linguistic considerations in the study of speech intelligibility. *J Acoust Soc Am* 1959;31:280–286.

Levi A, Eisenberg LS, Martinez AS, Schneider K. Performance comparisons between cochlear implant and platinum hearing aid user: case study. Presented at the 7th Symposium on Cochlear Implants in Children; Iowa City, IA, 1998.

Ling D. *Speech and the hearing impaired child: theory and practice.* Washington, DC: Alexander Graham Bell Association for the Deaf, 1976.

Mecklenburg D, Shallop J, Ling D. *Phonetic task evaluation.* Englewood, CO: Cochlear Corporation, 1987.

Mendel LL, Danhaeur JL. Test administration and interpretation. In: Mendel LL, Danhauer JL, eds. *Audiologic evaluation and management and speech perception assessment.* San Diego: Singular Publishing Group, 1997:15–58.

Miller GE, Nicely PE. An analysis of perceptual confusions among some English consonants. *J Acoust Soc Am* 1955;27:338–351.

Miyamoto RT, Kirk KI, Robbins AM, Todd S, Riley A. Speech perception and speech production skills of children with multichannel cochlear implants. *Acta Otolaryngol* 1996;116:240–243.

Miyamoto RT, Kirk KI, Robbins AM, Todd S, Riley A, Pisoni DB. Speech perception and speech intelligibility in children with multichannel cochlear implants. In: Honjo I, Takahashi H, eds. *Cochlear implant and related sciences update.* Basel: Karger, 1997:198–203. *(Advances in otorhinolaryngology, 52.)*

Miyamoto RT, Kirk KI, Svirsky MA, Sehgal ST. Communication skills in pediatric cochlear implant recipients. Presented at the Collegium Oto-Rhino-Laryngologicum Amicitiae Sacrum; Copenhagen, Denmark, 1998.

Miyamoto RT, Kirk KI, Todd SL, Robbins AM, Osberger MJ. Speech perception skills of children with multichannel cochlear implants or hearing aids. *Ann Otol Rhinol Laryngol* 1995;104:334–337.

Miyamoto RT, Osberger MJ, Robbins AM, Myres WA, Kessler K. Prelingually deafened children's performance with the Nucleus multichannel cochlear implant. *Am J Otol* 1993;14:437–445.

Miyamoto RT, Osberger MJ, Robbins AM, Myres WA, Kessler K, Pope ML. Longitudinal evaluation of communication skills of children with single- or multichannel cochlear implants. *Am J Otol* 1992;13:215–222.

Miyamoto RT, Osberger MJ, Robbins AM, *et al.* Comparison of sensory aids in deaf children. *Ann Otol Rhinol Laryngol* 1989;98:2–7.

Miyamoto RT, Osberger MJ, Todd SL, *et al.* Variables affecting implant performance in children. *Laryngoscope* 1994;104:1120–1124.

Miyamoto RT, Osberger MJ, Todd SL, *et al.* Speech perception skills of children with multichannel cochlear implants. In: Hochmair-Desoyer IJ, Hochmair ES, eds. *Advances in cochlear implants.* Wien: Manz, 1994:498–504.

Miyamoto RT, Robbins AM, Osberger MJ, Todd SL, Riley AI, Kirk KI. Comparison of multichannel tactile aids and multichannel cochlear implants in children with profound hearing impairments. *Am J Otol* 1995;16:8–13.

Miyamoto RT, Svirsky M, Kirk KI, Robbins AM, Todd S, Riley A. Speech intelligibility of children with multichannel cochlear implants. *Ann Otol Rhinol Laryngol* 1997;106:35–36.

Monsen RB. Toward measuring how well hearing-impaired children speak. *J Speech Hear Res* 1978;21:197–219.

Moog JS, Geers AE. *Early speech perception test for profoundly hearing-impaired children.* St. Louis: Central Institute for the Deaf, 1990.

Moog JS, Kozak VJ, Geers AE. *Grammatical analysis of elicited language—presentence level.* St. Louis: Central Institute for the Deaf, 1983.

Nilsson MJ, Soli SD, Sullivan JA. Development of the Hearing in Noise Test for the measurement of speech reception thresholds in quiet and in noise. *J Acoust Soc Am* 1994;95:1085–1099.

Osberger MJ. New directions in speech processing. I: Patient performance with simultaneous analog stimulation (SAS). Presented at the 7th Symposium on Cochlear Implants in Children; Iowa City, IA, 1998.

Osberger MJ, Fisher LM. Preoperative predictors of postoperative implant performance in children. Presented at the 7th Symposium on Cochlear Implants in Children; Iowa City, IA, 1998.

Osberger MJ, Fisher L, Zimmerman-Phillips S, Geier L, Barker MJ. Speech recognition performance of older children with cochlear implants. *Am J Otol* 1998;19:152–157.

Osberger MJ, Miyamoto RT, Zimmerman-Phillips S, *et al.* Independent evaluation of the speech perception abilities of children with the Nucleus 22-channel cochlear implant system. *Ear Hear* 1991; 12 [Suppl]:66S–80S.

Osberger MJ, Robbins A, Berry S, Todd S, Hesketh L, Sedey A. Analysis of the spontaneous speech samples of children with a cochlear implant or tactile aid. *Am J Otol* 1991;12[Suppl]:173–181.

Osberger MJ, Robbins AM, Miyamoto RT, *et al.* Speech perception abilities of children with cochlear implants, tactile aids, or hearing aids. *Am J Otol* 1991;12[Suppl]:105–115.

Osberger MJ, Robbins AM, Todd SL, Riley AI. Speech intelligibility of children with cochlear implants. *Volta Rev* 1994;96:169–180.

Osberger MJ, Robbins AM, Todd SL, Riley AI, Miyamoto RT. Speech production skills of children with multichannel cochlear implants. In: Hochmair-Desoyer IJ, Hochmair ES, eds. *Advances in cochlear implants.* Wien: Manz, 1994:503–508.

Osberger MJ, Robbins AM, Todd SL, Riley AI, Kirk KI, Carney AE. Cochlear implants and tactile aids for children with profound hearing impairment. In: Bess F, Gravel J, Tharpe AM, eds. *Amplification for children with auditory deficits.* Nashville, TN: Bill Wilkerson Center Press, 1996:283–307.

Osberger MJ, Todd SL, Berry SW, Robbins AM, Miyamoto RT. Effect of age at onset of deafness on children's speech perception abilities with a cochlear implant. *Ann Otol Rhinol Laryngol* 1991;100:883–888.

Otto S, Shannon RV, Brackmann DF, Hitselberger WE, Staller S, Menapace C. The multichannel auditory brain stem implant: performance in twenty patients. *Head Neck Surg* 1998;118:291–303.

Otto S, Staller S. Multichannel auditory brain stem implant: case studies comparing fitting strategies and results. *Ann Otol Rhinol Laryngol* 1995; 166[Suppl]:36–39.

Owens E, Kessler DK, Telleen CC, Schubert ED. The minimal auditory capabilities (MAC) battery. *Hear Aid J* 1981;9:32.

Owens E, Kessler DK, Raggio MW, Schubert ED. Analysis and revision of the minimal auditory capabilities (MAC) battery. *Ear Hear* 1985;6:280–290.

Parkinson AJ, Tyler RS, Woodworth GG, Lowder MW, Gantz BJ. A within-subject comparison of adult patients using the Nucleus F0F1F2 and F0F1F2B3B4B5 speech processing strategies. *J Speech Hear Res* 1996;39:261–277.

Peterson GE, Lehiste I. Revised CNC lists for auditory tests. *J Speech Hear Disord* 1962;27:62–70.

Pisoni DB, Geers AE. Working memory in children with cochlear implants: digits span and measures of spoken language. Presented at the 7th Symposium on Cochlear Implants in Children; Iowa City, IA, 1998.

Pisoni DB, Svirsky MA, Kirk KI, Miyamoto RT. Looking at the stars: a first report on the intercorrelations among measures of speech perception, intelligibility and language development in pediatric cochlear implant users. *Research on spoken language processing progress report no. 21.* Bloomington, IN: Speech Research Laboratory of Indiana University, 1997.

Quittner AL, Steck JT. Predictors of cochlear implant use in children. *Am J Otol* 1991;12[Suppl]:89–94.

Robbins AM. *Mr. Potato Head task*. Indianapolis: Indiana University School of Medicine, 1994.

Robbins AM, Kirk KI. Speech perception assessment performance in pediatric cochlear implant users. *Semin Hear* 1996;17:353–369.

Robbins AM, Osberger MJ. *Meaningful use of speech scale*. Indianapolis: Indiana University School of Medicine, 1991.

Robbins AM, Osberger MJ. *Nonsense imitative test of syllables*. Indianapolis: Indiana University School of Medicine, 1987.

Robbins AM, Renshaw JJ, Berry SW. Evaluating meaningful auditory integration in profoundly hearing-impaired children. *Am J Otol* 1991;12[Suppl]:144–150.

Robbins AM, Renshaw JJ, Miyamoto RT, Osberger MJ, Pope ML. *Minimal pairs test*. Indianapolis: Indiana University School of Medicine, 1988.

Robbins AM, Renshaw JJ, Osberger MJ. *Common phrases test*. Indianapolis: Indiana University School of Medicine, 1995.

Ross M, Lerman J. A picture identification test for hearing impaired children. *J Speech Hear Res* 1979;13:44–53.

Schindler RA, Kessler DK. The UCSF/Storz cochlear implant: patient results. *Am J Otol* 1987;8:247–250.

Schindler RA, Kessler DK. Clarion cochlear implant: phase I investigational results. *Am J Otol* 1993;14:263–272.

Schindler RA, Kessler DK, Barker M. Clarion patient performance: an update on the clinical trials. *Ann Otol Rhinol Laryngol* 1995;166[Suppl]:269–272.

Sehgal ST, Kirk KI, Svirsky M, Ertmer DJ, Osberger MJ. Imitative consonant feature production by children with multichannel sensory aids. *Ear Hear* 1998;19:72–84.

Sehgal ST, Kirk KI, Svirsky MA, Miyamoto RT. The effects of processor strategy on the speech perception performance of pediatric Nucleus multichannel cochlear implant users. *Ear Hear* 1998;19:149–161.

Shannon RV. Psychophysics. In: Tyler RS, ed. *Cochlear implants: audiological foundations*. San Diego: Singular Publishing Group, 1993:357–388.

Shipp DB, Nedelski JM. Prognostic indicators of speech recognition performance in adult cochlear implant users: a prospective analysis. *Ann Otol Rhinol Laryngol* 1995;166[Suppl]:194–196.

Shipp D, Nedzelski J, Chen J, Hanusaik L. Prognostic indicators of speech recognition performance in postlingually deafened adult cochlear implant users. In: Honjo I, Takahashi H, eds. *Cochlear implant and related sciences update. Advances in Otorhinolaryngology, 52*. Basel: Karger, 1997:74–77.

Simmons FB, Lusted H, Meyers T, Shelton C. Electrically induced auditory brainstem response as a clinical tool in estimating nerve survival. *Ann Otol Rhinol Laryngol* 1984;93[Suppl]:97–100.

Skinner MW, Fourakis MS, Holden TA, Holden LK, Demorest ME. Identification of speech by cochlear implant recipients with the Multipeak (MPEAK) and Spectral Peak (SPEAK) speech coding strategies. I. Vowels. *Ear Hear* 1996;17:182–197.

Skinner M, Holden L, Holden T, *et al*. Performance of postlingually deaf adults with the wearable speech processor (WSP III) and mini-speech processor

(MSP) of the Nucleus multi-channel cochlear implant. *Ear Hear* 1991;12:3–22.

Staller SJ, Beiter AL, Brimacombe JA, Mecklenberg D, Arndt P. Pediatric performance with the Nucleus 22-channel cochlear implant system. *Am J Otol* 1991;12:126–136.

Staller S, Menapace C, Domico E, *et al*. Speech perception abilities of adult and pediatric Nucleus implant recipients using Spectral Peak (SPEAK) coding strategy. *Otolaryngol Head Neck Surg* 1997;117:236–242.

Svirsky MA, Chin SB. Speech production by users of cochlear implants: a review. In: Waltzman S, Cohen NL, eds. *Cochlear implants*. New York: Thieme Medical Publishers (in press).

Svirsky MA, Sloan RB, Caldwell M, Miyamoto RT. Speech intelligibility of prelingually deaf children with multichannel cochlear implants. Presented at the 7th Symposium on Cochlear Implants in Children; Iowa City, IA, 1998.

Thielemeir MA, Tonokawa LL, Petersen B, Eisenberg LS. Audiological results in children with a cochlear implant. *Ear Hear* 1985;6[Suppl]:27S–35S.

Tillman TW, Carhart R. *An expanded test for speech discrimination utilizing CNC monosyllabics words. Northwestern University auditory test no. 6*. Brooks Air Force Base, TX: USAF School of Aerospace Medicine Technical Report, 1966.

Tobey E. Speech production. In: Tyler RS, ed. *Cochlear implants: audiological foundations*. San Diego: Singular Press, 1993:257–316.

Tobey E, Angelette S, Murchison C, *et al*. Speech production in children receiving a multichannel cochlear implant. *Am J Otol* 1991;12[Suppl]:164–172.

Tobey E, Hasenstab S. Effects of a Nucleus multichannel cochlear implant upon speech production in children. *Ear Hear* 1991;12[Suppl]:48S–54S.

Tobey E, Geers A, Brenner C. Speech production results: speech feature acquisition. *Volta Rev* 1994;96:109–130.

Tobey E, Pancamo S, Staller S, Brimacombe J, Beiter A. Consonant production in children receiving a multichannel cochlear implant. *Ear Hear* 1991; 12:23–31.

Tobey E, Staller S, Brimacombe J, Beiter A. Objective measures of speech production in children using cochlear implants. *Am Speech Hear Assoc* 1988;30:103.

Tye-Murray N, Kirk KI. Vowel and diphthong production by young users of cochlear implants and the relationship between the phonetic level evaluation and spontaneous speech. *J Speech Hear Res* 1993;36:488–502.

Tye-Murray N Tyler RS. Auditory and consonant word recognition skills of cochlear implant users. *Ear Hear* 1989;10:292–298.

Tye-Murray N, Tyler RS, Woodworth GG, Gantz BJ. Performance over time with a Nucleus or Ineraid cochlear implant. *Ear Hear* 1992;13:200–209.

Tyler RS. Speech perception by children. In: Tyler RS, ed. *Cochlear implants: audiological foundations*. San Diego: Singular Publishing Group, 1993:191–256.

Tyler RS, Gantz BJ, McCabe BF, Lowder MW, Otto SR, Preece JP. Audiological results with two single channel cochlear implants. *Ann Otol Rhinol Laryngol* 1985;94:133–139.

Tyler RS, Gantz BJ, Woodworth GG, Parkinson AJ,

Lowder MW, Schum LK. Initial independent results with the Clarion cochlear implant. *Ear Hear* 1996;17:528–536.

Tyler RS, Holsted BA. *A closed-set speech perception test for hearing-impaired children.* Iowa City: The University of Iowa, 1978.

Tyler RS, Lowder MW. Audiological management and performance of adults cochlear-implant patients. *Ear Nose Throat J* 1992;71:117–128.

Tyler RS, Preece J, Tye-Murray N. *The Iowa cochlear implant tests.* Iowa City, IA: The University of Iowa, Department of Otolaryngology—Head and Neck Surgery, 1983.

Tyler RS, Tye-Murray N, Moore B, McCabe B. Synthetic two-formant vowel perception by some of the better cochlear-implant patients. *Audiology* 1989;28:301–315.

Waltzman S, Cohen NL. Cochlear implantation in children younger than 2 years old. *Am J Otol* 1998;19:158–162.

Waltzman S, Cohen NL, Shapiro W. Effects of cochlear implantation on the young deaf child. In: Uziel AS, Mondain M, eds. *Cochlear implants in children.* Basel: Karger, 1995:125–128. *(Advances in otorhinolaryngology, 50.)*

Waltzman S, Cohen NL, Gomolin R, *et al.* Perception and production results in children implanted between two and five years of age. In: Honjo I, Takahashi H, eds. *Cochlear implant and related sciences update.* Basel: Karger, 1997:177–180. *(Advances in otorhinolaryngology, 52.)*

Whitford LA, Seligman PM, Everingham CE, et al. Evaluation of the Nucleus Spectra 22 processor and new speech processing strategy (SPEAK) in postlinguistically deafened adults. *Acta Otolaryngol* 1995;115:629–637.

Wilson BS. Signal processing. In: Tyler RS, ed. *Cochlear implants: audiological foundations.* San Diego: Singular Publishing Group, 1993:35–85.

Wilson BS, Lawson DT, Finley CC, Wolford RD. Coding strategies for multichannel cochlear prostheses. *Am J Otol* 1991;12[Suppl 1]:56–61.

Wilson BS, Lawson DT, Finley CC, Wolford RD. Importance of patient and processor variables in determining outcomes with cochlear implants. *J Speech Hear Res* 1993;36:373–379.

Zimmerman-Phillips S, Osberger MJ, Geier L, Barker M. Speech recognition performance of pediatric Clarion patients. *Am J Otol* 1997;18:S153–S154.

Zwolan TA, Zimmerman-Phillips S, Ashbaugh CJ, Hieber SJ, Kileny PR, Telian SA. Cochlear implantation of children with minimal open-set speech recognition. *Ear Hear* 1997;18:240–251.

Appendix 10A

Analyzing the Effects of Early Implantation and Results with Different Causes of Deafness:
Meta-analysis of the Pediatric Cochlear Implant Literature

André K. Cheng and John K. Niparko

Despite an extensive body of evidence documenting communicative benefit of cochlear implantation in profoundly deaf children, published results have engendered skepticism for some readers. For example, Lane (1995) has asserted that implanted prelingually deaf children "cannot" acquire open-set speech recognition and that testing of children with implants harbors "protocol bias."

A meta-analysis of reports on speech recognition in children with cochlear implants can address concerns about research methods and provide a systematic review of all relevant literature. Meta-analyses are particularly useful when large, randomized control trials are impractical, sample sizes of individual studies are too small, or studies disagree.

A. K. Cheng: Department of Otolaryngology—Head and Neck Surgery, The Johns Hopkins University, Baltimore, Maryland 21205.

J. K. Niparko: Department of Otolaryngology—Head and Neck Surgery, The Listening Center at Johns Hopkins, The Johns Hopkins University, Baltimore, Maryland 21205-1809.

When aggregate data can be pooled and compared, stronger conclusions may be drawn about effectiveness.

We analyzed published reports of the effect of age at implantation and cause and age at onset of deafness on speech perception benefit in children with cochlear implants and compared these results with previously unreported independent patient data sets. Even rigorously performed metanalyses may be subject to publication bias (Jeng *et al.*, 1995). Published data may misrepresent an intervention's impact by systematically failing to report inconclusive or negative outcomes (Oxman *et al.*, 1995).

METHODS

A MEDLINE search since 1966 of articles key worded by cochlear implant and cochlear implants yielded 1,916 citations. Additional searches using manufacturer names as key words and subcategories of deafness yielded no additional citations. Clinical results were reported in 577 (30.1%) of the citations. Speech perception was the subject matter in 421 (22.0%) of them, 218 of which pertained to children (younger than 18 years of age). Patient data with at least 1 year of follow-up were reported in 44 of the articles.

Unpublished results with at least 1 year of follow-up were obtained from clinical trial data submitted to the U.S. FDA in premarket applications submitted by Cochlear Corporation in 1990 ($n = 107$) and by Advanced Bionics Corporations in 1997 ($n = 53$). Data from 42 implanted children from The Listening Center at Johns Hopkins with at least 1 year of follow-up were also included in the unpublished data set.

The 44 published papers provided data on speech perception after implantation with multichannel cochlear implants ($n = 1,904$ children). However, many variables confounded direct comparison of results between studies. Variables included the use of different speech perception tests (because the children's ages and developmental stages differed), research design, patient factors

(*e.g.*, age at implantation, age at onset of deafness, cause of deafness), treatment variables (*e.g.*, device implanted, speech processing strategy), and data collection protocol. In contrast to the published data, individual patient data from the unpublished trials were collated and analyzed easily for the two variables of interest.

Eleven of the 44 papers provided speech perception data with respect to age at implantation (Waltzman *et al.*, 1997; Uziel *et al.*, 1993; Frachet *et al.*, 1995; Meyer *et al.*, 1995; Shea *et al.*, 1994; Tyler and Summerfield, 1996; Miyamoto *et al.*, 1994; Gantz *et al.*, 1994; Waltzman *et al.*, 1994; Waltzman *et al.*, 1995), although three were omitted because they reported duplicate results. Three articles reported patient data by age groupings, although the age groupings were different in the three articles (Meyer *et al.*, 1999; Waltzman *et al.*, 1997; Gantz *et al.*, 1994). In the remaining five studies, individual patient data were not presented, and the only extractable data was an average score (X) at an average age at implantation (Y) for a specified number of subjects (Z).

Nine articles provided data with respect to cause or age at onset of deafness (Gantz *et al.*, 1994; Waltzman *et al.*, 1994; Waltzman *et al.*, 1995; Bertram *et al.*, 1995; Uziel *et al.*, 1995; Miyamoto *et al.*, 1993; Osberger *et al.*, 1991; Waltzman *et al.*, 1992; Staller *et al.*, 1991). Three articles were omitted because they reported duplicate results.

The literature reported results of 22 different tests of receptive benefit in spoken communication. To provide a common measure to integrate results across studies, each test percentage score was translated into a Speech Perception Categories (Geers and Moog, 1987) ordinal score (Table 10A.1). The Speech Perception Categories provide an ordinal scale for five levels of speech perception that range across simple detection, pattern perception, inconsistent and consistent closed-set word recognition, and open-set word recognition. A sixth category was added to accommodate scores on open-set speech recognition tests that exceeded the

TABLE 10A.1. *Speech perception categories*

Speech Perception Categories

1	2	3	4	5	6
Detection	Pattern	Closed-set words		Open-set recognition	

```
ESP Pattern  50%----100
 MTS Stress  54%----100
ESP Spondee  33%-----50-------100
   ESP Mono  33%-----50-------100
   MTS Word  33%-----50-------100
  NU-CHIPS   36%-----50-------100
      WIPI   28%----------100
  GASP Word  16%---------25------100
   PBK Word   4%----------8--------100
   HHT Word  20%--------50-------100
GASP Sentences 20%--------30-------100
 CID Sentences  2%--------20-------100
```

ESP, Early Speech Perception Test; MTS, Median Trochee Spondee; NU-CHIPS, Northwestern University Childrens Perception of Speech Test; WIPI, Word Identification by Picture Identification; GASP, Glendonald Auditory Screening Procedure; PBK, Phonetically Balanced Kinderegarten word list; HHT, Hannover Hearing Test; CID, Central Institute for the Deaf.
[a]Speech perception categories are assigned to scores on different tests of receptive speech perception in children.
Adapted from Geers and Moog, 1987.

levels associated with older cochlear implant designs. This type of ordinal scale is representative of the range of spoken communication skills exhibited by implanted children in an educational setting.

EFFECTS OF AGE AT IMPLANTATION

There is concordance between the data reported in the literature compared with the data from unpublished clinical trials, arguing against systematic publication bias in the pediatric cochlear implantation field (Fig. 10A.1). The one exception is the reporting of higher scores in the literature for the oldest age group (>6 years) after 2 and 3 years of implant use. Of the eight published articles analyzed, six concluded that the earlier the age at implantation, the better were the results. A number of articles, however, stated this conclusion (or the opposite conclusion) without presenting any data. Although there was a trend toward better results with earlier implantation in the published literature, there was no statistically significant difference between subjects implanted at different age groups.

The published literature documents results in children with congenital deafness and deafness that is acquired over time. In the unpublished data set, the oldest group attained significantly lower scores after 2, 3, and 4 years of implant use than in the unpublished data set. There also seems to be no plateau of benefit over time, no matter what the age at implantation. This pattern is different than that reported for postlingually deafened adults, for whom earlier age at implantation correlates with better speech perception results, but results plateau after some period (NIH Consensus Conference, 1995).

EFFECTS OF CAUSE AND AGE AT ONSET OF DEAFNESS

Unpublished patient data show that congenitally deafened children score lower than children with acquired deafness during the first year after implantation (Fig. 10A.2). However, performance differences diminish over time and are not statistically significant 1 year after implantation. Pooling the literature results revealed no statistical difference in scores between the published and unpublished data for cause and age at onset of deafness. In published and unpublished data

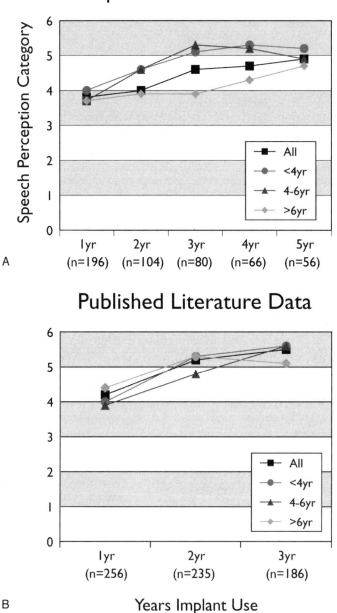

FIG. 10A.1. Mean speech perception category attained as a function of age at implantation. Curves on the left and right represent unpublished and published data sets, respectively. Changes in performance category should be considered in the context of different populations sampled at each time point.

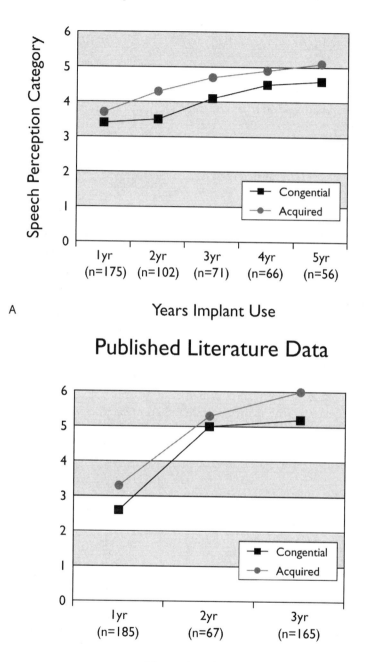

FIG. 10A.2. Mean speech perception category attained at the indicated year after implantation for congenital *(solid line)* and acquired *(dashed line)* causes of deafness. Curves on the left and right represent unpublished and published data sets, respectively. Changes in performance category should be considered in the context of different populations sampled at each time point.

sets, there seems to be no difference between subjects deafened from meningitis compared with other acquired causes of deafness.

Overall analysis of the benefits of cochlear implantation in children shows several results:

- Open-set speech understanding was observed in more than one-half of the reported implanted subjects within 2 years after implantation.
- Initial trends suggest that earlier implantation is associated with a greater trajectory of gains in speech recognition.
- There is no plateau in speech perception benefit over time.
- Differences in performance between congenital and acquired causes diminish over time and are not statistically significant.

Clinical results show little difference from published results, refuting the notion of publication bias in the pediatric cochlear implantation literature. However, because published data are pooled from literature representing an era of clinical practice that is rapidly evolving (*e.g.*, a diminishing age of implantation, technologic improvements in implants), the inclusion of older reports may increasingly misrepresent and underestimate the current benefit of childhood cochlear implantation.

Standardized reporting methods offer the best means of exploring overall treatment effects using cumulative metanalytic methods. Unfortunately, those methods cannot be applied to most pediatric cochlear implant reports. To eliminate the need for rescaling data for the purposes of combining results, future studies will hopefully report or have available individual patient data, including age at implantation, age at onset and cause of deafness, and speech perception scores yearly starting at a minimum of 1 year after implantation. Test protocols, which necessarily vary widely across pediatric populations, should be described explicitly. Adopting a unified approach to data reporting can provide a collective pool of data that that

can guide future management strategies and research.

REFERENCES

Bertram B, Lenarz T, Meyer V, Battmer RD, Hartrampf R. Performance comparisons in postmeningitic prelinguistic and congenitally deaf children. *Adv Otorhinolayngol* 1995;50:134–138.

Fisher LD, van Belle G. *Biostatistics: a methodology for the health sciences.* New York: John Wiley & Sons, 1993:310–321.

Frachet B, Minvielle E, Chouard CH, *et al.* Final report on 1992–1993 children's cochlear implant at the Assistance Publique-Hopitaux de Paris. *Adv Otorhinolayngol* 1995;50:102–107.

Gantz BJ, Tyler RS, Woodworth GG, Tye-Murray N, Fryauf-Bertschy H. Results of multichannel cochlear implants in congenital and acquired prelingual deafness in children: five-year follow-up. *Am J Otol* 1994;15[Suppl 2]:1–7.

Geers AE, Moog JS. Predicting spoken language acquisition of profoundly hearing impaired children. *J Speech Hear Disord* 1987;52:84–94.

Lane H. Letter to the editor. *Am J Otol* 1995;16:393–399.

Jeng GT, Scott JR, Burmeister LF. A comparison of meta-analytic results using literature vs individual patient data: paternal cell immunization for recurrent miscarriage. *JAMA* 1995;274:830–836.

Meyer V, Bertram B, Lenarz T. Performance comparisons in congenitally deaf children with different ages of implantation. *Adv Otorhinolayngol* 1995;50: 129–133.

Meyer V, Bertram B, Lenarz T. The influence of the age of implantation on the auditory speech perception of cochlear implantation in children. *(in press).*

Miyamoto RT, Osberger MJ, Robbins AM, Myres WA, Kessler K. Prelingually deafened children's performance with the Nucleus multichannel cochlear implant. *Am J Otol* 1993;14:437–445.

Miyamoto RT, Osberger MJ, Todd SL, *et al.* Variables affecting implant performance in children. *Laryngoscope* 1994;104:1120–1124.

NIH Consensus Conference. Cochlear Implants. *JAMA* 1995;274:1955–1961.

Osberger MJ, Todd SL, Berry SW, Robbins AM, Miyamoto RT. Effect of age at onset of deafness on children's speech perception abilities with a cochlear implant. *Ann Otol Rhinol* 1991;100:883–888.

Oxman AD, Clarke MJ, Stewart LA. From science to practice: meta-analyses using individual patient data are needed. *JAMA* 1995;274:845–846.

Shea JJ, Domico EH, Lupfer M. Speech perception after multichannel cochlear implantation in the pediatric patient. *Am J Otol* 1994;15:66–70.

Staller SJ, Beiter AL, Brimacombe JA, Mecklenburg DJ, Arndt P. Pediatric performance with the Nucleus 22-channel cochlear implant system. *Am J Otol* 1991;12:126–136.

Tyler RS, Summerfield AQ. Cochlear implantation: relationships with research on auditory deprivation and acclimatization. *Ear Hear* 1996;17[Suppl 3]:38S–50S.

Uziel AS, Reuillard-Artieres F, Mondain M, Piron J-P, Sillon M, Vieu A. Multichannel cochlear implantation in prelingually and postlingually deaf children. *Adv Otorhinolayngol* 1993;48:187–190.

Uziel AS, Reuillard-Artieres F, Sillon M, *et al.* Speech perception performances in prelingually deafened children with the Nucleus multichannel cochlear implant. *Adv Otorhinolayngol* 1995;50:114–118.

Waltzman SB, Cohen NL, Shapiro WH. Use of a multichannel cochlear implant in the congenitally and prelingually deaf population. *Laryngoscope* 1992;102:395–399.

Waltzman SB, Cohen NL, Gomolin RH, Shapiro WH, Ozdamar SR, Hoffman RA. Long-term results of early cochlear implantation in congenitally and prelingually deafened children. *Am J Otol* 1994;15[Suppl]:9–13.

Waltzman S, Cohen N, Shapiro W. Effects of cochlear implantation on the young deaf child. *Adv Otorhinolayngol* 1995;50:125–128.

Waltzman S, Cohen NL, Gomolin R, *et al.* Perception and production results in children implanted between 2 and 5 years of age. *Adv Otorhinolaryngol* 1997;52:177–180.

Appendix 10B

Music and Cochlear Implantation

Charles J. Limb

Spoken words are not the only complex sounds that can be used for communication. Although the primary goal of cochlear implantation is to support verbal communication, the improved ability to perceive music is an important potential benefit. Studies of the impact of cochlear implantation on musical perception have lagged behind studies on language skills, but evidence indicates that some implant users can hear and appreciate music (Gfeller and Lansing, 1991; Eisenberg, 1982). Anecdotal experiences with implant patients suggest that a person's response to music after cochlear implantation may span a broad range, with some patients enjoying music but others finding it less pleasant. Although the degree to which the components of music can be perceived is limited, even prelingually deaf implant patients with only modest performance in speech perception have been reported to enjoy music (Eisenberg, 1982).

The term music describes a series of complex sound waves that are presented to the listener in an organized fashion. The organization of musical sound contains pitch (frequency) and rhythmic (temporal) components. Although different musical forms vary in their tonal and rhythmic content, these components are two of the definitive attributes of all music. Although the ability of implant patients to process frequency and temporal information is undoubtedly critical for music perception, there are several other important variables. Individual preferences may determine to a large extent the rhythmic or harmonic qualities of the music to which a person listens. A patient's musical background, the processing strategies employed, and type of cochlear implant all affect to a significant degree how an implanted individual responds to music (Gfeller *et al.*, 1997; McDermott and McKay, 1997). It has also been reported that younger age correlates strongly with an implanted patient's performance on certain musical perception tasks (Gfeller and 1997).

Spoken language, like music, is composed of organized sound waves with frequency and temporal features. As a consequence of these shared aspects, language comprehension and musical reception demand a number

C. J. Limb: Department of Otolaryngology, Indiana University, Indianapolis, Indiana 46202.

of similar mechanisms for processing acoustic inputs. However, there are significant differences between language and music that have implications for implant-mediated listening. Several intrinsic aspects of speech aid comprehension. Speech tends to organize around particular frequencies, known as formants, combinations of which can be used to produce all vowel sounds. Although the exact frequencies of formants are specific to each individual, acoustic relationships between formants are consistent across individuals. Discrimination between formants is especially important for language comprehension. Listening to speech involves decoding a wide variety of cues within the speech wave itself. For example, even the basic phonemes contain many acoustic cues (in addition to formant frequencies) that can be used for understanding a vocal utterance. These cues provide a form of redundancy within speech that helps to overcome acoustic distortion and to reduce ambiguity.

When a person speaks, many extrinsic cues are also available to aid comprehension. Lip movements, facial expressions, body gestures, linguistic context, and grammatical rules provide important clues that help a listener understand what is being said. Even though the overall range of possible vocalizations has a broad frequency spectrum, the human voice has a relatively limited frequency distribution at any one time. Conversational language usually involves only a single sound source (the speaker) to which a listener must attend. Although the perception of a given vowel within a word is altered by other sounds (*e.g.*, fricatives) within the word, language does not usually require the synchronous processing of multiple independent sound sources.

Instrumental music generally lacks the redundant features of speech that provide cues for listening. Music is not organized around formants; music instead spans a broad frequency spectrum that corresponds to bass or low-pitched instruments, treble or high-pitched instruments, and instruments such as the piano or harp that generate a wider range

of pitches. Visual cues are largely unavailable to the music listener, especially in the case of prerecorded music (live musical performances are a clear exception). Unlike language, musical information is often presented to the listener simultaneously, with multiple instruments of widely ranging timbral characteristics playing an assortment of frequencies and rhythms at the same time. These unique attributes of music described previously should be kept in mind when considering improving the abilities of implant users to hear music.

How is it possible that we experience emotion, such as joy or sadness, in response to music? Music provides daily enjoyment to countless individuals worldwide. One of the main features of music is its ability to evoke a wide range of emotions. As we listen to music, the human mind endows sounds with significance such that they symbolize something beyond pure sound (Sloboda, 1985).

Unlike language, which is representational, music is primarily abstract. Musical notes do not convey a predefined meaning the way that words do. Although musical pitch is based on the absolute frequency with which a sound wave vibrates (*e.g.*, 256 Hz is equal to a middle C), the emotional qualities of music are derived mainly from relationships between notes. One note in a melody gains meaning from its musical interaction with other notes in the melody. This explains why, for example, a musical note played in the song Ode to Joy has a very different connotation from the identical note played in a funeral dirge. Melodies can be transposed from one key to another without modifying their overall melodic quality. However, if the relative intervals between pitches of a given melody are revised, the melody itself has been rewritten. Ode to Joy played with different notes is no longer Ode to Joy.

Music, like spoken language, is inextricably linked to time. The moment after a sound is produced, it disappears. We cannot freeze a song and linger over it the way we can stare intently at a painting. We can, however, appreciate a temporal series of musical events as rhythm, which is one of the most integral components of music. Like pitch, rhythm is perceived on an entirely relative scale, so that each component of a rhythm only had significance in the context of its other components. If the timing of a component is disturbed, the rhythm itself has been fundamentally altered. A 10 second drum roll stretched out over 10 minutes becomes a slow metronome.

Pitch and rhythm are two critical elements of music and language, and they are likely the sources of pleasure (or any other emotion) and meaning we derive from musical sounds. For the recipient of a cochlear implant to hear and appreciate music in the same way a normally hearing person does, he or she must be able to discriminate between different frequencies. The temporal fidelity of incoming signals through the implant must be maintained. It appears that many implant users can perform discriminations of pitch patterns and of rhythm, especially when electrical pulse stimuli are applied (Gfeller *et al.*, 1998; Pijl, 1997; McDermott and McKay, 1997). However, pitch and timbre information transmitted through speech processors is not always perceived with precision. One study of two subjects with single bipolar intracochlear electrode pairs reported that pitch information was largely unavailable to them when musical stimuli were processed through speech processors (Pijl, 1997). For electrical pulse stimuli, the accuracy of pitch interval judgments decreases as the intervals between pitches become larger (McDermott and McKay, 1997). Implant recipients appear to be better at distinguishing rhythmic patterns than melodic or harmonic patterns (Gfeller and Lansing, 1991 and 1992).

It appears that discerning rhythms with a cochlear implant is easier than identifying musical notes. Such aspects of implant mediated listening reveal the challenges of perceiving music in its fullness through an implant. More importantly, they point toward areas requiring further investigation, with the ultimate goal of improved perception of all acoustic information. Future advances in processing schemes that improve speech representation for cochlear implant listeners may also add a dimension of improved comprehension of other complex stimuli, such as music. With continued research, even those with profound hearing impairment may one day hear music at its clearest.

REFERENCES

Eisenberg LS. Use of the cochlear implant by the prelingually deaf. *Ann Otol Rhinol Laryngol Suppl* 1982;91:62–66.
Gfeller K, Woodworth G, Robin DA, Witt S, Knutson JF. Perception of rhythmic and sequential pitch patterns by normally hearing adults and adult cochlear implant users. *Ear Hear* 1997;18:252–260.
Gfeller K, Knutson JF, Woodworth G, Witt S, DeBus B. Timbral recognition and appraisal by adult cochlear implant users and normal-hearing adults. *J Am Acad Audiol* 1998;9:1–19.
Gfeller KE, Lansing C. Melodic, rhythmic, and timbral perception of adult cochlear implant users. *J Speech Hear Res* 1991;34:916–920.
Gfeller KE, Lansing C. Musical perception of cochlear implant users as measured by the primary measures of music audiation: an item analysis. *J Music Ther* 1992;29:18–39.
McDermott HJ, McKay CM. Musical pitch perception with electrical stimulation of the cochlea. *J Acoust Soc Am* 1997;101:1622–1631.
Pijl S. Labeling of musical interval size by cochlear implant patients and normally hearing subjects. *Ear Hear* 19967;18:364–372.
Sloboda J. *The musical mind: the cognitive psychology of music.* Oxford: Oxford University Press, 1985.

11

Outcomes of Cochlear Implantation: Assessment of Quality of Life Impact and Economic Evaluation of the Benefits of the Cochlear Implant in Relation to Costs

John K. Niparko, André K. Cheng, and
Howard W. Francis

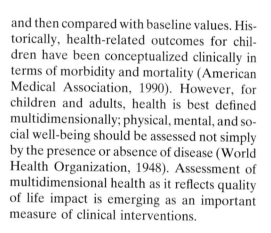

Management of sensorineural hearing loss is most often assessed in terms of audiologic benefit. In this context, *benefit* is most clearly defined by enhanced speech understanding. Other approaches evaluate effects on other life attributes in addition to restored sensory function. Trends in clinical research have increasingly emphasized the importance of assessing the impact of a medical treatment on an individual's daily life (Drummond and Maynard, 1993). Called *outcomes research*, these methods survey an intervention's performance in real life, when implemented by many professionals on broad populations of individuals.

Outcomes research continues to garner interest in shaping health care policy. Several perspectives of outcomes may be considered

and then compared with baseline values. Historically, health-related outcomes for children have been conceptualized clinically in terms of morbidity and mortality (American Medical Association, 1990). However, for children and adults, health is best defined multidimensionally; physical, mental, and social well-being should be assessed not simply by the presence or absence of disease (World Health Organization, 1948). Assessment of multidimensional health as it reflects quality of life impact is emerging as an important measure of clinical interventions.

APPLYING OUTCOMES RESEARCH TO COST-EFFECTIVENESS

Market forces at work in today's rapidly changing and competitive health care industry have induced medical care providers, from sole practitioner to large health maintenance organizations, to justify interventions based not only on safety and efficacy, but also on cost-effectiveness. This is particularly true when new technologies are considered, because medical technology probably has become one of the system's most important cost driver (Samuel, 1988). HMO's and insurance companies are not considered as factors.

J. K. Niparko: Department of Otolaryngology—Head & Neck Surgery, The Listening Center at Johns Hopkins, The Johns Hopkins University, Baltimore, Maryland 21205-1809.

A. K. Cheng: Department of Otolaryngology—Head & Neck Surgery, The Johns Hopkins University, Baltimore, Maryland 21205.

H. W. Francis: Department of Otolaryngology—Head & Neck Surgery, The Listening Center at Johns Hopkins, The Johns Hopkins University, Baltimore, Maryland 21205-1809.

Methods of assessing cost-effectiveness evaluate health interventions based on the relation between the resources consumed (costs) and the resultant health outcomes (effects). Such analyses provide a quantified assessment of the value provided and seek to describe the impact of an intervention in terms of benefit and cost. An outcome can be practically assessed with respect to the costs for the care, rehabilitation, and maintenance associated with a particular treatment. Such research provides the basis for solving problems of medical economics, rating the effectiveness of interventions, and optimizing use of health care dollars.

The effectiveness of an intervention may be evaluated in the context of its cost in several ways. These methods differ in the manner in which outcomes are valued. In *cost-benefit analysis,* outcomes are valued in financial terms [reported in U.S. dollars ($)], usually with respect to future health care expenditures saved.

Cost-benefit ratio =

$$\frac{\text{Net costs (cumulative evaluation, treatment, maintenance in \$)}}{\text{Net monetary effects (in \$)}}$$

In *cost-effectiveness analysis,* outcomes are measured in natural units of clinical effects. Clinical effects are often expressed in life years saved, but depending on the study, effects may be expressed in any unit of measure deemed clinically significant. For example, in comparing different antihypertensive intervention strategies, millimeters of mercury of blood pressure reduction may be an appropriate unit of measure. The key feature of cost-effectiveness analysis is that a person does not need to assign a dollar value to the outcome.

Cost-effectiveness ratio =

$$\frac{\text{Net costs (cumulative evaluation, treatment, maintenance in \$)}}{\text{Net effects (in units of clinical effects)}}$$

A form of cost-effectiveness analysis that rates outcome in terms of generic changes in life expectancy and quality of life is *cost-utility analysis.* The unit of outcome measure is *quality-adjusted life-years* (QALYs). In this approach, life-years are converted into QALYs by a quality of life factor called *health utility.* This conversion factor represents a quantitative valuation of a person's quality of life expressed on a scale from 0.00 (death) to 1.00 (perfect health).

Cost-utility ratio =

$$\frac{\text{Net costs (cumulative evaluation, treatment, maintenance in \$)}}{\text{Net effects (in QALYs)}}$$

For example, although treatments for hearing rehabilitation have little impact on longevity, they commonly result in improved awareness and possibly in enhanced communication. These factors change one's quality of life, and cost-utility therefore provides an appropriate measurement tool for rating effects relative to associated costs.

Because QALYs incorporate generic changes in life expectancy and quality of life resulting from an intervention, cost per QALY of diverse interventions can be compared. Substantial improvement in the quality of life resulting from an intervention decreases the cost incurred per QALY. The lower the cost per QALY, or the greater the number of QALYs obtained at a given cost, the greater is the cost-effectiveness of an intervention.

Properly performed cost-utility analyses entail methodologic considerations related to cost and effect to yield a cost-utility ratio (Fig. 11.1).

Cost determinations include the following features:

- Cumulative costs for diagnosis and prognostication, medical and surgical treatment, rehabilitation, maintenance, and follow-up are determined.
- A comprehensive analysis requires the inclusion of costs associated with potential complications, replacements, and warranties.

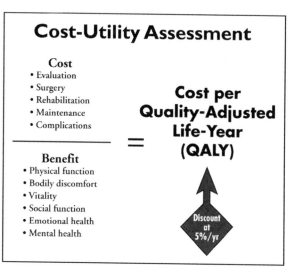

FIG. 11.1. The utility of a medical intervention is measured in cost per quality-adjusted life-years (QALYs), which is the ratio of cost and benefit discounted at 5% per year to provide a value in today's dollars.

• If appropriate, the morbidity associated with a surgical intervention, for example, is accounted for by an estimate of a temporary reduction in quality of life.

Benefit determinations include the following factors:

• Benefit is analyzed according to the concept of *utility*.
• *Utility* is basic to systems of commerce and trade, and it represents the perceived value of a particular good or service.
• *Health utility* represents the perceived value of a person's health, expressed as a numerical valuation of a person's quality of life on a 0.00 (death) to 1.00 (perfect health) scale.
• Benefit analysis seeks to describe changes in health status with methods that are sensitive to the condition and a change in the condition with the intervention under study.
• Ideally, this analysis evaluates attributes of the treatment that are applicable to cost-effectiveness relative to other treatments.
• The most useful methods of assessing quality of life effects are those that are compact, reproducible, valid, and generalizable and

that appropriately weigh the multiple factors that determine overall health status.

The following are examples of assessment instruments:

• Medical Outcomes Study Shortform-36: surveys patient perception of physical function, discomfort, vitality, social function, and emotional and mental health (Ware and Sherboune, 1992)
• Ontario Health Utility Index: measures patient perception of vision, hearing, speech, emotion, ambulation, dexterity, cognition, self-care, and pain (Feeny *et al.*, 1992)
• Quality of Well-being Scale: broadly measures patient perception of physical activity, mobility, discomfort, social interaction, and mental, emotional, and sexual health (Kaplan *et al.*, 1976)

The cost-utility yield can be determined as follows:

• Health utility resulting from an intervention is measured in QALYs, which provide the denominator in cost-utility ratios.
• The cost per QALY represents the utility of a particular intervention relative to its cost. Costs and utility dollar figures are dis-

counted at 5% to provide a result that is valued in today's dollars (Fig. 11.1).

- Duration of therapeutic benefit is incorporated in the QALY measure.
- Sustained improvement in the quality of life resulting from an intervention diminishes the cost per QALY. Because QALYs incorporate generic changes in life expectancy and quality of life produced by a health care intervention, cost per QALY of diverse interventions can be compared. The lower the cost per QALY, or the greater the number of QALYs obtained at a given cost, the greater is the cost-utility.

COST-UTILITY OF COCHLEAR IMPLANTATION IN ADULTS

Because hearing rehabilitation presumably improves audition and communication and has little impact on longevity, cost-utility analysis provides an appropriate measure of hearing rehabilitation. Seventeen cost-utility studies have been performed to assess cochlear implantation in adults (Palmer et al., 1999; Fugain et al., 1998; Wyatt et al., 1996; Wyatt et al., 1995a; Wyatt et al., 1995b; Wyatt and Niparko, 1995; Harris et al., 1995; Evans et al., 1995; Lea and Hailey, 1995; Summerfield et al., 1995; six studies in Summerfield and Marshall, 1995; Lea, 1991).

Ten of these studies used models of cost and benefit, although four report duplicate results. Seven of the studies tracked actual costs and performed outcome measurements in cohorts of patients. Costs per QALY for the cochlear implant in adult users were determined using clinical cost data accumulated through preoperative, operative, and postoperative phases of cochlear implantation. Benefits were determined by measuring health utility before and after implantation; the difference in health utility values was then translated into an increased number of QALYs associated with cochlear implantation. Generally, these studies have reported the following:

- Patient data on adults (>18 years) with bilateral, postlingual, profound deafness

- A decrement in health utility associated with profound deafness on a scale from 0.00 (death) to 1.00 (perfect health) (Fig. 11.2A)
- A subsequent gain in health utility after cochlear implantation (Fig. 11.2B)
- Cost-utility value assessed in terms of $/QALY (Fig. 11.3)

These studies provide information that sheds light on the impact of cochlear implantation and that may help to further understand the impact of acquired profound hearing impairment on quality of life.

Pooled results from adults with profound deafness ($n = 619$) yielded a decrement in health utility of -0.46 (95% CI: -0.44 to -0.48) from a perfect health score of 1.00 (i.e., $1.00 - 0.46 =$ health utility of 0.54) (Table 11.1). Most of these studies have concluded that the cochlear implant compares favorably with other accepted health interventions, but the reported range of results is considerable. Health utility gains varied from +0.07 to +0.41, yielding cost-utility values of $7,405 to $31,177/QALY. Pooled results from seven studies ($n = 511$) indicated a health utility gain from cochlear implantation of +0.26 (95% CI: +0.24 to +0.28), yielding an improvement from the profoundly deaf health utility of 0.54 to 0.80 (Table 11.2). This resulted in a weighted average cost-utility figure from cochlear implantation of $12,787/QALY (Table 11.3). This cost-utility value compares favorably to that of other medical and surgical interventions (Fig. 11.4).

One limitation of these studies relates to the difficulty in comparing the health utility gain from those who receive a cochlear implant to controls who do not. Controls are defined as adults with bilateral, postlingual, profound deafness who have not received a cochlear implant. They may be on the waiting list to receive an implant, rejected as an implant candidate for medical or insurance reasons, or may not wish to receive an implant. Only one study incorporated the use of controls. Palmer et al. (1999) followed 14

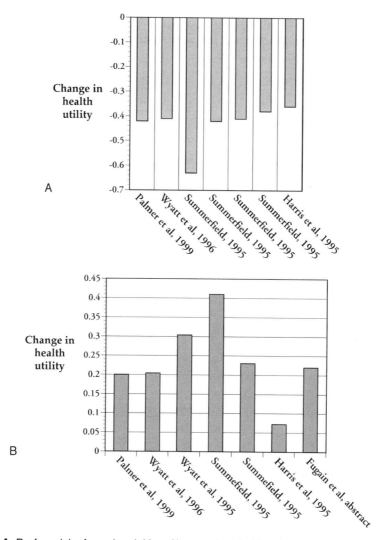

FIG. 11.2. A: Profound deafness in adulthood is associated with a decline in health utility. **B:** Cochlear implantation is associated with an increase in healthy utility in deaf adults.

control patients prospectively for 1 year along with 37 implanted patients. Whereas there was a +0.20 increase in health utility (0.58 to 0.78) in the implanted group, the control group reported the same baseline health utility with no change after 1 year (0.58 and 0.58, respectively).

Most cost-utility analyses used the Visual Analog Scale (VAS) or the Ontario Health Utilities Index (HUI) to determine health utility values. The VAS is a feeling thermometer rating scale with which patients simply rate their own health on a scale from 0 to 100. The HUI is a multiattribute health survey that incorporates into its scale a health utility loss for blind or deaf or mute of −0.40 (*i.e.*, 1.00 − 0.40 = health utility of 0.60), a value derived by the time tradeoff method from a sample of the general population in Ontario, Canada. For two disparate health utility methods, the HUI (−0.42; time tradeoff applied to general population) and the VAS (−0.47; rating scale applied to patients with deafness) derive similar valuations of

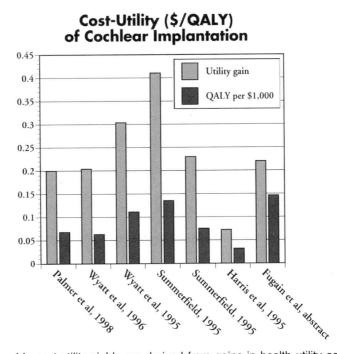

FIG. 11.3. Favorable cost-utility yields are derived from gains in health utility associated with cochlear implantation.

health utility effects of profound deafness. The subsequent health utility gain from cochlear implantation is less similar between the HUI (+0.20) and VAS (+0.31). The VAS has been criticized for overestimating losses in health utility from mild diseases because the respondent is not forced to make a choice under conditions of uncertainty (Torrance *et al.*, 1995; Torrance *et al.*, 1996). However, the HUI can be faulted for attaching a value to profound deafness based on responses of people who have never experienced deafness. With the VAS, patients derive the valuation of their own health because they have experienced normal hearing and profound deafness in their lives.

TABLE 11.1. *Loss in health utility from profound deafness in adults*

Study	Instrument	Patients	N	Utility loss	SD	95% CI
Palmer et al, in press	HUI	Implanted	40	−0.42	0.17	(−0.37, −0.47)
Palmer et al, in press	HUI	Controls	14	−0.42	0.20	(−0.32, −0.52)
Wyatt et al, 1996	HUI	Controls	32	−0.41	0.32	(−0.30, −0.52)
Niparko, unpublished	VAS-without	Implanted	229	−0.47	0.26	(−0.42, −0.53)
Summerfield, 1995	VAS-without	Implanted	105	−0.63	0.26	(−0.58, −0.68)
Summerfield, 1995	VAS-before	Implanted	103	−0.42	0.21	(−0.38, −0.46)
Summerfield, 1995	VAS	Controls	52	−0.41	0.26	(−0.34, −0.48)
Summerfield, 1995	VAS	Controls	37	−0.38	0.25	(−0.30, −0.46)
Harris et al, 1995	QWB	Implanted	7	−0.36	0.12	(−0.27, −0.45)
			619	−0.46[a]	0.23	(0.44, 0.48)

HUI, Ontario Health Utility Index, Mark II; VAS, Visual Analog Scale; VAS-without, patient rates health utility if the cochlear implant was taken away; VAS-before, patient rates health utility before implantation; QWB, Quality of Well-Being Scale.
[a]This represents a health utility loss of 0.46 from a "perfect health" score of 1.00 (i.e., 1.00 − 0.46 = 0.54). Weight = 1 ÷ variance.

TABLE 11.2. *Gain in health utility from cochlear implantation in adults*

Study	Instrument	Study design	N	Utility gain	SD	95% CI
Palmer et al, in press	HUI	Prospective	37	+0.20	0.17	(0.15, 0.25)
Wyatt et al, 1996	HUI	Cross-sectional	229	+0.204	0.237	(0.17, 0.24)
Wyatt et al, 1995	VAS-without	Retrospective	229	+0.304	0.239	(0.27, 0.34)
Summerfield, 1995	VAS-without	Retrospective	105	+0.41	0.26	(0.36, 0.46)
Summerfield, 1995	VAS-before	Retrospective	103	+0.23	0.26	(0.18, 0.28)
Harris et al, 1995	QWB	Prospective	7	+0.072	0.119	(−0.02, 0.16)
Fugain et al, abstract	Not specified	Retrospective	30	+0.22	0.25	(0.13, 0.31)
			511	+0.26[a]	0.23	(0.24, 0.28)

HUI, Ontario Health Utility Index, Mark II; VAS, Visual Analog Scale; VAS-without, patient rates health utility if the cochlear implant was taken away; VAS-before, patient rates health utility before implantation; QWB, Quality of Well-Being Scale.

[a]This represents a health utility gain of 0.26 from the above "profoundly deaf" score of 0.54 (i.e., 0.54 + 0.26 = 0.80). Weight = 1 ÷ variance.

Taken together, these observations suggest that severe to profound hearing loss has an impact on quality of life that is substantial and measurable and that cochlear implantation is associated with marked improvement in self-rated measures of quality of life. The cochlear implant produces effects that favorably influence cost-effectiveness ratios, and cochlear implantation appears to represent an effective use of health care dollars.

OUTCOME MEASURES OF COCHLEAR IMPLANTS IN CHILDREN

As an intervention that uniquely bridges the medical and educational aspects of rehabilitation in childhood deafness, cochlear implantation should be assessed for its costs and communication-related outcomes and

for the level of audiologic benefit. The benefits of pediatric cochlear implantation can be assessed with broad measures that are probably interrelated:

- Traditional measures of auditory outcomes, including performance on tests of speech perception, intelligibility, and complexity of speech production, and linguistic competence
- Educational performance and use of special educational and rehabilitative resources
- Perceived changes in quality of life

Financial constraints on health care and special education services at the federal, state, and local levels increasingly mandate assessments of outcomes. Such assessments are likely to be important in shaping policy to-

TABLE 11.3. *Cost-utility of cochlear implantation*

Study	Instrument	Country	N	Utility	$/QALY
Palmer et al, in press	HUI	U.S.	37	+0.20	$14,670
Wyatt et al, 1996	HUI	U.S.	229	+0.204	$15,928
Wyatt et al, 1995	VAS-without	U.S.	229	+0.304	$9,000
Summerfield, 1995	VAS-without	U.K.	105	+0.41	$7,405
Summerfield, 1995	VAS-before	U.K.	103	+0.23	$13,200
Harris et al, 1995	QWB	U.S.	7	+0.072	$31,711
Fugain et al, abstract	Not specified	France	30	+0.22	$6,848
			511	+0.26	$12,787[a]

HUI, Ontario Health Utility Index, Mark II; VAS, Visual Analog Scale; VAS-without, patient rates health utility if the cochlear implant was taken away; VAS-before, patient rates health utility before implantation; QWB, Quality of Well-Being Scale; $/QALY, cost-utility determination.

[a]Weight = 1 ÷ variance.

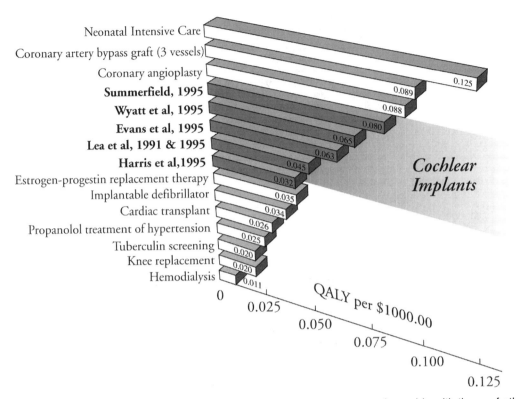

FIG. 11.4. The cost-utility of cochlear implantation in adults compares favorably with those of other medical and surgical interventions.

ward treatment of childhood hearing impairment. For example, outcomes analysis for childhood cochlear implantation can further inform discussions of universal screening of hearing in newborns. Early identification likely impacts the subsequent evaluation and management of candidates for cochlear implantation. Evaluating the impact of age of identification on cochlear implant results provides key outcomes data in the appraisal of different options for screening hearing in young children. An ongoing analysis of a variety of outcomes can also contribute constructively to the social discourse on the appropriateness of cochlear implantation in children (see Chapter 14).

Until the long-term effects of the cochlear implant on educational achievement and vocational outcome are known, the assessment of educational independence, verbal language skills, and literacy can serve as prelimi-

nary outcome measures. Measures that reflect the development of these skills have been shown to predict educational and vocational outcome in hearing-impaired children (Trybus and Karchmer, 1977; Saur *et al.*, 1986; Kasen *et al.*, 1990; Holt, 1993).

Several skill sets directly impact scholastic performance. For speech and language-impaired populations, the development of an aural concept of language is critical to the development of visual language comprehension (reading) and expression (writing) skills. For example, mathematical computational ability among 15-year-old hearing-impaired individuals lies below the seventh-grade level, whereas the average ability of 15-year-old hearing students is at the tenth-grade level (Holt, 1993). Even more striking is the disparity in reading comprehension. Mean reading comprehension ability among the hearing impaired is at the third-grade level, whereas the mean ability among 15-year-old hearing students is at the tenth-grade level.

Auditory perception appears to be critical to a number of cognitive processes. Tests of attention reveal that hearing-impaired children have deficits in their selective visual attention, suggesting that auditory input affects the development of attention skills (Quittner *et al.*, 1991). Profoundly hearing-impaired children who receive a cochlear implant demonstrate improved visual attention skills that eventually match those of age-matched peers with less severe hearing impairments who are able to use hearing aids. Fundamental cognitive domains such as attention reasonably can be expected to exert a broad impact on quality of life. However, measurement of such effects represents a considerable challenge in clinical research.

Special Education

In the United States, special education is defined as unconventional instruction for children who do not benefit optimally from conventional educational practices or have impaired access to conventional instruction caused by disability (Lloyd *et al.*, 1991; Mastropieri and Scruggs, 1987; Smith and Lockerson, 1992; Snell, 1993). These services are delivered to those with physical and communication handicaps, sensory disabilities (blindness and deafness), differences in intellectual capacity (gifted and mentally retarded), emotional or behavioral disturbances, and learning disabilities. Education of the hearing-impaired student often draws on all aspects of special education to foster receptive and expressive communication skills, particularly when verbal communication is the objective. Special instructional services typically include individualized teaching techniques, materials, equipment, facilities, and related support services.

Mandates derive from laws of compulsory education. Legislative action in the United States, particularly the Education for All Handicapped Children Act of 1974, defined specific requirements for schooling students with disabilities, including the hearing impaired. These mandates compel systems of education to avail students with disabilities, at no cost, a public education in the least-restrictive environment—one that approximates as closely as possible that experienced by nondisabled students. To address the specific needs of disabled children, this legislation stipulates the following:

- Individualized education plans must faithfully reflect a student's educational needs.
- The educational options that are provided to disabled students cannot be constrained by their handicap.

Compliance with legal standards poses a considerable demand for special education services in the United States (Lloyd *et al.*, 1991). During the 1989–1990 school year, more than 4.5 million children received these services. About 85% of these children and youths were of school age, making up about 10% of all school-aged children, and they required approximately 15,000 special education teachers. Such demand entails steep expenditures by systems of education. Given the substantial costs associated with special education, an analysis of patterns of usage of educational resources is a logical first step in analysis of the cost-effectiveness of technologies such as the cochlear implant that may impact educational placement.

The costs associated with education constitute only one of many considerations in developing programs of special education. Special education for hearing-impaired children should be carefully crafted to meet the child's individual needs (Northern and Downs, 1991; Vergera *et al.*, 1993). Highly differentiated programs of instruction with appropriately trained professionals and the requisite support services remain the primary objective. Such a program should include special activities beyond the regular curriculum, careful monitoring of academic and maturational progress, and frequent consideration of the child's emotional health and self-esteem.

Consideration of a hearing-impaired

child's educational needs is multifaceted. For example, a self-contained classroom may provide more focused remediation of educational deficits but also provides limited access to models of spoken language. Such language models can enhance language acquisition for hearing-impaired children (McCormick and Schiefelbusch, 1990).

Placement and Speech and Language Rehabilitative Services

When children with disabilities can benefit from participation with nondisabled children, they are often enrolled in a program offered by a neighborhood school (Lloyd *et al.*, 1991). Mainstreaming, inclusion, or integration is conceptually consistent with the legal mandate for education in a minimally restrictive environment. In the United States, two-thirds of students with disabilities receive most of their instruction in regular education classes.

The appropriateness of mainstreaming hearing-impaired children is highly debatable (Northern and Downs, 1991). For most children with disabilities in the United States, a comprehensive program of services different from conventional instruction is not provided. Instead, those features of the educational program from which the child cannot benefit are modified and designated in the individualized education plan. In general, the lesser the degree of disability, the fewer special education services are required, and the more likely it is that these services will be provided in a mainstream setting. For the hearing-impaired child, placement in a mainstream setting often introduces demands for related support services to enhance speech understanding.

Limitations in the reception and expression of English language often constitute the primary factor in determining educational placement and the need for speech and language services for hearing-impaired children. When deficits in a language base preclude mainstreaming, special education may be provided in a separate classroom for part of the school day. For children with severe speech and language delays, schooling in a self-contained special education room is often needed for the entire school day.

The Educational Resource Matrix (ERM)

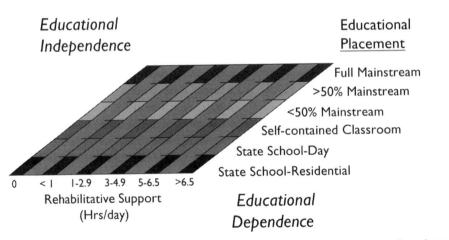

Educational Resource Matrix

Educational Independence

Educational Placement

Full Mainstream
>50% Mainstream
<50% Mainstream
Self-contained Classroom
State School-Day
State School-Residential

0   < l   l-2.9   3-4.9   5-6.5   >6.5
Rehabilitative Support
(Hrs/day)

Educational Dependence

FIG. 11.5. The educational resource matrix (ERM) plots classroom placement *(ordinate)* against the number of hours per day of rehabilitative support *(abscissa)*. Movement toward the left upper corner of the ERM is associated with a gain in educational independence.

for hearing-impaired children tracks the pattern of resource use associated with classroom placement (Fig. 11.5). Greater educational independence (as evidenced by movement toward a mainstream environment with less need for supportive services) is mapped as movement toward the upper left-hand corner of the matrix. However, initial observations suggest that progress into mainstream settings is more likely to be associated with greater use of special services such as speech and language rehabilitation early on. These needs then appear to diminish with time. This pattern is modeled in the ERM as movement to the upper right hand corner of the matrix illustration.

In addition to placement alternatives, specialized support services are an intervention mainstay in most special education settings. Interpreters, speech language pathologists, itinerant teachers of the deaf, instructional assistants, and academic tutors provide services to augment classroom instruction in our region. Provision of these services is determined by the educational needs of the child and by logistical issues such as availability of appropriate professionals, budgetary limitations, and legislative requirements. These factors often affect a child's placement more than educational needs. Moreover, the family's psychosocial status and support play a critical role in the child's rehabilitation and probably affect placement (Quittner *et al.*, 1991).

After a deaf child has developed a foundation of communication skills, a mainstream classroom teacher may work with an interpreter, speech and language pathologist, or deaf educator to provide the child with access to classroom instruction and provide individualized instruction to compensate for the child's language and speech delays. In many cases, increased intervention is required for subjects requiring mastery of abstract thinking and reasoning skills. The level of support required may correspond with the relative linguistic demands of different school subjects. Although the deaf child may have communication abilities that are adequate for some subjects, subjects that involve greater abstract thinking require higher-order English language skills and may entail more intensive support services.

In the United States, more than 90% of special education takes place in regular public schools, with the remainder provided in special day or residential schools, hospitals, and home schooling (Lloyd *et al.*, 1991; Mastropieri and Scuggs, 1992; Smith and Lockerson, 1992). Similarly, school programs for teaching the hearing impaired and options for mainstreaming vary markedly with geographic location in the United States. In the mid-Atlantic region, for example, an oral-language private school for the deaf is not available. Options for educational services range from a residential school employing predominantly manual strategies to public school programs that use a range of strategies for developing oral language.

Clinical investigators have preliminarily analyzed the impact of cochlear implantation on school placement (Koch *et al.*, 1997; Nottingham Paediatric Cochlear Implant Programme, 1997; Francis *et al.*, 1999). These investigations found mainstreaming rates of 58% after 2 years of implant experience (Nottingham Paediatric Cochlear Implant Programme, 1997) and 75% after 4 years of implant experience (Francis *et al.*, 1999). These rates exceed the (control) rates of mainstreaming of unimplanted children with similar levels of baseline hearing by fivefold (Nottingham Paediatric Cochlear Implant Programme, 1997) to twofold (Francis *et al.*, 1999). However, such figures ignore the large numbers of variables affecting placement and greater detail of analysis is required. Moreover, given the variability in educational placement and services, models that track the use of educational resources by hearing-impaired children are likely to be regionally specific.

Educational Resource Matrix

The ERM (Fig. 11.5) has been developed to map educational placement and the use of rehabilitation resources by hearing-impaired children (Koch *et al.*, 1997). The ERM serves as a model recognizing that programs, services, and policies related to the education of hearing-impaired children vary markedly across the United States but offers a basis on which to begin appraisal of the cost-benefit of cochlear implants in these children.

The ERM stratifies qualitative aspects of school setting and levels of rehabilitative support based on the experience of the rehabilitation team at the Johns Hopkins University Cochlear Implant Program (The Listening Center at Johns Hopkins). The school environment is monitored by the cochlear implant rehabilitation team, affording the observation of classroom placement and use of special educational services over years. Because of variability in the resources and policies of school districts, changes in classroom placement by an implanted child is not a sufficient indication of progress in educational independence. Most noticeable was the observation that a change in classroom placement was often accompanied by changes in the need for support services. The ERM makes it possible to follow placement and resource usage over time to provide a first approximation of educational independence. Through school visits, teacher and parent interviews, and review of individual education plans, trends in educational independence in implanted children are compared with those of unimplanted severely to profoundly hearing-impaired students. Assigning real costs to coordinates on the ERM enables estimates of cost-benefit ratios associated with levels of educational independence (Koch *et al.*, 1997; Francis *et al.*, 1999).

Educational Placement

Stratification of educational placement reflects a continuum from full mainstream placement (within the child's local school) to residential placement at a state school for the deaf (Fig. 11.5). Typically, public school districts often incorporate partial main-streaming into programs of deaf education. Educational setting is indexed according to the degree of student independence according to six categories:

1. Full mainstream in regular classroom and school
2. More than 50% of the school day spent in a regular classroom and school; less than 50% of the school day spent in a special education classroom
3. Less than 50% of the school day spent in a regular classroom and school; more than 50% of the school day spent in a special education classroom
4. Full-time placement in a special education classroom in a regular school
5. State school for the deaf: day student
6. State school for the deaf: residential student

Rehabilitative Support Services

Specialized support includes the use of related services designed to enhance communication. The ERM reflects the range of specialty services often required by hearing-impaired students. Teachers of the hearing impaired, itinerant special educators, speech and language pathologists, educational audiologists, interpreters (*e.g.*, sign language, cued speech, oral), occupational therapists, and instructional assistants may be required. Use of these services is based on a 6.5-hour school day and are averaged over a 5-day week. When the child attends a half-day program, divisions are based on percentage of total time spent in school. Support services vary along a continuum, which can be divided as follows:

1. No support services
2. Less than 1 hour per day
3. 1 to 2.9 hours per day
4. 3 to 4.9 hours per day
5. 5 to 6.5 hours per day
6. More than 6.5 hours per day

Determining the pattern of educational resource use of populations of implanted children in the ERM requires long-term follow-up. Given the length of time needed for implanted children to acquire receptive (Boothroyd *et al.*, 1991; Osberger *et al.*, 1991; Fryhauf-Bertschy *et al.*, 1992) and expressive (Hasenstab and Tobey, 1991; Tye-Murray *et al.*, 1995) skills of oral language, measurable changes in the use of educational resources may not be evident until 24 months or longer after implantation in young children. Prior communication mode, duration of device use, and performance on scales of intelligence may further contribute to variance in educational progress (Quittner and Steck, 1991).

In the Mid-Atlantic region, self-contained classrooms in neighborhood schools are staffed in such a manner as to markedly lower the ratio of students to teachers from that of a regular classroom. State schools for the deaf in the Mid-Atlantic region maintain similarly low ratios of students to staff. Lower ratios of student to staff contribute to higher educational costs. Conversely, movement on the ERM toward greater mainstream placement is accompa-

nied by reduced educational costs. However, the cost reductions associated with changes in placement are likely to be offset in initial years by an increased need for support services to optimize instruction in mainstream settings.

Observed Trends in Educational Placement and Resource Use

In a study of 35 implanted school-age children from the Johns Hopkins Cochlear Implant Program, a positive correlation between the length of implant experience and the incidence of placement in mainstream classrooms was observed (Fig. 11.6). Although classroom placement remained static in the first 2 years of implantation, the rate of mainstream placement increased to 30% in the second 2 years of implant experience, and 75% among children with over 4 years of experience (Fig. 11.7). For an age-matched group of nonimplanted children, there was also a positive trend toward increased mainstream placement, although at older ages and

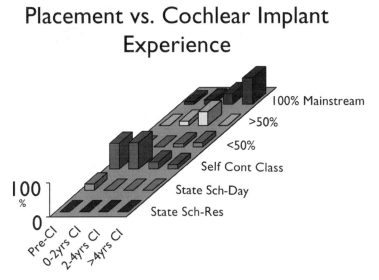

FIG. 11.6. Educational placement is compared with the length of cochlear implant experience. Whereas educational placement was minimally changed in the first 2 years compared with the status before implantation, rates of full-time placement in mainstream classrooms increased thereafter to a high of 76% for children with more than 4 years of implant experience. CI, cochlear implantation; Sch, school; Res, residential.

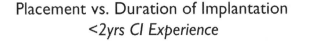

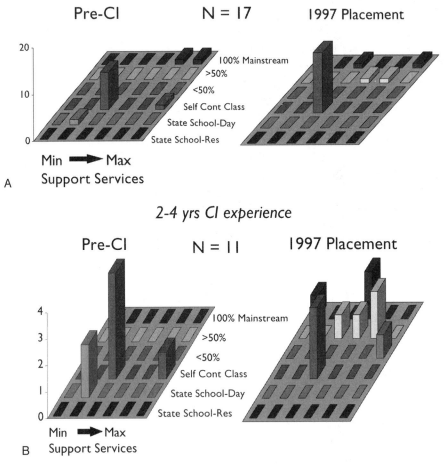

FIG. 11.7. A gradual increase in educational independence is evident in the before and after cochlear implantation use of educational resources by children with less than 2 years of implant experience **(A)**, 2 to 4 years of implant experience **(B)**, and more than 4 years of implant experience **(C)**.

at lower rates compared with the implanted group. There was also a decline in the use of support services by fully mainstreamed implanted children with increasing implant experience. When compared with an age-matched group of nonimplanted fully mainstreamed hearing-impaired children, implanted children used one-fourth the number of support hours. More so than the trend toward mainstream placement itself, this decline in the use of special education services

suggests a substantial evolution in language skills and educational independence by implanted children within the first 4 yours of their implant experience.

In the third and fourth years of implant experience, as children began their transition toward mainstream placement, 4 of 10 children demonstrated an increase in the use of support services, whereas others showed a decline. The variable use of special support services by implanted children in transition

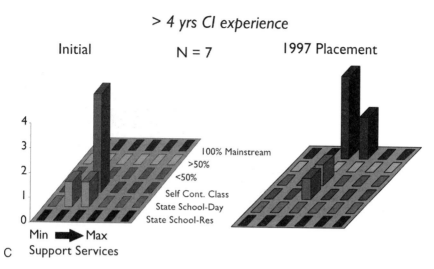

> 4 yrs Cl experience

Initial   N = 7   1997 Placement

4
3
2
1
0

100% Mainstream
>50%
<50%
Self Cont. Class
State School-Day
State School-Res

Min ➡ Max
C   Support Services

FIG. 11.7. *(Continued)*

speaks to a complex array of factors that may influence the path of educational migration by a cochlear implanted child, including the presence of concomitant learning disabilities, the effectiveness of preimplantation intervention, the age at implantation, and the resources and policies of the school.

Cost-Benefit Considerations for Children

The ERM should not be construed as a measure of implant-mediated scholastic performance, nor can the ERM be used to determine educational prognosis. Several other clinical instruments have been offered to rate and predict educational success with implants (Northern and Downs, 1991; Boothroyd *et al.*, 1991; Hellman *et al.*, 1991). However, because cost data can be assigned to location points within the ERM, it can be used to generate longitudinal data on relative costs of education. This is critical in calculating cost-benefit ratios concerning multichannel cochlear implants (Wyatt *et al.*, 1995a).

Educational costs can be assigned to variables in the ERM based on actual budgetary data. For example, costs used to assess the impact of observed educational trends on the cost-benefit of multiple channel implantation

(Fig. 11.8) were derived from the 1995 State of Maryland Department of Education Budget (Francis *et al.*, 1999). The lower right corner of the ERM represents one extreme of the matrix, the cost of full-time education in a state school for the deaf at $42,000/year. The upper left corner represents the other extreme, the cost of the education of a fully mainstreamed child who does not require support, at $6,106/year. Hourly costs associated with speech and language support were derived from salary figures for public school speech pathologists and interpreters for the 1995–1996 school year and was estimated at $23/hour for the state of Maryland. Cost figures for cochlear implantation should include the cost of evaluation, placement of the implant, rehabilitation, device maintenance, and allowances for potential complications as previously described (Wyatt *et al.*, 1995a). This was estimated to be $43,000 based on 1997 cost data from The Listening Center at Johns Hopkins.

A cost-benefit analysis was performed with financial projections covering the 13-year period of education for children implanted at 3 and 5 years of age (Fig. 11.8 and Table 11.4) (Francis *et al.*, 1999). The analysis was performed for four educational scenar-

Educational Resource Matrix

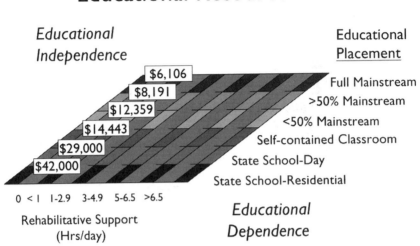

FIG. 11.8. Educational resource matrix labeled with associated educational placement costs based on 1995 budget projections from the Maryland Department of Education.

ios that reflect observed trends in the use of educational resources by implanted children. Because of the lack of data on the use of educational resources by implanted children in high school, an assumption was made that patterns of placement and use of support services remained static from middle school into high school. The cost of implantation and a kindergarten to 12th grade education was compared with the educational costs associated with observed trends in the use of educational resources by a nonimplanted

TABLE 11.4. *Scenarios of educational migration by children with profound hearing impairment*

Cochlear implant at 3 years of age	**Scenario IA** 2 y: > 50% mainstream placement, 2.63 h/d support services 11 y: 100% mainstream, 1 h/d support services Net present cost = $145,196	**Scenario IB** 2 y: 100% self-contained classroom, 0.5 h/d support services 2 y: 100% mainstream classroom, 2 h/d support services 9 y: 100% mainstream classroom, 1 h/d support services Net present cost = $147,200
Cochlear implant at 5 years of age	**Scenario IC** 2 y: 100% self-contained classroom, 0.5 h/d support services 2 y: >50% mainstream placement, 2.63 h/d support services 9 y: 100% mainstream classroom, 1 h/d support services Net present cost = $150,382	**Scenario ID** 2 y: 100% self-contained classroom, 0.5 h/d support services 2 y: 100% mainstream classroom, 2 h/d support services 9 y: 100% mainstream classroom, 1 h/d support services Net present cost = $143,203
Conventional amplification	**Scenario IIA** 5 y: 100% self-contained classroom, 0.5 h/d support services 8 y: 100% mainstream classroom, 4.44 h/d support services Net present cost = $177,324	**Scenario IIB** 13 y: State school for the deaf, day student Net present cost = $247,087 Residential student Net present cost = $342,033

age-matched cohort (Fig. 11.8 and Table 11.4). Future costs and savings were discounted at 5% per annum to accurately reflect the time value of money: $1 today is worth more than $1 tomorrow.

Educational costs for a 3-year-old child who receives a cochlear implant may be compared with that of nonimplanted children in a regular public school or a residential state school for the deaf. Cost savings associated with cochlear implantation from this perspective range from $30,000 to $200,000. There is a similar cost savings associated with cochlear implantation at 5 years of age, even in the scenario where progression to full-time mainstream placement is the most delayed ($27,000 to $192,000 cost savings).

Cost-benefit projections based on observed advancement toward educational independence and very conservative cost figures indicate an extremely favorable net present value of the implant. The ERM illustrates that small increases in educational independence can result in annual savings in educational expenses that, when generalized to populations of implanted children, probably results in an overall cost savings associated with increased educational independence.

The ERM seeks to describe the baseline and longitudinal trends of educational placement of children implanted with multichannel cochlear implants. Such information appears to be useful in determining cost-benefit ratios associated with the cochlear implant, particularly as it affects special education needs. However, these cost-benefit projections must be supplemented with measures of the impact on quality of life to determine the overall cost-effectiveness of cochlear implants in children.

Cost-Effectiveness Considerations for Children

Cost-effectiveness ratios of cochlear implants in children must incorporate a range of considerations that extend beyond cost-benefit analyses (Wyatt *et al.*, 1995a; Hutton *et al.*, 1995). Broad measures of benefit in pediatric cochlear implantation may be measured in terms of communication outcomes, educational benefit, and perceived quality of life as reflected by social adjustment and by physical, mental, and emotional health states.

Determining the quality of life associated with cochlear implantation in children presents a substantial challenge. There are difficulties in assessing quality of life changes in children across developmental phases, because methods for assessing quality of life in children are not as well established as in the adult population. Most measures rely on parental opinion or reporting, which reflect the change in quality of life as perceived by the parent. In one such study, Cunningham (1990) examined the impressions of parents of 3-M single-channel device users. Parents reported subjective improvements in speech, language, and attention; 98% responded that they would recommend the device to other parents. Along with parental reports, objective evaluation of language-related and quality of life measures are needed to generate robust measures of pediatric implant outcomes.

Quality of life impact greatly affects perceived benefit as indicated by self-ratings, and it is not valid to assume that this impact will match that seen in postlingual adults with cochlear implants (see the section on Cost-Utility of Cochlear Implantation in Adults). Because many of the costs of an intervention such as the multichannel cochlear implant are up-front and are tied to surgical treatment and initial audiologic and rehabilitative services, the device appears to be more cost-effective in children than in adults because of the longer periods of use in children. Cost-effectiveness of an intervention is greatly enhanced by durability because sustained benefits effectively diminish the cost per QALY. However, predictions of long-term cost-effectiveness cannot be based on expected period of use alone. For example, it may be that the perceived decrement in quality of life for prelingual childhood deafness is considered less than that for postlingual adult deafness.

Systematic study of the cost-effectiveness of pediatric cochlear implantation with respect to quality of life impact has several requirements:

- Analysis of the impact of sensorineural hearing impairment on quality of life of children and their families stratified by severity, pattern, time of onset of hearing impairment, and communication or educational strategy
- Appraisal of existing scales of quality of life and general health perception for sensitivity to hearing-related changes in children
- Determination of the effects of auditory rehabilitation interventions on these measures

Studies are assessing the longitudinal quality of life impact of profound deafness and cochlear implantation in children. This information allows expression of benefit in terms of units of clinical effect: increments of perceived quality of life (cost-effectiveness analysis) and QALYs (cost-utility analysis). The degree to which implant-mediated speech perception and production (Osberger *et al.*, 1991) can yield language benefits, reading comprehension, and other functional capabilities should be addressed. The true measure of cost-effectiveness of cochlear implants in profoundly deaf children can be determined only after longitudinal study of an array of measures of maturation and development (Hutton *et al.*, 1995). The impact of changes in scholastic performance on vocational options also requires longitudinal study. Future cost-benefit and cost-utility of implants in children are likely to be influenced by factors beyond educational success.

SUMMARY

Studies of the cost-utility of the cochlear implant in postlingual adults have assessed

multiple attributes of quality of life and health status to determine utility gained from the multichannel cochlear implant. The precise cost-utility results varied between studies, probably because of differences in methods used to value benefit, the level of benefit actually obtained, and differences in costs associated with the intervention. Nonetheless, these appraisals consistently indicate that the multichannel cochlear implant occupies a highly favorable position in terms of its cost-effectiveness relative to other medical and surgical interventions employed within the United States. Such studies are also important in analyzing the needed components of programs of rehabilitation and future directions for clinical intervention. Third-party payers, consumers, and health care providers need to make decisions based on economic and health outcomes data. These studies shed new light on the importance of access to hearing care.

Current research in pediatric cochlear implantation is focused on measuring benefit in ways that can complement traditional audiologic outcomes: educational benefit and perceived quality of life. This allows the expression of cost-benefit, cost-effectiveness, and cost-utility ratios that assess the larger personal and societal impact of the cochlear implant on childhood deafness.

REFERENCES

American Medical Association. *Profiles of Adolescent Health Series,* vol I: *American adolescents: how healthy are they?* Chicago: American Medical Association, 1990.
Boothroyd A, Geers A, Moog J. Practical implications of cochlear implants in children. *Ear Hear* 1991; 12[Suppl 4]:81S–89S.
Cunningham J. Parents evaluation of the effects of the 3M/House cochlear implant on children. *Ear Hear* 1990;1:375–381.
Drummond M, Maynard F. Purchasing and providing cost-effective health care. Edinburgh: Churchill Livingstone, 1993.
Evans AR, Seeger T, Lehnhardt M. Cost-utility analysis of cochlear implants. *Ann Otol Rhinol Laryngol Suppl* 1995;104[Suppl 166, Pt 2]:S239–S240.

Feeny D, Furlong W, Barr R, Torrance G, Rosenbaum P, Weitzman S. A comprehensive multiattribute system for classifying the health status of survivors of childhood cancer. *J Clin Oncol* 1992;10: 923–928.

Francis HW, Koch ME, Wyatt JR, Niparko JK. Trends in educational placement and cost-benefit consideration in children with cochlear implants. *Arch Otolaryngol Head Neck Surg (in press)*.

Fryhauf-Bertschy H, Tyler RS, Kelsay DM, Gantz BJ. Performance over time of congenitally deaf and post-lingually deafened children using a multichannel cochlear implant. *J Speech Hear Res* 1992;35: 913–920.

Fugain C, Ouayoun MC, Meyer B, Chouard CH. Advantages and limits of QALY for cost-effectiveness measurement of cochlear implant. Abstract from *4th Pediatric Cochlear Implantation*. 'S Hertogenbosch, the Netherlands, 1998;170.

Harris JP, Anderson JP, Novak N. An outcomes study of cochlear implants in deaf patients: audiologic, economic and quality of life changes. *Arch Otolaryngol Head Neck Surg* 1995;121:398–404.

Hasenstab MS, Tobey EA. Language development in children receiving Nucleus multichannel cochlear implants. *Ear Hear* 1991;12:55S–65S.

Hellman S, Chute P, Kretschmer R, Nevins M, Parisier S, Thurston L. The development of a child's implant profile. *Am Ann Deaf* 1991;136:77–81.

Holt J. Stanford achievement test, 8th ed: reading comprehension subgroup results. *Am Ann Deaf* 1993; 138:172–175.

Hutton J, Politi C, Seeger T. Cost-effectiveness of cochlear implantation of children. In: Uziel AS, Mondain M, eds. *Cochlear implants in children. Advances in Otorhinolaryngology, 50*. Basel: Karger, 1995: 201–206.

Kaplan R, Bush J, Berry C. Health status: types of validity and the index of well-being. *Health Serv Res* 1976;11:478–507.

Kasen S, Ouellette R, Cohen P. Mainstreaming and postsecondary educational and employment status of a rubella cohort. *Am Ann Deaf* 1990;135: 22–26.

Koch ME, Wyatt JR, Francis HW, Niparko JK. A model of educational resource use by children with cochlear implants. *Otolaryngol Head Neck Surg* 1997;117:1–6.

Lea AR, Hailey DM. Cochlear implants. *Med Prog Technol* 1995;21:47–52.

Lea AR. Cochlear implants. *Health care technology, series 6*. Canberra: Australian Institute of Health, 1991.

Lloyd JW, Singh NN, Repp AC. The regular education initiative: alternative perspectives on concepts, issues, and models. Sycamore Publishing Company, 1991.

Mastropieri MA, Scruggs TE. Effective instruction for special education. In: McCormick L, Schiefelbusch R, eds. *Early language intervention*. New York: Macmillan, 1987.

Northern JL, Downs MP. Education of hearing-impaired children. In: *Hearing in children*. Baltimore: Williams & Wilkins, 1991:323–354.

Nottingham Paediatric Cochlear Implant Programme. Outcomes for paediatric cochlear implantation in Nottingham: safe, effective, efficient. MRC-INR, Her Majesty's Stationary Office. Progress report, May 1997.

Osberger MJ, Miyamoto R, Zimmerman-Phillips S, et al. Independent evaluation of the speech perception abilities of children with the Nucleus 22-channel cochlear implant system. *Ear Hear* 1991;12[Suppl 4]: 66S–80S.

Palmer CS, Niparko JK, Wyatt JR, Rothman M, De-Lissovoy G A prospective study: cost-utility of the multichannel cochlear implant. *Arch Otolaryngol Head Neck Surg (in press)*.

Paul L. Programming peer support for functional language. In: Warren S, Rogers-Warren A, eds. *Teaching functional language*. Baltimore: University Park Press, 1985:289–308.

Quittner A, Steck J. Predictors of cochlear implant use in children. *Am J Otol* 1991;12[Suppl]:89–94.

Quittner AL, Stech JT, Rouiller RL. Cochlear implants in children: a study of parental stress and adjustment. *Am J Otol* 1991;12[Suppl]:95–104.

Samuel F. Technology and costs: complex relationship. *Hospitals* 1988;62:72.

Saur R, Coggiola D, Long G, Simonson J. Educational mainstreaming and the career development of hearing-impaired students: a longitudinal analysis. *Volta Rev* 1986;88:79–88.

Smith D, Lockerson R. *Introduction to special education*. Allyn & Bacon, 1992.

Snell M. *Systematic instruction of people with severe disabilities*, 4th ed. Merrill Publishing Company, 1993.

Summerfield AQ, Marshall DH. *Cochlear implantation in the UK 1990–1994*. London: MRC-INR, Her Majesty's Stationery Office, 1995.

Summerfield AQ, Marshall DH, Davis AC. Cochlear implantation: demands, costs, and utility. *Ann Otol Rhinol Laryngol Suppl* 1995;104[Suppl 166, Pt 2]:S245–S248.

Torrance GW, Feeny DH, Furlong WJ, Barr RD, Zhang Y, Wang Q. Multiattribute utility function for a comprehensive health status classification system: health utilities index mark 2. *Med Care* 1996;34: 702–722.

Torrance GW, Furlong W, Feeny D, Boyle M. Multiattribute preference functions: health utilities index. *Pharmacoeconomics* 1995;7:503–520.

Trybus R, Karchmer M. School achievement scores of hearing impaired children: national data on achievement status and growth patterns. *Am Ann Deaf* 1977;122:62–69.

Tye-Murray N, Spencer L, Woodworth GG. Acquisition of speech by children who have prolonged cochlear implant experience. *J Speech Hear Res* 1995; 38:327–337.

Vergera KC, Oller DK, Eilers R, Balkany T. Curricula objectives for educators of children with cochlear implants. In: Fraysse B, Deguine O, eds. *Cochlear implants: new perspectives*. Basel: Karger, 1993: 216–221.

Ware JE Jr, Sherboune CD. The MOS 36-item short-form health survey (SF-36). I. Conceptual framework and item selection. *Med Care* 1992;30:473–483.

World Health Organization. World Health Organization Constitution. In: *Basic documents*. Geneva: World Health Organization, 1948.

Wyatt JR, Niparko JK, Rothman ML, DeLissovoy G. Cost-effectiveness of the multi-channel cochlear implant. *Am J Otol* 1995a;16:52–62.

Wyatt JR, Niparko JK, Rothman ML, DeLissovoy GV. Cost-effectiveness of the multichannel cochlear implant. *Ann Otol Rhinol Laryngol Suppl* 1995b; 104[Suppl 166, Pt 2]:S248–S250.

Wyatt JR, Niparko JK. Evaluating the cost effectiveness of hearing rehabilitation. In: Cummings CW, Harker LA, Schuller DE, eds. *Otolaryngology—head and neck surgery*, 2nd ed. St. Louis: Mosby—Year Book, 1995:112–125.

Wyatt JR, Niparko JK, Rothman M, DeLissovoy G. Cost utility of the multichannel cochlear implant in 258 profoundly deaf individuals. *Laryngoscope* 1996;106:816–821.

Cochlear Implants: Principles & Practices, edited by John K. Niparko, Karen Iler Kirk, Nancy K. Mellon, Amy McConkey Robbins, Debara L. Tucci, and Blake S. Wilson. Lippincott Williams & Wilkins, Philadelphia © 2000.

Language Learning and Cochlear Implant Rehabilitation

12

Language Acquisition

Nancy K. Mellon

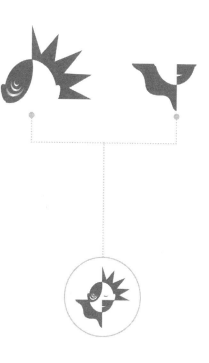

The study of how children learn a language is not only fascinating in its complexity, but also important in addressing the needs of children with language disabilities. The complexity of learning a language arises from a synthesis of the many influences and activities that enable a child to become linguistically engaged. For example, children learn language by developing and assembling together four systems of skills. The pragmatics of interaction, the phonology of sound production, the semantics (meaning), and the rules of grammar are separate but interrelated systems that comprise the foundation of language acquisition (Rescorla and Mirak, 1997). Except for the semantic system, acquisition of each of these systems is subject to a critical period after which full mastery of language is unlikely (Crystal, 1997; Hurford, 1991; Lenneberg, 1967).

Because these systems are developing in a parallel, simultaneous fashion and not in well-delineated discrete stages, use of the term milestone is not appropriate for describing language development overall (Crystal,

1997). Eventual mastery of language entails a timely convergence of the systems of skills. Mastery in each system must be achieved in order for the child to develop communicative competence (Rice, 1989). With the development of the systems of skills that support language, there develops a symbolic dimension of language that reflects social and cultural conventions. Despite the tremendous complexity of this symbolism, even the very young listener assimilates this information.

The first year begins to crystallize experience, behavior, and innate perceptual abilities to provide a framework for later acquisition of more refined language. Because speech production is not yet manifest, hearing-impaired children are likely to go undiagnosed during this period and may remain isolated from early linguistic experiences in speech or sign (Marschark, 1997). Unfortunately, the delay in exposure to appropriate language models is often reflected in poor language outcomes (Yoshinaga-Itano *et al.*, 1998). Age of acquisition affects language outcomes regardless of modality, because signed and spoken languages are subject to a critical period (Mayberry and Fischer, 1989; Newport, 1988; Newport, 1990; Mayberry, 1993; Padden and Ramsey, 1998). If language is introduced after this period, deaf children

N. K. Mellon: The Johns Hopkins University, The Listening Center at Johns Hopkins, Baltimore, Maryland 21287.

typically must be painstakingly taught language instead of effortlessly acquiring language through environmental exposure (Bench, 1992). This process is less efficient and less effective. Consequently, most hearing-impaired children are unable to fully overcome the linguistic, social, and cognitive deficits associated with delayed exposure to language (Vernon and Wallrabenstein, 1984; Vaccari and Marschark, 1997; Furth, 1966; Schum, 1991).

Cochlear implants can improve access to ambient language but are typically provided at age 2 and older, after much of the early development of language systems has already occurred. Ordinarily, by the age of 3 years, a child is capable of understanding three-fourths of the language that will comprise everyday conversation for the rest of his life (White, 1979). By the age of 4 years, a child typically achieves sufficient mastery of the grammatical, phonologic, and pragmatic systems to be considered a native speaker or signer (Crystal, 1997). For the hearing impaired child who is just beginning to hear speech, language delay poses developmental challenges across social, cognitive, behavioral, and linguistic domains.

To understand the problems hearing-impaired children confront in acquiring spoken language, it is necessary to appreciate the complexity of natural language acquisition and the neurobiologic underpinnings of language development. The intent of this chapter is to provide a functional synthesis of the basic elements of spoken language acquisition in children with hearing. These basic elements are presented in four parts. The first part concerns the experience children normally gain as listeners. As in all other realms of perception, sensory experience sculpts the neural template to begin the process of learning. The second part relates language acquisition to its social context—speech production and language develop as consequences of an infant's drive to communicate. The third section examines how various processes combine to enable language acquisition. The fourth part concerns the

neural basis for language acquisition and the timing of acquisition and language modality on brain development.

Children with hearing impairment often evidence significant departures in acquisition of the systems of skills needed to develop language optimally. These departures are described in the relevant sections.

AUDITORY EXPERIENCE

Innate Perceptual Abilities

Although infants are born into a myriad of language environments, they share a common pattern of phonemic perception (Kuhl et al., 1997) (Fig. 12.1). The ability to perceive these universal patterns suggests that human infants possess at birth an innate language structure (Marler, 1994). This structure guides the complex process of acquiring language. Given the requisite perceptual abilities, infants begin to adopt the phonetic repertoire of the language heard early in life. Over time, linguistic experience refines the infant's perceptual abilities to reflect the regularities of the ambient language. By the age of 2 years, a child's speech bears an indelible imprint of their native language.

Skinner (1957) articulated the behaviorist view of language development in his book, *Verbal Behavior*. This text examined the many dynamics that underlie verbal behaviors. In Skinner's view, culture and individual experience dominate language development, while a genetic framework provides the minimal underpinnings for learning (Marler, 1994).

Chomsky (1957) argued that the complexities of language development could only be explained by innate mechanisms unique to the human brain. In his view, infants possess a neural template for mental grammar that specifies possible sentence patterns, enabling the child to speak and understand sentences. Pinker (1994) attributed a dimension of creativity to an innate mental grammar in developing language. Creativity is inherent in a

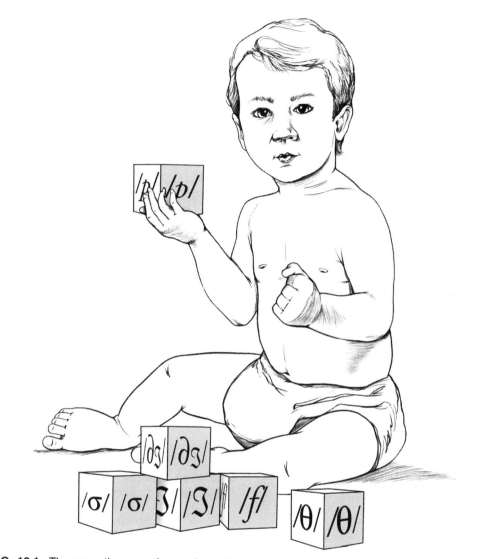

FIG. 12.1. The acoustic space for newborns is partitioned by natural auditory boundaries. These boundaries are universal, enabling discrimination of all phonetic contrasts possible in the world's languages. (Adapted from Kuhl, 1994.)

young child's ability to understand and construct sentences he or she has never heard.

Pinker and Bloom (1990) attribute language development to natural selection. Evolutionary theory, they assert, offers criteria for traits acquired through natural selection. These are a complex design for some function and the lack of alternative processes capable of explaining such complexity. Human language meets these criteria.

Two areas of study support the notion of an innate mental grammar. First, deaf children deprived of exposure to sign language models create their own system of gestures. These systems of gesture known as homesigns incorporate organizational features common to spoken languages (Mohay, 1982; Goldin-Meadow and Mylander, 1984, 1990). Second, critical periods for language learning have been observed beyond which true language competence cannot be achieved (Lenneberg, 1967; Marcotte and Morere, 1990; Hurford, 1991).

In the 1990s an integrative position on language acquisition emerged (Marler, 1994). This perspective holds that linguistic experience can promote optimal language learning only when the proper elements of nature are in place (Jackendoff, 1994). Accordingly, a child with normal perceptual abilities acquires language after being exposed to appropriate language stimulation during a critical period.

The Fetal Environment: Implications for Perception

The human infant has a relatively mature auditory system by 32 weeks' gestational age (Cooper and Aslin, 1989). The intrauterine environment includes sounds generated by the rush of the mother's blood, her digestive system, and her heartbeat. Some aspects of the external speech signal probably penetrate the fetal environment. Studies suggest that intrauterine dampening makes low- to moderate-intensity sound inaudible and attenuates sounds at frequencies greater than 1,000 Hz, which includes most of the higher formant content of speech sounds (Kuhl, 1994). However, low-frequency, intense (>80 dB) sounds can penetrate the womb. These sounds convey suprasegmental aspects of speech: the prosodic (rhythmic) patterns of speech and the intonation and rhythm of the speaker. Fundamental frequencies of the voice may be perceived as well. Sound patterns transmitted to the fetus differ in ways particular to the language of the speaker (Kuhl, 1994). A newborn brings to the process of learning language a familiarity with the ambient language.

Prenatal auditory experience with the suprasegmental aspects of the mother's voice influences early auditory preferences (Cooper and Aslin, 1989). Neonates consistently demonstrate auditory preferences for familiar over unfamiliar stimuli (DeCasper and Fifer, 1980; Panniton and DeCasper, 1984;

DeCasper and Spence, 1986; Jusczyk et al. 1993).

Preferences for familiar language are evidenced even before birth. DeCasper et al. (1986) demonstrated that, at 38 weeks' gestational age, the fetus responds differentially to familiar and unfamiliar stories. DeCasper used a fetal monitor to detect a drop in fetal heart rate in response to a familiar story, and increased heart rate to a novel story (DeCasper et al., 1986). Infants also demonstrate preferences for certain voiced stimuli:

- The sound of the mother's voice over another female voice (DeCasper and Fifer, 1980)
- The sounds of maternal heartbeat over a male voice or silence (Panniton and DeCasper, 1984; Cooper and Aslin, 1989)
- Stories read to them prenatally over novel stories (DeCasper and Spence, 1986)
- Familiar over novel melodies, varying only in melodic contour (Cooper and Aslin, 1989)

These studies suggest that human infants are able to make distinctions based on auditory experience within a remarkably short time. Which aspects of an infant's neural template contribute to the language learning process? What kind of linguistic experience can best nurture language development?

Infant-Directed Talk: Facilitating Language Acquisition

Early experience with sound may set parameters for speech perception. For example, exposure to the sounds of speech prenatally may bias the infant to attend to the suprasegmental aspects of the speech stream (Cooper and Aslin, 1989). "Motherese" or infant-directed talk (IDT) uniquely exploits the acoustic aspects of the speech signal. IDT consists of speech with pitch and temporal characteristics naturally modified for very young children. Not surprisingly, infants as young as 4 weeks old exhibit a preference for IDT (Cooper and Aslin, 1989; Werker and McLeod, 1989; Fernald and Simon, 1984; Fernald and Mazzie, 1991).

Werker and McLeod (1989) demonstrated that IDT elicits greater attentional and affective response than adult-directed speech, regardless of the gender of the speaker. Infants prefer IDT even after low pass filtering to remove lexical information (Fernald and Kuhl, 1987). After filtering, the exaggerated pitch contours of speech remain, retaining the temporal aspects of the melody of language. Similarly, deaf infants appear to prefer sign motherese. Masataka (1998) reported greater attentional and affective responsiveness in 6-month old deaf infants for Japanese sign language directed to infants than to adult directed signing (Masataka, 1998). In a later study, hearing infants demonstrated the same preference. These results suggest that infants are prepared to detect characteristics of motherese in sign even without prior experience in the modality (Masataka, 1998).

Language acquisition occurs in a social context and contains substantial information regarding the affect of the speaker (Locke, 1996). Because language is used to establish and maintain social relationships, engaging the infant in interactions that nurture language development also promotes social and emotional development. Mothers use IDT to involve the infant in early conversational exchanges. Parents speaking to infants naturally accentuate pitch contours, using rising contours to attract attention and a rising-falling contour to maintain attention (Cooper and Aslin, 1989). IDT has been found to stimulate vocal imitation in infants, to improve the salience of speech in noise, and to highlight target syllables (Werker and McLeod, 1989, Kuhl and Meltzoff, 1982).

Cross-cultural studies reveal consistencies in the acoustic properties of speech addressed to young infants. Speech directed to children is consistently higher in fundamental frequency, accentuated in pitch contours, and slower in cadence (Kuhl et al., 1997). Parents in the United States, Russia, and Sweden employ a common strategy of hyperarticulating vowels in their speech to infants (Kuhl et al., 1997). Hyperaticulation serves

to stretch the vowel space presented to the infant, enhancing the contrasts between vowels. Modification of speech in IDT may enhance language learning by making key features of the speech signal more accessible to infants. In this case, exaggerated vowels enable infants to better sort vowels into discrete vowel categories. This categorization is an important precursor to word learning.

IDT also facilitates the segmentation of the speech stream into meaningful units for processing. Mothers using IDT to speak to 14-month-old infants consistently place key words on exaggerated pitch peaks in word-final position, acoustically highlighting the stressed word or syllable (Fernald and Mazzie, 1991). Speech prosody alerts the infant to language structure by emphasizing units for attention, such as words, clauses, and phrases. Taken together, research indicates that the exaggerated pitch contours, repetition, slowed cadence, elongated vowels, and simplified semantic and syntactic structure of IDT facilitate language acquisition and emotional development (Fernald and Simon, 1984; Werker and McLeod, 1989; Kuhl et al., 1997).

Infant Auditory Preferences

Infants display auditory preferences as newborns reflect prenatal sound experience. At birth infants demonstrate through behavioral responses a preference for the utterances of their native language to those of foreign languages (Moon et al., 1993). For example, 4-day-old infants can discriminate native-language utterances from those of a nonnative language (Mehler et al., 1988). This ability relies at least in part on prior exposure to the elements of the native language that are critical for recognition. This conclusion is supported by the fact that the same infants fail to discriminate between the utterances of two unfamiliar languages (Mehler et al., 1988).

Although many characteristics of early speech acquisition appear to be language specific, certain processing abilities in infants are common across linguistic environments. Adults do not share these commonalties across cultures (Aslin *et al.*, 1983). Consequently, infants exhibit similarities in representing speech despite wide differences in the phonologies of human languages. These observations suggest that initial processing strategies present in infancy are modified by linguistic experience with the parental language (Miller and Jusczyk, 1989, Kuhl, 1994; Elmas, 1981; Werker and Tees, 1983). Examining infant auditory perceptual development helps to define the role that linguistic experience plays in modifying initial auditory capabilities (Kuhl *et al.*, 1992, Kuhl, 1994, Werker and Tees, 1984; Werker and Polka, 1993).

Perceptual Tuning in the First 6 Months

What is the nature of the change in early perceptual abilities resulting from linguistic experience with a specific language? A neonate's natural auditory boundaries are universal (Polka and Bohn, 1996). Similar perceptual boundaries also exist in other species and may even be similar across species; animals such as macaques (Kuhl and Padden, 1983) and chinchillas (Kuhl and Miller, 1975) share similar perceptual boundaries within acoustic space. These observations suggest that the experience of hearing provides a set of natural psychophysical boundaries that may guide the selection of the infant's phonetic repertoire (Kuhl and Padden, 1983).

Young infants between 1 and 4 months of age demonstrate a consistent ability to discriminate most or all of the phonetic contrasts that exist in human languages (Miller and Jusczyk, 1989; Aslin *et al.*, 1983; Eimas *et al.*, 1987; Werker and Tees, 1983). In contrast, adults often have difficulty discriminating nonnative phonetic contrasts (Polka, 1995; Werker and Tees, 1983; Iverson and Kuhl, 1996; Miller and Eimas, 1983; Tees and Werker, 1984). For example, English speakers can easily distinguish between the sounds /r/ and /l/ because in English they belong to two distinct phonetic categories (Iverson and Kuhl, 1996). In contrast, the

Japanese language does not contain the contrastive /r/ and /l/ sounds found in English. Although Japanese infants can routinely discriminate between these phonemes, Japanese adults often fail to make this distinction. (Kuhl, 1994). These observations are supported by electrophysiologic and behavioral tests revealing no response or deficient response to /r/ and /l/ sounds in Japanese adults (Buchwald *et al.*, 1994). Lack of exposure to specific contrasts during a sensitive period in childhood may result in a lack of responsiveness to these sound patterns as adults.

Research suggests that a functional reorganization between 4 and 6 months results in a decline in the infant's ability to discriminate acoustic variability between stimuli within the same phonetic category (Kuhl, 1993; Pegg and Werker, 1997). The perceptual decline occurs earlier for vowels than for consonants (Polka and Werker, 1994). By the time an infant is 12 months old, universal patterns of perception are replaced by perceptual boundaries that conform to native language regularities (Kuhl, 1994; Kuhl *et al.*, 1997). These findings suggest that speech perception capabilities are modified by exposure to the phonologic system of the native language during the first 6 months of life.

Kuhl (1993) offers an explanation for this phenomenon in the native language magnet (NLM) theory. The theory holds that development of speech perception includes built-in and learned components. In the first phase of development, the infant segments the sound stream into gross categories separated by natural auditory boundaries (Fig. 12.2). The ability to partition the acoustic space underlying phonetic distinctions is independent of linguistic experience (Kuhl, 1979; Kuhl, 1994; Jusczyk and Betoncini, 1988).

In the second phase, language-specific magnet effects are exhibited. After repeated exposure to repetitive vowel sounds, infants store in memory a representation mirroring the vowel system of the ambient language. The best exemplar of the stored vowel becomes a prototype. Nearby nonprototypes

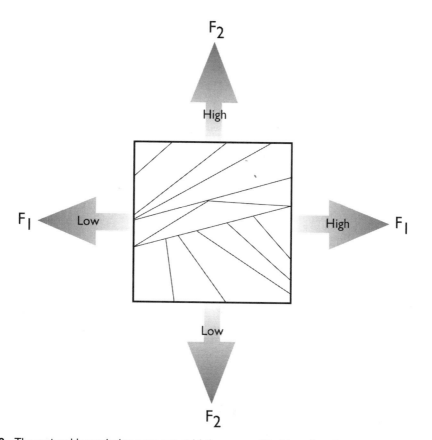

FIG. 12.2. The natural boundaries present at birth are modified to reflect language-specific magnet effects *(dots)*. Infants fail to discriminate phonetic contrasts that lack salience within their linguistic environment. (Adapted from Kuhl, 1994.)

are drawn to the best exemplar through a perceptual magnet effect (Fig. 12.3). This effect corresponds to the establishment of phonemic boundaries encompassing a variety of allophones. Linguistic experience alters perceived differences between speech stimuli warping the perceptual space underlying speech.

In phase three, the magnet effect minimizes acoustic differences near magnet attractors and maximizes those near the boundaries between two magnets (Fig. 12.3). The infant's perceptual space is rearranged to incorporate magnet placement. This restructuring functionally erases some boundaries that are present in the language-general perceptual map. Thereafter, the infant can easily distinguish the boundary between two

phonetic categories but cannot easily discriminate sounds within the same phonetic category. The language-general perceptual abilities of the neonate become the language-specific skills of the older infant.

Perceptual magnet effects may explain how exposure to ambient language reduces the infant's ability to discriminate between speech sounds that do not differentiate between words in the native language. To test this hypothesis, Kuhl *et al.* (1992) studied phonetic perception in 6-month-old Swedish and English infants using native and foreign-language sounds. American and Swedish babies were trained and tested with the English /i/ prototype and the Swedish /y/ prototype. American infants perceived the English /i/ prototype as identical to its vari-

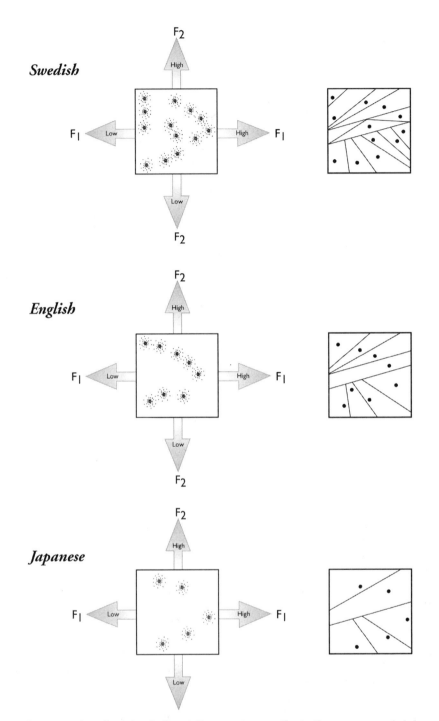

FIG. 12.3. By 6 months, the infant's linguistic experience affects the way speech information is stored in memory. The distributional properties of vowels in three different languages are shown. (Adapted from Kuhl, 1994.)

ants two-thirds of the time. In contrast, they perceived the Swedish /y/ as identical to its prototype in only one-half of the trials. Swedish infants demonstrated the opposite effect. These results indicate that linguistic experience in the first 6 months of life alters infant perception of speech sounds.

Similar conclusions have been derived using different research methodologies exposed to other native languages. For instance, Cheour *et al.* (1998) demonstrated the development of language-specific electrophysiologic responses that correlated with phonemic perception in Finnish and Estonian children younger than the age of 12 months. Measurements of mismatch negativity (MMN), reflective of the ability to perceive phonetic contrasts such as those resulting from F2 differences, revealed an inability to discriminate nonnative vowels. Finnish and Estonian infants demonstrated greater MMN amplitudes associated with phonemic contrasts for their respective phonemes only. Nonnative phonetic contrasts failed to generate the same amplitude of MMN. These data were interpreted as the first neurophysiologic evidence for the development of brain memory traces for native speech sounds.

The NLM offers one possible explanation as to why young children are better language learners than adults are. Perceptual tuning to native language regularities occurs during a critical period in early development and may explain the difficulty experienced by adults in learning a second language. Adults who are unable to perceive many of the phonetic contrasts in the nonnative language are unlikely to develop unaccented, fluent speech.

Segmenting the Speech Stream: 6 to 9 Months

Young children hear an estimated 20,000 to 40,000 words each day (Kuhl, 1994). Development between 6- and 9-months enables the infant to partition the sound patterns embedded in continuous speech (Jusczyk *et al.*, 1992). This aspect of development occurs within the framework of infant directed talk that highlights words, clauses and phrases.

An understanding of the prosodic structure of words in the infant's native language is present before word learning (Juscyzk *et al.*, 1992). For example, English words tend to have stressed (strong) initial syllables. Nine-month-old, but not 6-month-old, infants learning English have exhibited a preference for words that follow this strong-weak pattern (Jusczyk *et al.*, 1993). Nine-month-old, but not 6-month-old, infants also demonstrate preferences for lists of nonwords that contain highly frequent phonetic patterns (high-probability patterns) to nonwords with phonetic patterns occurring infrequently in the native language (Jusczyk *et al.*, 1994).

American infants in this age group have been observed to listen longer to words with English sound patterns than to words with Dutch sound patterns (Jusczyk *et al.*, 1993). Dutch children show the opposite preference. A 9-month-old child, but not a 6-month-old infant, exhibits sensitivity to the acoustic correlates of major phrasal units in English (Jusczyk *et al.*, 1992). They prefer speech with pauses at the usual phrasal boundaries to artificially segmented speech in which pauses do not coincide with natural boundaries.

Juscyzk and Hohne (1997) demonstrated a preferential response to familiar words, revealing an ability to store in memory sound patterns of words that occur frequently in fluent speech. Eight-month-old infants listened to recordings of stories for 10 days during a 2-week period. Two weeks later, listening times for the list of story words, words that had appeared repeatedly in the stories, were significantly higher than those for foil words words that never appeared in the stories.

Between 6 and 9 months, infant attention prioritizes the sound patterns specific to their native language. This development arises at a time when infants show a diminishing ability to discriminate phonetic contrasts that do not appear in their native language (Werker and Tees, 1984). A loss of flexibility in discriminating phonetic contrasts precedes focused attention to the encoding and representation of sound patterns in the ambient language.

Speech Perception as Intermodal Event

Perceptual capabilities develop in concert with visual and motor inputs. Speech perception is multimodal: auditory, visual, and motor inputs contribute to speech understanding. A study by Kuhl and Meltzoff (1982) showed that 4-month-old infants could recognize the correspondence between auditory and visual presentation of speech sounds. Infants were presented with a face producing a vowel sound and auditory stimuli that matched or did not match the lip movements. Infants exhibited greater attention to a face that matched the spoken vowel 73% of the time, rather than to a mismatched pair. This observation suggests that infants understand the bimodal equivalences of speech.

Altered speech signals can provide clues as to the speech elements that contribute to infant speech perception. When auditory stimuli were modified to remove identifying spectral information but preserve temporal characteristics, mean fixation time for the matched face dropped to chance. These results indicate that infants rely on spectral information to match auditory and visual cues.

Kuhl and Meltzoff (1982) speculate that young infants appreciate auditory-motor equivalences and that this style of representing speech may enable vocal learning. Infants may be predisposed to store speech representations with the corresponding visual information. This finding suggests that combining visual and tactile information about speech may aid in language learning.

The Transition to Word Learning: Listening for Meaning

A second reorganization of functional pathways accompanies the transition to word learning. Infants shift their attention from the prosodic features and phonetic detail in the sound patterns of language and begin to attach meaning to specific patterns stored in memory.

Stager and Werker (1997) demonstrated that infants listen for more phonetic detail in speech perception tasks than in word learning tasks. Fourteen-month-old and 6-month-old infants were taught to associate dissimilar nonsense words with their referents during a habituation phase. The stimuli used, *bih* and *dih*, differed only in the initial consonant. After presentation of same word-object combination (*i.e.*, same trial), the infants were presented with the same words and objects but a switch in the word-object pairing (*i.e.*, switch trial). Fourteen-month-old infants failed to detect a switch in the word-object pairs. However, 6-month-old infants did notice the switch in the word-object pairing and looked significantly longer during the switch trial.

Why do older infants fail at a perceptual task they excelled at earlier on? Stager and Werker (1997) attribute this phenomenon to the different approaches used by the two groups. Six-month-old infants may perform the task as a simple sound-discrimination task while older infants may approach the task as a word learning task. The investigators hypothesize that failure to attend to fine phonetic detail when attempting word learning may result from functional reorganization. Inattention to fine detail may aid word learning by freeing attention for the more demanding task of mapping sound onto meaning. The decrease in the amount of detail used by infants may be analogous to an infant's decline in ability to discriminate non-native contrasts. In both transitions, a decline in perceptual performance marks developmental change.

SPEECH PRODUCTION

Language learning begins with the infant's orientation to the communicative behaviors of others (Locke, 1997). Human infants possess neural mechanisms dedicated to processing information regarding faces and voices and their related activities (Locke, 1997). Together, these mechanisms comprise a specialization in social cognition that orients the infant toward the source of linguistic information. Vocal learning and early word production are facilitated by the infant's disposition to take vocal turns with a partner and to orient to and imitate prosody. Infants must also learn to use gesture communicatively, to assimilate native language phonetic patterns, and to seek to understand and alter the thoughts and feelings of conversational partners (Locke, 1997). Given appropriate perceptual experience and motor development, these abilities enable infants to function as conversational partners in the ambient language despite their relative linguistic immaturity.

Speech and Language Development: Social Influences

A speaker makes approximately five selections per second from a lexicon of up to 50,000 words. The rapidity of this process belies its complexity. Spoken communication entails an intricate interaction between the semantics and grammar of language, modulation of inflection, pitch and volume, and facial expression (Bench, 1992). The complexity inherent in the delivery of speech is matched by equally complex behaviors in the listener. Perceiving and producing speech and language requires simultaneous processing and serial processing (Bench, 1992).

Speaking and listening are bound up with social skills (Locke, 1997). Communication entails an appreciation of what the listener is gleaning from what is heard and sensitivity to possible misunderstandings. It also requires attention to the mood and the nonverbal cues of the conversational partner. Appraisal of communication skills in hearing-impaired children often revolves around speech perception and production on what is being heard and the intelligibility of what is being produced. However, conversation

functions in context, on a plane beyond mere word understanding.

The goal of communication is to add to, change, or mold the recipient's perceptions; to effect such a change it is necessary to discern the thoughts, beliefs, and intentions of the communicative partner. Deaf children often have great difficulty making these kinds of inferences about communication partners (Vacccari and Marschark, 1997). Their difficulty with theory of mind and with reading emotional expression has been ascribed to a lack of exposure to conversation about mental states (Peterson and Siegal, 1995; Schum, 1991). Differences between deaf and hearing children in this regard may also stem from differences in language mode.

Studies examining emotional processing and expression in deaf children and adults need to consider the dual role that facial expression plays in communication between deaf mothers and infants (Reilly and Bellugi, 1996). Mothers all use facial expression to convey information reflecting emotional state (Vaccari and Marschark, 1997). However, deaf mothers also use specific facial gestures in prescribed ways as grammatical markers in American sign language (ASL). The affective and grammatical demands of facial expression may be placed in competition. Reilly and Bellugi (1996) propose a shift from affective use of facial expression to grammatical use at around the time of the child's second birthday. Deaf children, who are reading facial gestures as grammatical cues and not as affective cues, are likely to display differences in processing and expressing emotion.

Successful communication relies on an array of cues beyond the specific words or phrases chosen by the speaker. Effective communicators automatically tailor their communication differently for particular listeners and settings (Bench, 1992). It is during early conversational exchanges, typically with the parents, that such skills are modeled and nurtured. Deaf children of hearing parents often contend with a lack of a full communication system, changing, and often limiting their communication with their child.

Vocal Imitation

Language development is motivated by a drive to communicate with others (Rescorla and Mirak, 1997). Speech production is a principal outcome of this motivation. Locke (1996) views infant speech development as an unintended consequence of social exchange. This exchange is primarily affective and is critical to normal development across many domains. Vocal imitation is important to spoken language development because it enables the infant to become a conversational partner.

Kuhl and Meltzoff (1996) identify five stages in vocal development:

1. *Reflexive phonation* (0 to 2 months) is dominated by reflexive or vegetative sounds such as coughing or sneezing.
2. In *cooing* (1 to 4 months), infants produce vowel-like sounds.
3. *Expansion* (3 to 8 months) is marked by the appearance of fully resonant clear vowels.
4. Canonical *babbling* (5 to 10 months) entails production of consonant-vowel syllables, such as "mamama."
5. In *meaningful speech* (10 to 18 months), long intonated utterances blending babbling and true words are produced.

Speech development is related to the infant's physical development and is guided by linguistic experience. Hearing allows the infant to access spoken language models and to monitor self-produced speech (Kuhl, 1996); both inputs are necessary for refinement of vocal production. Vocal imitation allows infants to monitor their own attempts at reproducing sounds they hear in the environment and to map speech sounds onto the motor abilities that produce them (Kuhl, 1996; Locke, 1993; Kuhl and Meltzoff, 1996). For example, cooing allows infants to learn to associate articulatory movements with auditory consequences.

Like hearing children, deaf children produce babble, but the range of their phonetic inventories is typically constrained. The repertoire of speech sounds produced by the deaf infant is usually limited to sounds that are easily seen on the lips, such as /ba/ and /ma/ (Kuhl and Meltzoff, 1996). Because hearing-impaired children often cannot rely on auditory feedback to monitor their speech, they may depend on their visual, tactile, or kinesthetic senses instead (Bench, 1992). Fluent speech is difficult to achieve through exclusive feedback from these senses, because they provide less precise feedback than hearing. The experience of hearing the ambient language and the ability to hear one's own early attempts at speech are needed to construct an auditory-articulatory map (Kuhl and Meltzoff, 1996).

The time frame for acquiring practice in listening and speaking is important to achieving normal development. Hearing language early in life shapes a person into a native speaker (Kuhl, 1996). Very young infants fail to exhibit effects of language environment in their vocalizations, but by 10 to 12 months, differences in linguistic environments are reflected in speech production (Locke, 1997; Rescorla and Mirak, 1997). Two- and three-year-old infants from different cultures show clear differences in phonemic repertoire. Children who learn language before age 7 are most adept at vocabulary nuances and acquire perfection in accent (Marler, 1994).

Early attempts at mirroring speech targets are refined by motor maturation and linguistic experience. Kuhl and Meltzoff (1996) have characterized developmental changes in speech production in 12-, 16-, and 20-week-old infants. Infant vocalizations in response to speech were analyzed using spectrographic analyses. At 12 weeks, infants produced vowel categories that overlapped in acoustic space. Over time, infant vowel categories became progressively more discrete because of tighter clustering of vowels in each category. By 20 weeks, distinct vowel sounds were produced. Whether the observed developmental shift results from maturation in the infant's articulatory abilities or from vocal learning has not been resolved (Kuhl and Meltzoff, 1996). Kuhl suggests that stored representations guide speech production by serving as *targets* that infants try to match when producing speech. Refinements in motor control enable greater accuracy at reaching for targets.

Speech production relies on integration of visual, auditory, and motor inputs and requires mapping of perceived speech sounds onto vocal outputs. However, speech and language are not synonymous. Language is a system of arbitrary symbols for ideas, mutually transparent to users of that language that exists for the purpose of social communication and internal regulation. Spoken language employs speech to convey these ideas. However, meaning is not inherent in the sounds and cues that comprise speech but relies on an association between speech and the objects and concepts referred to. The infant must learn to associate meaning with particular sound patterns. This process begins in childhood but extends throughout life as new meanings continue to be incorporated into the lexicon.

NORMAL LANGUAGE ACQUISITION

Language acquisition involves the development of four interrelated systems: the pragmatic system, the phonologic system, the semantic system, and the grammatical system (Rice, 1989; Rescorla and Mirak, 1997). Given a common communication mode with the parent, children acquiring language in sign or speech proceed through similar stages and acquire linguistic competence at approximately the same ages. Unfortunately, delays in diagnosing hearing loss and degraded auditory inputs often preclude the hearing-impaired child's early access to speech or sign models. Consequently, the hearing-impaired child's first language develops more like a second language, depending heavily on learning and very little on the normal processes of language acquisition (Bench, 1992).

Pragmatic Development

Certain behaviors are required for a child to initiate and maintain discourse. Pragmatic development includes the infants engagement in turn-taking, mutuality, and contingent interaction with a communicative partner (Rescorla and Mirak, 1997). At around 9 months, infants begin to point out objects in the environment and employ eye gaze and vocalizations to elicit a response from the communicative partner. The infant's activities establish joint attention whereby the child and the parent attend to the same event or topic. Joint attention promotes language development by establishing a context for sound-object or sound-meaning associations (Crystal, 1997). By 12 to 15 months, infants use a variety of vocalizations to request, command, question, comment, or respond to the parent's communications. These exchanges comprise a negotiation of meaning in which sound-meaning associations can be clarified and reinforced (Rescorla and Mirak, 1997).

Children between the ages of 2 and 4 emerge as true conversational partners, having mastered conversational strategies. Children at this stage are able to initiate conversation and to anticipate and repair communication breakdowns with clarification, repetition, or requests for explanation. They are also more adept at social conventions and turn-taking.

Phonologic Development

Phonologic development refers to the infant's ability to detect, produce, and manipulate the 42 vowel-consonant combinations (phonemes) used in the English language. Receptive mastery of phonology is virtually complete by 4 to 6 months, whereas expressive mastery is not fully complete until age 6 or 7 (Rescorla and Mirak, 1997). By 10 months of age, sounds that are most regularly produced in the infant's repertoire comply with the conventions of the infant's native language. At 1 year, most children can perceive the distinctions between sounds used by adults to express differences in meaning, but they are limited in their ability to produce these sounds (Crystal, 1997). Phonologic development is thought to be critical to reading ability because hearing children use phonologic awareness to develop a speechlike code they can apply to decode written English (Bench, 1992).

Semantic Development

Semantic development is the most apparent feature of early language acquisition. At 1 year, most children have begun to acquire their first words. Unlike phonologic and grammatical development, semantic development is not complete by puberty (Crystal, 1997). The process of acquiring new vocabulary and meaning continue across the lifespan. Rates of vocabulary acquisition vary widely and are linked to later linguistic ability (Locke, 1997).

By 9 months of age, most hearing infants begin to comprehend and produce words. The mean age for comprehending 10 words is 10.5 months, and the mean age for producing 10 words is 15.1 months (Kuhl *et al.*, 1991). Speech production lags behind and is bolstered by speech perception. By 18 months, children can generally produce about 50 words and can understand five times as many (Crystal, 1997). Many children experience a vocabulary spurt at about 18 months, during which the rate of vocabulary acquisition increases from 1 or 2 words a week to 8 to 10 words per week (Rescorla and Mirak, 1997).

By age 2, children typically possess a spoken vocabulary in excess of 200 words (Crystal, 1997). During the preschool years, children learn to comprehend more than 14,000 words (Rice, 1989). Children manage this rapid learning by a process referred to as *fast mapping*, whereby they quickly absorb new words that they encounter in meaningful context (Rice, 1989). Children fast map words they have encountered only once or twice in conversational exchanges and form an initial, partial sense of a word's meaning based on a quick survey of possible meanings. Incorporating the new word involves reorganization of words in storage and the underlying cognitive domain (Rice, 1989). Fast mapping ability is critical to overall language development and helps lay a foundation for later reading ability. Language-delayed children demonstrate limited ability to fast map new words.

Children vary widely in their rate of vocabulary acquisition. A survey of the lexical usage of German children used tape recordings to monitor the number of words produced in children's speech over a 12-hour period. The study revealed great variability between children. One 2-year-old child in the study produced more than 20,000 words each day, and a 3.5-year-old child produced nearly twice as many (Crystal, 1997). In comparison, some older children produced words numbered in the 20,000s.

Children who are beginning to attach meaning to sounds often exhibit three types of errors during the second and third year: overextension, underextension, and mismatch (Crystal, 1997). A child using overextension may lump together objects sharing a common property such as color, shape, or size under the same word heading. For example, a child may apply the word dog to other animals. In contrast, a child may underextend the use of the word dog by using it to refer to the family pet and not to other dogs outside the home. Mismatch results from misidentification of a word-meaning association. Hearing-impaired children make many of the same errors in developing sign-meaning associations (Bench, 1992).

Grammatical Development

The first phase of grammatical development is most noticeable between 12 and 18 months and is composed of single-word utterances (Crystal, 1997). About 60% of the words at this stage have a naming function, an additional 20% refer to actions. The infant may also produce utterances such as "allgone," which are used as single units. During this phase, single words sometimes function as sentences; intonation and gesture help clarify the intent of the communication.

Around 18 months, infants typically begin to use two-word phrases such as "more juice" or "shut door." By 2 years, the child may begin to produce sentences that are three or four words long, assembling them into a variety of grammatical constructions. The 30-month infant may use telegraphic sentences, such as "this my cup" (Rescorla and Mirak, 1997), which omits grammatical words and word endings yet conveys meaning. Between 20 and 37 months, children begin to regularize irregular word forms (Locke, 1997). Deaf children using sign language exhibit an ability to modify word forms by 36 months (Marschark, 1997). Similarly, by 36 months, grammatical words and endings appear in the speech of hearing children, and a major grammatical advance in the form of sentences composed of multiple clauses also appears at this time (Crystal, 1997).

By 48 months, children exhibit mastery of negation and the use of the past tense in speech and sign. At 4 years of age, children can use sentences appropriately to describe complex situations and to anticipate future occurrences (Rescorla and Mirak, 1997; Marschark, 1997). Similarly, children achieve mastery of verb agreement, semantic relations, and complex use of verbs of motion and location in speech and sign at the same ages (Locke, 1997). Hearing children continue to refine their mastery of complex constructions of English grammar until the age of 10 or 11 years (Crystal, 1997).

Late learners of a first language are particularly disadvantaged with respect to grammatical competence. For example, even deaf individuals who were first exposed to sign in adolescence, despite an average of 42 years of signing experience, continue to evidence departures in processing patterns (Mayberry and Fischer, 1989). Nonnative signers evidence significant differences in terms of sign production and comprehension. Although native speakers and signers disregard the surface form of language to extract meaning when processing language (Mayberry and

Fischer, 1989), nonnative language users fail to progress beyond the surface form of language to fully acquire language structure (Singleton *et al.*, 1998). Language competence is contingent on mastery of language structure. Deaf children who are not exposed to language models in any modality because of delayed diagnosis or inappropriate intervention may be at risk for poor language competence in any language.

Some aspects of language acquisition develop in stages that are not modality specific (Schlesinger and Meadow, 1972), but acquiring language structures such as syntax may depend on modality-specific mechanisms (Klima and Bellugi, 1979). Transfer from one language to another may prove difficult. Such transfers may be particularly problematic when they involve a change in the mode of transmission, as is required in the switch from sign to spoken English. This is evidenced in the generally poor reading and writing attainment of hearing-impaired children (Bench, 1992).

Reading and Writing

Despite technologic and educational advances, the language and academic achievement of the average deaf high school graduate remains below that of the average fourth-grade hearing student (Holt, 1994; Yoshinaga-Itano *et al.*, 1998). Knowledge of English grammar and vocabulary and the ability to access even minimal amounts of residual hearing are the factors most predictive of literacy for deaf adults (Moores and Sweet, 1990).

Children using sign language often face a significant challenge in reading and writing, because these skills rely on a knowledge of English syntax, phonologic awareness, and semantics (Bench, 1992). ASL grammar differs significantly from English grammar in terms of morphology and syntax, which are expressed through visuospatial rather than sequential auditory parameters (Crystal, 1997). Difficulty in transferring skills based in a manual language such as ASL to spoken language skills may lie in the fundamental differences inherent in language processing specific to each communication mode.

Whereas processing in ASL involves simultaneous sign modulations, spoken language generally employs processing strategies based on temporal and sequential organization (Crystal, 1997). For example, ASL uses visuospatial relations to convey semantic contrasts of aspect, such as completeness, habituality, or continuousness. In contrast, spoken English relies on lexicon and word order to communicate the same information. Similarly, ASL uses distinctive facial gestures to mark some types of phrases and clauses. Decoding communication entails simultaneous processing of facial gesture and sign (Mayberry and Fischer, 1989).

Reduced capabilities for reading and writing in deaf children have been linked to a lack of inner speech (Bench, 1992; Paul and Quigley, 1984). Providing a framework for developing inner speech, which normally unfolds through exposure to spoken language is critical to developing literacy. Hearing children exhibit mastery of English grammar in early childhood (Crystal, 1997). Grammatical errors in syntax and morphology are sorted and mastered by hearing children by about the age of 4 years (Crystal, 1997). At an early age, familiarity with connected speech in English enables hearing children to recognize possible sentence constructions. This knowledge can be used to guide reading and writing. In contrast, hearing-impaired children and adults exhibit idiosyncratic use of grammar in their writing (Bench, 1992). Difficulty in mastering English grammar likely engenders difficulty in reading and writing (Bench, 1992).

Studies suggest that children who rely on sign language use different strategies for decoding written English (Bench, 1992). Although hearing children use a speechlike code to decode written letters, many deaf children use a visual code when beginning to read, storing and coding words as visual sequences of letters. Retaining an inner speech, particularly for phonology, is associated with better reading, speech-reading, language competence, and speech intelligibility in hearing-impaired children (Bench, 1992). Children use a variety of strategies when reading, of which phonologic coding is only one. However, any strategy whose development relies on listening experience is likely less well developed in a hearing-impaired child.

In reading, deaf children are asked to recognize a language to which they have limited exposure. Consequently, deaf children cannot decode unfamiliar written words into a known vocabulary; they instead must memorize each word in association with its meaning (Schaper and Reitsma, 1993). The total lexicon for ASL is approximately 4,000 signs (Crystal, 1997), and most words the young reader encounters therefore are likely to be unfamiliar.

NEURAL BASIS OF LANGUAGE

Neurolinguistic Theory of Language Acquisition

Locke's (1997) theory of neurolinguistic development divides language acquisition into four phases and is based on traditional concepts of brain compartmentalization (Fig. 12.4). The first phase is primarily affective; the infant attends to the human face and voice, learning suprasegmental vocal characteristics. The second phase is affective and social; the infant collects utterances that it processes in the right hemisphere. The third phase is analytic and computational and is served by the left hemisphere. The infant begins to sort stored utterances into syllables and segments and, in the process, discovers regularities that are integrated into a set of grammatical rules. The fourth phase is integrative and elaborative; this phase facilitates lexical learning.

Locke's theory suggests that mental grammar is acquired during development to solve the problem of memory overloads of lexical information. Locke holds that the analytic mechanism responsible for linguistic grammar is subject to a sensitive period, after

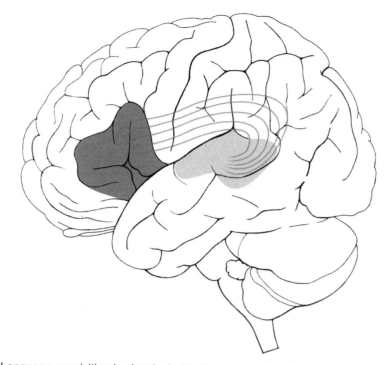

FIG. 12.4. Language acquisition is closely tied to the segregation of unique regions of the cerebral cortex. Areas of specialization critical to language are Broca's area, the motor-speech area adjacent to the (presylvian) areas of the motor strip of the cerebral cortex *(dark shaded region)*, and Wernicke's area, an area subserving language reception *(light shaded region)*. These areas of specialization were initially postulated on the basis of clinical findings. Observing a patient with an anterior, left-sided brain lesion who could understand spoken language but could not speak, Pierre Paul Broca observed that "Nous parlons avel l'hemisphere gauche" in 1864. This concept introduced the principle of specialized brain function. Three years later, Carl Wernicke described a patient with deficits in comprehension associated with injury of postsylvian regions of the superior temporal lobe. Wernicke's area subserves comprehension in audition and reading. Wernicke also synthesized the information of his era to generate theories about the brain's representation of language. He held that complex mental functions such as language arise from neural interactions of motor and perceptual areas and are mediated by neural pathways such as the arcuate fasciculus *(stippled lines)* that connect Wernicke's and Broca's areas. Classically, these regions were thought to subserve receptive and expressive verbal communication, respectively, but they represent areas of specialization for similar functioning in written and signed communication, although the degree of lateralization differs between spoken and signed language. Lateralization is also subject to sensitive periods. In hearing and deafness, most processing occurs in left hemisphere structures only if language is acquired early in life.

which full and grammatical use of language does not develop. This analytic mechanism is triggered when stores of lexical information reach a critical level. If the infant fails to capture the requisite number of stored utterances, the mechanism fails to activate, and linguistic processing switches to homologous right hemisphere language areas.

Locke (1997) asserts that the use of right hemisphere structures increases anatomic symmetry. Further, right hemisphere structures are not optimal for language acquisition because they are not specialized for phonologic encoding or decoding. Locke's theory offers a possible explanation for the lack of hemispheric asymmetry observed in language-learning–disabled populations. Approximately 99% of right-handed and

66% of left-handed people exhibit left hemisphere lateralization for language (Damasio and Damasio, 1992). Language areas in the left hemisphere, particularly the planum temporale, are already larger in the fetus (Locke, 1997). However, in language-learning–disabled populations, particularly in dyslexic populations, neuroimaging studies have found symmetry between left and right hemisphere language areas. For a time, the left hemisphere regions were thought to be smaller in the language disabled, but volumetric measures from magnetic imaging studies revealed that the right perisylvian area, including planum temporale and superior temporal gyrus, are actually larger in dyslexic children (Plante *et al.*, 1991; Petersen *et al*, 1988). These regions in the left hemisphere have been implicated in the processing of phonemes and auditory information. Reduced volume in the left perisylvian region is associated with lower verbal IQ (Semrud-Clikeman, 1997).

Hearing infants typically experience a period of rapid word learning after approximately 50 words have been acquired (Rescoral and Mirak, 1997). The vocabulary spurt corresponds with the emergence of meaningful speech and may trigger the analytic mechanism through which infant's extract grammatical rules from stored lexical information (Locke, 1997). Because activation of the analytic mechanism is subject to a sensitive period, failure to acquire a large enough lexicon to trigger activation may constrain grammatical development. Locke (1997) holds that lexicon delayed may be grammar denied. Deaf children who remain undiagnosed during this period often possess no lexicon at all leaving them at risk for departures in grammatical development.

Neurobiologic Basis of Speech Perception

Few studies have examined brain activation in children performing language tasks. One study directly pertinent here relates to phonetic processing. Dehaene-Lambertz and Dehaene (1994) used evoked response po-
tentials (ERPs) to measure the speed and cerebral correlates of syllable discrimination in 2- and 3-month-old infants. Infants were presented with strings of syllables, either /ba/ or /ga/, whose first consonants differed in place of articulation. Two processing stages were identified and localized to the temporal lobes. Peak 1 at 220 milliseconds appeared insensitive to the acoustical differences between the syllables, but there was recovery for the deviant syllable by peak 2 at 390 milliseconds. These results suggest that infants can discriminate a single instance of a deviant syllable in less than 400 milliseconds. ERP amplitudes of peak 1 and peak 2 were significantly larger over left hemisphere posterior electrodes than over the right, possibly indicating a functional asymmetry for processing short syllables in the left hemisphere.

Ojemann (1983) developed a model for brain organization for language. This model was based on data derived from electrical stimulation mapping of language-related areas in epileptic patients. All subjects exhibited left hemisphere lateralization for language. Ojemann elicited brain activity with language tasks—naming, reading, short-term verbal memory, mimicry of orofacial movements, and phoneme identification—during neurosurgical procedures under local anesthesia. Ojemann identified a common perisylvian cortex for motor and language functions in the left hemisphere, including sites common to identification of phonemes and sequencing of movements. The finding of a common cortical area subserving orofacial mimicry and phonemic identification provides evidence for a link between perceptual mechanisms and speech-motor functions (Ojemann, 1983). These results lend support to Kuhl's contention that an auditory-articulatory blueprint guides speech development. If infants use motor feedback to guide vocal imitation, the examiner would expect to see common cortical areas for speech perception and speech motor.

Other research examines processing of single words. A child's expressive vocabulary at 20 months has been correlated with later linguistic ability (Locke, 1997). Children who have large vocabularies at 20 months *i.e.,* high producers) are likely to exhibit better linguistic ability in maturity than children who are low producers. Mills *et al.* (1993) elicited ERPs on normal 20-month-old children as they listened to lists of known, unknown, and backward words. For both groups, unknown words selectively activated the right hemisphere, while known words selectively activated the left hemisphere. Known and unknown words were discriminated in the right and left hemisphere. High producers exhibited more subtle ERPs in the temporal and parietal areas, while low producers demonstrated a more significant response over frontal, temporal, and parietal lobes. These results suggest that greater linguistic ability may be represented by more subtle neural responses to the same stimulus.

Results of imaging studies and electrical mapping suggest that there is substantial individual variability in the exact locations of sites related to a particular language function. This variability is at least partly related to the individual's gender and overall language ability and may be modified by language experience (Ojemann, 1983). Ojemann (1983) suggests an inverse relationship between language proficiency on a particular task and the cortical areas needed to perform that function. Over time, a simple processes such as naming use smaller primary cortical areas. The exact cortical sites subserving language may show flexibility over time even in adults and may be altered by facility with a particular function. Taken together these studies suggest that language experience may modify perceptual abilities and underlying neural structures.

Lateralizing the Left Hemisphere for Language

The left hemisphere of the brain is specialized for language in deaf and hearing persons who are skilled in language (Corina *et al.,* 1992). There is some debate in the literature regarding the basis for this asymmetry

(Hickok *et al.,* 1996). The debate centers on whether left hemisphere specialization for processing linguistic information may reflect a specialization for more general functions that enable language processing. The basis of lateralization has been proposed to be processing of rapid changes in temporal information (Tallal *et al.,* 1993), processing of complex motor patterns (Hickok *et al.,* 1996), or the symbolic properties of language (Corina *et al.,* 1992).

Researchers have been interested in comparing how signed and spoken languages are processed in the brain, because the peripheral sensory, motor channels, and symbolic properties of the two language systems are so different (Mayberry and Fischer, 1989). Tallal *et al.* (1993) assert that left hemispheric dominance for speech developed from a specialization for fast temporal processing of auditory information. Spoken language entails the processing of rapid transitions between linguistically relevant inputs, some as short as 40 milliseconds (Tallal *et al.,* 1993). In contrast, the shortest linguistically relevant transition in sign is approximately 200 milliseconds (Hickok *et al.,* 1996).

Signed languages depend on vision and manual articulation and use spatial relations to convey systematic differences in meaning (Hickok *et al.,* 1996). In contrast, spoken language relies on audition and oral articulation (Mayberry and Fischer, 1989). If hemispheric lateralization for language processing relied on physical characteristics of the linguistic signal or motor processes, the neural organization in native signers and speakers should be different (Hickok *et al.,* 1996). However, studies suggest that the left hemisphere is the base for linguistic processing, regardless of the sensory modality (Hickok *et al.,* 1996; Bellugi *et al.,* 1989; Emmorey and Corina, 1993).

A study by Hickok *et al.* (1996) examined the linguistic abilities of deaf signers with unilateral lesions in the left or right hemisphere. Signers with left hemisphere damage performed well on visuospatial tasks but poorly in all areas of language competence. Right hemisphere damaged signers showed the opposite pattern, performing well on tests of language competence but demonstrating impaired visuospatial performance. These results suggest that at the hemispheric level the neural organization of sign and spoken language is the same. The investigators suggest that left hemisphere dominance for language is driven by higher-order properties of the system and not by more general sensory or motor processes. Visuospatial abilities and sign language abilities were concluded to belong to largely independent cognitive domains in deaf signers.

Visuospatial information that is not linguistically relevant may be processed in the right hemisphere in native signers. Bellugi *et al.* (1989) examined two uses of space in ASL: spatial syntax and spatial mapping. *Spatial syntax* refers to the active manipulation of spatial loci to represent grammatical functions. *Spatial mapping* refers to the topographic use of space, such as the use of space to describe actual spatial arrangements of objects. Bellugi *et al.* (1989) observed that the two uses of space in ASL were differentially affected by brain damage. Syntactic relations were disrupted by left hemisphere damage, and spatial relations were impaired as a result of right hemisphere damage.

Corina *et al.* (1992) compared the lateralization of spoken language, signed language, and nonlinguistic gesture in deaf and hearing individuals. Because nonlinguistic gesture and sign language are transmitted in the same modality, this comparison allowed separate analysis of the skilled motor movement and linguistic components of sign language. Differences in right-hand interference patterns for linguistic and nonlinguistic gestures were observed, indicating that left hemisphere asymmetry honors a distinction between linguistic and nonlinguistic input presented in the same modality. No evidence of hemispheric asymmetry was found for symbolic or arbitrary gestures in hearing or deaf individuals.

Emmorey and Corina (1993) tested the hypothesis that left hemisphere specialization for language is independent of modality by examining neurologically intact deaf signers. The investigators examined hemispheric specialization in normal deaf signers for forms of ASL signs and English words. Concrete (imageable) items differed in their site of processing from abstract items. Deaf and hearing subjects showed a left hemisphere advantage for abstract lexical items. Deaf signers evidenced a right hemisphere advantage for imageable concrete signs, whereas English speakers showed no asymmetry for imageable words. These results confirm prior studies suggesting that the left hemisphere is specialized for language regardless of modality, but they also suggest a possible difference in degree of lateralization between signed and spoken language based on imageability, with some categories of signs processed in the right hemisphere.

Effects of Language Modality on Hemispheric Specialization

Neville and Lawson (1987) employed ERPs to examine attention to visual stimuli in normal-hearing subjects who were born to deaf parents and whose first language was ASL. These results were compared with normal-hearing and congenitally deaf subjects who used speech and sign respectively. All three groups performed similarly during attention to central stimuli. However, deaf subjects displayed attention effects to peripheral stimuli over the occipital regions of both hemispheres that were several times larger than those displayed by hearing subjects in either group. Deaf subjects and hearing subjects born to deaf parents detected the direction of target motion better when it occurred in the right visual field. Hearing subjects showed the opposite effect. Accordingly, the amplitude of attention related increases in ERPs were larger in the left hemisphere for deaf and hearing subjects born to deaf parents. Hearing subjects showed amplitude increases in the right hemisphere.

These results suggest that aspects of the visual system that are organized symmetrically in the two hemispheres are affected by early auditory deprivation. Acquisition of a visual language and auditory deprivation since birth appear to have different effects on the development of cortical specialization in humans. The investigators speculate that the left hemisphere is initially biased to subserve language acquisition but that critical parameters of the language acquired may help determine other functions that the left and right hemisphere will mediate.

Two other studies also suggest that specific processing requirements of the language acquired may in part determine neural organization. Bavelier *et al.* (1998) used functional magnetic resonance imaging (fMRI) to examine cerebral organization during sentence processing tasks in English and ASL in hearing and deaf subjects. Both groups activated classic left hemisphere language structures when processing their native language. Deaf and hearing native signers recruited right hemisphere structures when processing ASL.

Neville *et al.* (1998) also employed fMRI to examine cerebral organization during sentence processing in English and ASL. Hearing and deaf subjects processing in their native language activated left hemisphere structures. In contrast, deaf subjects reading in English did not display activation in left hemisphere regions. The investigators concluded that expression of the bias for these areas to mediate language processing depends on early acquisition of a natural language. This was evidenced by extensive activation of homologous right hemisphere regions in hearing and deaf native signers.

Auditory experience may be critical to the development of some aspects of cortical specialization in humans (Szelag and Wasilewski, 1992). In a study of perception of emotional and nonemotional faces, Szelag and Wasilewski (1992) observed that hearing children displayed cerebral asymmetry in recognizing faces expressing emotion. In contrast, deaf children failed to display cerebral asymmetry for any kind of emotion expressed in displayed faces. The investigators suggest that hemispheric specialization depends specifically on auditory experience and not on linguistic input. These results may also reflect differences in affective mentoring and the use of facial expression in spoken and signed languages.

A study by Neville *et al.* (1992) further documented differences in neural processing of linguistic information between deaf and hearing subjects. The researchers elicited ERPs for two categories of English words in hearing and deaf adults. The subjects were presented with words that provide semantic information (*i.e.*, open-class words) and words that provide grammatical information (*i.e.*, closed-class words). The investigators speculated that acquisition of grammatical processes is an important factor in the development of cerebral asymmetries. They observed that deaf individuals who acquire ASL as a first-language and learn English later evidence difficulty with English grammar but not with vocabulary. They expected deaf subjects to exhibit marked differences in the processing of closed-class, but not open-class English words. Although ERPs for semantic processing were nearly identical in deaf and hearing subjects, ERPs for grammatical processing were markedly different. These results provide neurobiologic support for the hypothesis that early exposure to and acquisition of grammatical structure is a critical factor in specializing the neural systems subserving language processing.

Taken together, these studies suggest that specialization of the left hemisphere for language requires early exposure to language, regardless of modality. Late language exposure may result in abnormal cerebral specialization for linguistic functions. For example, children who are congenitally deaf or who acquire deafness before the age of 3 years have been found to exhibit anomalous cerebral representation for speech (Marcotte and Morere, 1990). Deprivation studies also support the notion of a critical period for lateralization of language functions. Children with normal hearing who have been deprived of exposure to language until puberty display right hemisphere lateralization for language and nonlanguage functions (Fromkin *et al.*, 1974).

Normal language acquisition occurs with early exposure to language (Newport, 1990; Johnson and Newport, 1989). Language exposure beginning later in life shows a corresponding linear decline in language competence with age (Mayberry, 1993). The timing of first-language acquisition has been found to effect later language processing skills, regardless of whether the language learned is spoken or signed (Mayberry, 1993). Late first-language learners demonstrate difficulty in acquiring language structure. Moreover, lexical identification, an overburdened working memory and an underdeveloped lexicon are associated with delayed language acquisition, regardless of modality.

CONCLUSIONS

Several basic principles underlie language acquisition:

- Multiple systems of skills undergo development.
- This pattern of development is subject to a critical period—an optimal time for refining the nervous system's perceptual capabilities for salient features.
- Systems develop simultaneously rather than in series.
- Receptive capabilities lay the foundation for production and grammatical development.
- Language acquisition depends on innate and experiential factors.
- The timing of first-language acquisition effects linguistic competence.
- Specific processing requirements of the language acquired may determine cerebral organization for language.

Developments during the first year sculpt the child's perception and production of language, given the ability to access the language environment. Language competence is the byproduct of a complex interplay between the infant's innate abilities and the language environment. Infants may carry a bias to seek out linguistic cues in the environment, to select them for further processing, and to prioritize them for memory encoding.

Infant perceptual abilities appear to be subject to a critical period during which the brain structures that subserve language are activated. Exposure to language during this period is required and serves to validate neural structures (Chapter 1). Specific processing requirements of the language acquired may differentially activate neural structures subserving language.

Children who lack the perceptual acuity to access the language environment and whose language mentors do not share the same communication mode are denied the normal exposure to a sophisticated language system in any modality. This form of linguistic deprivation poses a significant challenge to the child's development across domains. Language acquisition is critical to further development, because children use language to establish their social identity and to reach out to the wider world.

REFERENCES

Aslin R, Pisoni D, Jusczyk P. Auditory development and speech perception in infancy. In: Haith M, Campos J, eds. *Carmichael's handbook of child psychology: infancy and developmental psychology*. New York: Wiley, 1983:573–687.

Bavelier D, Corina D, Jezzard P, *et al.* Hemispheric specialization for English and ASL: left invariance-right variability. *Neuroreport* 1998;9:1537–1542.

Bellugi U, Poizner H, Klima E. Language, modality and the brain. *Trends Neurosci* 1989;12:380–388.

Bench R. *Communication skills in hearing-impaired children*. San Diego: Singular Publishing, 1992.

Buchwald J, Guthrie D, Schwafel J, Erwin R, Lancker D. Influence of language structure on brain-behavior development. *Brain Lang* 1994;46:607–619.

Cheour M, Ceponinene R, Lehtokoski A, *et al.* Development of language-specific phoneme representations in the infant brain. *Nat Neurosci* 1998;1:351–353.

Chomsky N. *Syntactic structures*. The Hague: Mouton, 1957.

Cooper R, Aslin R. The language environment of the young infant: implications for early perceptual development. *Can J Psychol* 1989;43:247–265.

Corina D, Vaid J, Bellugi U. The linguistic basis of left hemisphere specialization. *Science* 1992;255:1258–1260.

Crystal D. *The Cambridge encyclopedia of the English language*, 2nd ed. Cambridge: Cambridge University Press, 1997.

Damasio AR, Damasio H. Brain and language. *Sci Am* 1992;267:88–95.

DeCasper A, Spence M. Newborns prefer a familiar story over an unfamiliar one. *Infant Behav Dev* 1986;9:133–150.

DeCasper A, Fifer W. Of human bonding: newborns prefer their mothers' voices. *Science* 1980;208:1174–1176.

Dehaene-Lambertz G, Dehaene S. Speed and cerebral correlates of syllable discrimination in infants. *Nature* 1994;370:292–295.

Eimas P. Infants, speech, and language: a look at some connections. *Cognition* 1981;10:79–84.

Eimas P, Miller P, Jusczyk P. On speech perception and the acquisition of language. In: Harnad S, ed. *Categorical perception: the groundwork of cognition.* New York: Cambridge University Press, 1987:161–195.

Emmorey K, Corina D. Hemispheric specialization for ASL signs and English words: differences between imageable and abstract forms. *Neuropsychologia* 1993;31:645–653.

Fernald A, Mazzie C. Prosody and focus in speech to infants. *Dev Psychol* 1991;27:209–221.

Fernald A, Simon T. Expanded intonation contours in mothers' speech to newborns. *Dev Psychol* 1984;20:104–113.

Flege J, Munro M, Fox R. Auditory and categorical effects on cross-language vowel perception. *J Acoust Soc Am* 1994;95:3623–3641.

Furth H. *Thinking without language: psychological implications of deafness.* New York: Free Press, 1966.

Goldin-Meadow S, Mylander C. The role of parental input in the development of the morphological system. *J Child Lang* 1990;17:527–563.

Goldin-Meadow S, Mylander C. Gestural communication in deaf children: the effects and noneffects of parental input on early language development. *Monogr Soc Res Child Dev* 1984;49:3–4.

Hickok G, Bellugi U, Klima E. The neurobiology of sign language and its implications for the neural basis of language. *Nature* 1996;382:699–702.

Holt J. Classroom attributes and achievement test scores for deaf and hard of hearing students. *Am Ann Deaf* 1994;139:430–437.

Hurford J. The evolution of the critical period for language acquisition. *Cognition* 1991;40:159–201.

Iverson P, Kuhl P. Influences of phonetic identification and category goodness on American listeners perception of /r/ and /l/. *J Acoust Soc Am* 1996;99:1130–1140.

Jackendoff R. *Patterns in the mind: language and human nature.* New York: Basic Books, 1994.

Johnson J, Newport E. Critical period effects in second language learning: the influence of maturational state on the acquisition of English as a second language. *Cogn Psychol* 1989;21:60–99.

Jusczyk P, Bertoncini J. Viewing the development of speech perception as an innately guided learning process. *Lang Speech* 1988;31:217–238.

Jusczyk P, Cutler A, Redanz N. Infants preference for the predominant stress patterns of English words. *Child Dev* 1993;64:675–687.

Jusczyk P, Friederici A, Wessels J, Svenkerud V, Jusczyk A. Infant's sensitivity to the sound patterns of native language words. *J Memory Lang* 1993;32:402–420.

Jusczyk P, Hirsh-Pasek K, Nelson D, Kennedy L, Woodward A, Piwoz J. Perception of acoustic correlates of major phrasal units by young infants. *Cogn Psychol* 1992;24:252–293.

Jusczyk P, Hohne E. Infants memory for spoken words. *Science* 1887;277:1984–1986.

Jusczyk P, Luce P, Charles-Luce J. Infants sensitivity to phonatactic patterns in native language. *J Memory Lang* 1994;33:630–645.

Kuhl P, Andruski J, Christovich I, *et al.* Cross-language analysis of phonetic units in language addressed to infants. *Science* 1997;277:684–686.

Kuhl P, Meltzoff A. Infant vocalization in response to speech: vocal imitation and developmental change. *J Acoust Soc Am* 1996;100(Pt 1):2425–2438.

Kuhl P, Meltzoff A. The bimodal perception of speech in infancy. *Science* 1982;218:1138–1141.

Kuhl PK, Miller JD. Speech perception by the chinchilla: voiced-voiceless distinction in alveolar plosive consonants. *Science* 1975;190:69–72.

Kuhl P, Padden D. Enhanced discriminability at the phonetic boundaries for the place feature in macaques. *J Acoust Soc Am* 1983;73:1003–1010.

Kuhl P, Williams K, Lacerda F, Stevens K, Lindblom B. Linguistic experience alters phonetic perception in infants by 6 months of age. *Science* 1992;255:606–608.

Kuhl P. Developmental speech reception: implications for models of language impairment. *Ann NY Acad Sci* 1993;682:248–263.

Kuhl P. Learning and representation in speech and language. *Curr Opin Neurobiol* 1994;4:812–822.

Kuhl P. Speech perception in early infancy: perceptual constancy for spectrally dissimilar vowel categories. *J Acoust Soc Am* 1979;66:1668–1679.

Lenneberg E. *The biological foundation of language.* New York: Wiley, 1967.

Locke J. A theory of neurolinguistic development. *Brain Lang* 1997;58:265–326.

Locke J. Why do infants begin to talk? Language as an unintended consequence. *J Child Lang* 1996;23:251–268.

Locke J. *The child's path to spoken language.* Cambridge: Harvard University Press, 1993.

Marcotte A, Morere D. Speech lateralization in deaf populations: evidence for a developmental critical period. *Brain Lang* 1990;39:134–152.

Marler P. Born to talk? *Nat Hist* 1994;10:70–72.

Marschark M. *Raising and educating a deaf child.* New York: Oxford University Press, 1997.

Masataka N. Perception of motherese in Japanese sign language by 6-month-old hearing infants. *Dev Psychol* 1998;34:241–246.

Mayberry R. First-language acquisition after childhood differs from second-language acquisition: the case of American Sign Language. *J Speech Hear Res* 1993;36:1258–1270.

Mayberry R, Fischer S. Looking through phonological shape to lexical meaning: the bottleneck of non-native sign language processing. *Memory Cogn* 1989;17:740–754.

Mehler J, Jusczyk P, Lambertz G, Halsted N, Bertoncini J, Amiel-Tison C. A precursor of language acquisition in young infants. *Cognition* 1988;29:143–178.

Miller J, Jusczyk P. Seeking the neurobiological bases of speech perception. *Cognition* 1989;33:111–137.

Miller J, Eimas P. Studies on the categorization of speech by infants. *Cognition* 1983;13:135–165.

Mills D, Coffey-Corina S, Neville H. Language acquisition and cerebral specialization in 20-month-old infants. *J Cogn Neurosci* 1993;5:317–334.

Mohay H. A preliminary description of the communication systems evolved by two deaf children in the absence of a sign language model. *Sign Lang Studies* 1982:34:73–90.

Moores D, Sweet C. Factors predictive of school achievement. In: Moores DF, Meadow-Orlans KP, eds. *Educational and developmental aspects of deafness.* Washington, DC: Gallaudet University Press, 1990.

Neville H, Bavelier D, Corina D, *et al.* Cerebral organization for language in deaf and hearing subjects: biological constraints and effects of experience. *Proc Natl Acad Sci USA* 1998;95:922–929.

Neville H, Mills D, Lawson D. Fractionating language: different neural subsystems with different sensitive periods. *Cereb Cortex* 1992;2:244–258.

Neville H, Lawson D. Attention to central and peripheral visual space in a movement detection task. III. Separate effects of auditory deprivation and acquisition of a visual language. *Brain Res* 1987;405:284–294.

Newport E. Constraints on learning and their role in language acquisition: studies of the acquisition of American Sign Language. *Lang Sci* 1988;10:147–172.

Newport E. Maturational constraints on language learning. *Cogn Sci* 1990;14:11–28.

Ojemann G. Brain organization for language from the perspective of electrical stimulation mapping. *Behav Brain Sci* 1983;6:189–230.

Padden C, Ramsey C. Reading ability in signing deaf children. *Top Lang Disord* 1998;18:16–29.

Panneton R, DeCasper A. Newborns prefer an intrauterine heartbeat sound to a male voice. *The International Conference on Infant Studies,* New York 1984.

Paul P, Quigley S. *Language and deafness.* San Diego: Singular Publishing, 1994.

Pegg J, Werker J. Adult and infant perception of two English phones. *J Acoust Soc Am* 1997;102:3742–3753.

Petersen S, Fox P, Posner M, Mintun M, Raichle M. Positron emission tomographic studies of the cortical anatomy of single-word processing. *Nature* 1988;331:585–589.

Peterson C, Siegal M. Deafness, conversation and theory of mind. *J Child Psychol Psychiatry* 1995;36:459–474.

Pinker S, Bloom P. Natural language and natural selection. *Behav Brain Sci* 1990;13:797–784.

Pinker S. *The language instinct.* New York: William Morrow, 1994.

Plante E, Swisher L, Vance R, Rapcsak S. MRI findings in boys with specific language impairment. *Brain Lang* 1991;41:52–66.

Polka L, Bohn O. A cross-language comparison of vowel perception in English-learning and German-learning infants. *J Acoust Soc Am* 1996;100:577–592.

Polka L. Linguistic influences in adult perception of non-native vowel contrasts. *J Acoust Soc Am* 1995; 97:1286–1296.

Reilly J, Belllugi U. Competition on the face: affect and language in ASL motherese. *J Child Lang* 1996; 23:219–239.

Rescorla L, Mirak J. Normal language acquisition. *Semin Pediatr Neurol* 1997;4:70–76.

Rice M. Children's language acquisition. *Am Psychol* 1989;44:149–156.

Schaper M, Reitsma P. The use of speech-based recording in reading by prelingually deaf children. *Am Ann Deaf* 1994;138:46–54.

Schum R. Communication and social growth: a developmental model of social behavior in deaf children. *Ear Hear* 1991;12:320–327.

Skinner BF. Verbal behavior. New York: Appleton-Century-Crofts, 1957.

Stager C, Werker J. Infants listen for more phonetic detail in speech perception than in word-learning tasks. *Nature* 1997;388:381–382.

Tallal P, Miller S, Fitch R. Neurobiological basis of speech: a case for the preeminence of temporal processing. *Ann NY Acad Sci* 1994;682:27–47.

Tees R, Werker J. Perceptual flexibility: maintenance or recovery of the ability to discriminate non-native speech sounds. *Can J Psychol* 1984;38:579–590.

Vaccari C, Marschark M. Communication between parents and deaf children: implications of socio-emotional development. *J Child Psychol Psychiatry* 1997;38:793–801.

Vernon M, Wallrabenstein J. The diagnosis of deafness in a child. *J Commun Disord* 1984;17:1–8.

Werker J, McLeod P. Infant preference for both male and female infant-directed talk: a developmental study of attentional and affective responsiveness. *Can J Psychol* 1989;43:230–246.

Werker J, Tees R. Developmental changes across childhood in the perception of non-native speech sounds. *Can J Psychol* 1983;37:278–286.

Werker J, Tees R. Phonemic and phonetic factors in adult cross-language speech perception. *J Acoust Soc Am* 1984;75:1866–1878.

Werker J, Tees R. The organization and reorganization of human speech perception. *Annu Rev Neurosci* 1992;15:377–402.

White B. The special importance of hearing ability in the development of infants and toddlers. In: Simmons A, Calvert DR, eds. *Parent-infant intervention: communication disorders.* New York: Grune & Stratton, 1979:55–61.

Yoshinaga-Itano C, Sedey A, Coulter D, Mehl A. Language of early- and later-identified children with hearing loss. *Pediatrics* 1998;102:1161–1171.

Appendix 12A

Reading and Deafness

Betty Schopmeyer

Deaf and hard of hearing students have well-documented deficits in reading. Paul (1998) cites two general findings: the reading level of the average 18- and 19-year-old student with a severe to profound hearing impairment is no better than that of the normally hearing 9- to 10-year-old student, and the reading progress rate of the hearing impaired student is approximately one-half of one school grade per year, with a plateau at third or fourth grade for most.

Reading involves a complex integration of processes that must be described in more detail before examining the problem of reading ability in the deaf. Reading may be broken down into text-based, reader-based, and task-based components (Paul, 1998). Text-based considerations include sound-symbol correspondence, word meanings, syntax, and written language conventions such as punctuation. Reader-based factors refer to aspects of comprehension: prior knowledge, metacognitive skills, literal and inferential understanding, comprehension of connected discourse, drawing conclusions, and obtaining the main idea. Task-based factors include the environment in which reading takes place and the evaluation methodology used to determine comprehension. Students with profound hearing impairments typically experience difficulty in all three areas.

Although clearly integrated in practice, the components of the reading process have been examined separately in the literature in attempts to identify their relative weight in deaf readers' performance.

TEXT-BASED FACTORS

Sound and Symbol Correspondence

The ability of a reader to decode a word by associating its letters with an internal phonologic system is referred to as a phonetic assembly or "bottom-up" style of word recognition. The use of this strategy in the reading process implies that the reader is employing phonologic recoding strategies in which printed text is translated into previously mastered acoustic units. Phonologic recoding may be used to decode words for initial identification or for storing words in memory once identified (Treiman and Hirsh-Pasek, 1983). A review of some phonologic code studies with deaf students reveals that they may make some use of a phonologic coding strategy to decode words. The phonology of the deaf reader appears to derive from a combination of lip-reading, finger-spelling, articulation, and exposure to writing (Marschark, 1997). The lack of access to the phonemes of spoken language, however, results in decreased opportunity for deaf individuals to master the alphabetic system in the way that hearing students do (Treiman and Hirsh-Pasek, 1983) and forces them to rely more on visual and whole word recognition strategies during reading (Marschark, 1997). Hearing-impaired students who have some access to the sounds of language through residual hearing tend to be better readers than their profoundly deaf peers. The use of speech-based coding strategies appears to be associated with better perfor-

B. Schopmeyer: Cochlear Implant Rehabilitation, The Listening Center at Johns Hopkins, The Johns Hopkins University, Baltimore, Maryland 21287.

mance in reading tasks (Schaper and Reitsma, 1993), as do skills in speech production (Marschark 1997; Geers and Moog, 1989), although Moores and Sweet (1990) found speech ability to be less important than text-based factors for literacy. Phonologic recoding is also thought to provide a more durable basis for retaining words in working memory (Hung *et al.*, 1981; Treiman and Hirsh-Pasek, 1983; Marschark, 1997).

Although phonology is one deficit area for many deaf readers, a significant portion of deaf children's observed reading problems appear to stem from sources other than their inability to hear the sounds of the language. After a word is recognized through phonologic or visual strategies, the issue of meaning is introduced.

Knowledge of Vocabulary and Syntax

Of all the subcomponents of the reading process, deaf students demonstrate the most differences in vocabulary, including signed, spoken, and written forms (Geers and Moog, 1989; Chaikof, 1996; Marschark, 1997). Deaf children typically know fewer words than their hearing peers and tend toward mastery of concrete nouns and familiar verbs rather than words representing abstract concepts (Marschark 1997). Vocabulary deficits may impact reading by "tying up" processing capacity at the expense of higher-level syntactic and text comprehension abilities (Hung *et al.*, 1989; Marschark, 1997). The importance of vocabulary in reading skill is emphasized by the findings of Yurkowski and Ewoldt (1986) that a firm semantic base enables processing of complex syntax, an area in which deaf students typically lag behind their hearing peers. Competence in this area is correlated with successful reading (Geers and Moog, 1989).

READER-BASED FACTORS

Children bring prior knowledge about the world to early reading experiences. Much of this knowledge is acquired through the child's exposure to various experiences and to the language that accompanies them. Direct parental conversation and explanation, as well as incidental learning, contribute to this knowledge. Deaf children of hearing parents may be severely impacted by the commonly observed factors of language "mismatch" between parent and child, late diagnosis, and inability to take advantage of incidental learning opportunities. The inability to overhear conversation and narrative discourse, for example, impedes the child's ability to comprehend connected language structure, the main idea, and associative relationships between events. Literacy begins at a young age for children growing up in homes in which knowledge about books and reading conventions, reading stories aloud, and conversation about these stories are common. Deaf children, even if diagnosed very early, are frequently in a situation in which there is a parent-child communication barrier that may preclude access to the ongoing literacy exposure typically given to young children (Maxwell, 1986). They may enter school without the kinds of early experiences that foster easy access to literacy.

Inferential and Metacognitive Factors

Deaf children appear to have deficits in drawing inferences and comprehending figurative language in verbal or nonverbal modes (Rittenhouse and Stearns, 1990). Erickson (1987) refers to deaf readers' inability to master literal and nonliteral reading tasks at an adequate level and to deficits in using metacognitive strategies to monitor their own ongoing comprehension during reading. These characteristics may be directly related to the tendency of hearing parents and professionals to focus on the concrete in linguistic interactions with deaf children.

Reading is linked to short-term memory, attention, and vocabulary. A reciprocal causation factor operates as well: children who read more increase these skills through reading, and children with better skills and better reading competence tend to read more (Marschark 1997). In comparison to hearing children, deaf children gain less vocabulary from the reading experiences, which perpetuates the cycle of less reading leading to less ability to read.

TASK-BASED FACTORS

Home Environment

Deaf children of deaf parents generally read at levels higher than deaf children of hearing parents (Marschark, 1997; Padden and Ramsey, 1998; Kuntze, 1998; Moores and Sweet, 1990). A study done in 1978 by Jensema and Trybus compared families with two deaf parents for whom ASL was the primary language with families with one deaf parent for whom spoken English was the primary language. In comparing children from both these conditions with deaf children with hearing parents, they found that children with one deaf parent read better than those with hearing parents, and those with two deaf parents did best of all. It has been suggested that children who have deaf parents are more likely to have a hereditary form of deafness unaccompanied by other subtle handicapping conditions that may be present in the wider pool of deaf children born to hearing parents (Padden and Ramsey, 1998). The later diagnosis of deafness in children of hearing parents and the resulting delays in intervention are also likely to contribute to the more severe language and reading delays observed in this population.

Research (Padden and Ramsey, 1998; Prinz and Strong, 1998) has focused on identifying the nature of the connection between early immersion in a fluent ASL environment and later development of English literacy. According to Padden and Ramsey (1998), it is not just knowing ASL that leads to literacy in English, but rather the child's ability, given explicit guidance, to capitalize on specific components of ASL that appear to foster associative relationships between ASL and English. These components are exposure to finger-spelling and initialized signs within the context of ASL syntactic structure. Finger-spelling, which comprises about

15% of ASL discourse, has a basis in English alphabetic principle and is presented to deaf children by deaf adults in regularized ways (e.g., chaining, sandwiching) that have evolved within the deaf community for the purpose of cracking the code of written language. Innovative teaching methods employing specific cross-modality bilingual principles are beginning to impact ASL students with positive literacy results. Some researchers contend that strong ASL skills may be used in specific ways to form a "bridge" to printed English, hypothesizing that the path to English literacy for deaf children is a unique one (Singleton *et al.*, 1998.)

School Environment

The school environment of many deaf children is less than optimal in terms of language modeling. Even in total communication classes, the level of teacher sign use is often not high (Woodward and Allen, 1987), and teachers may omit from their signed communication 20% to 50% of the words they speak (Marschark, 1997). A study by Howarth *et al.* (1981) looked at differences in how reading instruction was carried out for deaf and hearing children. They observed that deaf children were stopped significantly more frequently than hearing children to discuss vocabulary and to receive instruction in other aspects of language. These interruptions result in lack of cohesive text presentation that may contribute to comprehension problems for connected discourse.

Assessment Methods

Deaf children typically have difficulty understanding question forms (LaSasso, 1990). Poor question comprehension affects learning and imposes limitations on a child's ability to demonstrate what he or she has learned from formal educational and incidental experiences. The ways in which deaf students are tested for purposes of evaluating their reading skill may therefore impose an additional level of difficulty onto the basic comprehension task (LaSasso, 1980.)

Comprehension is typically assessed through questions, which may not be understood by the deaf student, even when the basic text has been processed.

EDUCATIONAL PROGRAMMING

Although there is general agreement that reading abilities of deaf students are far from optimal, there is less consensus about solutions to the problem. Methodologies using ASL as a first language with incorporation of specific techniques such as sign gloss systems to develop reading skills in English have claimed positive results (Prinz and Strong 1998; Nelson, 1998). Marschark (1987) recommends use of ASL and an English-based system of signs or cued speech as the best way to encourage literacy in deaf children. Oral programs rely on maximum use of spoken English skills to facilitate literacy.

READING FOR CHILDREN WITH COCHLEAR IMPLANTS

Ninety percent of deaf children have hearing parents, and although some of them provide early exposure to ASL, there are many practical, emotional, and cultural reasons why most of these children are not raised in a rich ASL environment. The cochlear implant offers access to auditory information to children who receive little or no benefit from hearing aids. Language and phonologic development in implanted children has been shown to exceed that of similar children using hearing aids (Chapter 11). This increased access, combined with appropriate intervention, may provide the young implanted child with a better chance of developing more quickly and easily the sound-symbol relationships, oral language abilities, improved vocabulary, and mature syntax that correlate with better reading. Although other viable routes to improved reading may also be identified and should continue to be researched, the cochlear implant appears to be of significant benefit in obtaining the universally desired goal of increased literacy for deaf chil-

dren. Little research has been done on reading skills in children with cochlear implants. This is a critical area that must be investigated, particularly as young children with implants approach school age with perhaps 3, 4, or more years of implant experience.

REFERENCES

Allen TE, Woodward J. Teacher characteristics and the degree to which teachers incorporate features of English in their sign communication with hearing impaired students. Am Ann Deaf 1987;132:61–7.

Chaikof MK. Reading—a more attainable horizon for CI children. CICI Contact 1996;Fall:17–20.

Erickson ME. Deaf readers reading beyond the literal. Am Ann Deaf 1987;10:291–293.

Geers A, Moog J. Factors predictive of the development of literacy in profoundly hearing-impaired adolescents. Volta Rev 1989;91:69–86.

Howarth SP, Wood DJ, Griffiths AJ, Howarth CI. A comparative study of the reading lessons of deaf and hearing primary school children. Br J Educ Psychol 1981;51:156–162.

Hung DL, Tzeng OJL, Warren DH. A chronometric study of sentence processing in deaf children. Cogn Psychol 1981;13:583–610.

Jensema C, Trybus R. Communication patterns and educational achievement of hearing-impaired students. Series T, Number 2 Office of Demographic Studies, Gallaudet College, Washington.

Kuntze M. Literacy and deaf children: the language question. Top Lang Disord 1998;18:1–15.

LaSasso C. Developing the ability of hearing-impaired students to comprehend and generate question forms. Am Ann Deaf 1990;135:409–412.

LaSasso C. The validity and reliability of the cloze procedure as a measure of readability for prelingually, profoundly deaf students. Am Ann Deaf 1980;125:559–563.

Marschark M. Raising and educating a deaf child. New York; Oxford University Press, 1997.

Maxwell MM. Beginning reading and deaf children. Am Ann Deaf 1986;131:14–20.

Moores DF, Sweet C. Factors predictive of school achievement. In: Moores DF, Meadow-Orleans KP, eds. Educational and developmental aspects of deafness. Washington, DC: Gallaudet University Press, 1990.

Nelson KE. Toward a differentiated account of facilitators of literacy development and ASL in deaf children. Top Lang Disord 1998;18:73–88.

Padden C, Ramsey C. Reading ability in signing deaf children. Top Lang Disord 1998;18:30–46.

Paul P. Reading for students with hearing impairments: research review and implications. Volta Rev 1998; 99:73–87.

Prinz PM, Strong M. ASL proficiency and English literacy within a bilingual deaf education model of instruction. Top Lang Disord 1998;18:47–60.

Rittenhouse RK, Stearns K. Figurative language and

reading comprehension in American deaf and hard-of-hearing children: textual interactions. *Br J Disord Commun* 1990;25:369–374.

Schaper MW, Reitsma P. The use of speech-based recoding in reading by prelingually deaf children. *Am Ann Deaf* 1993;138:46–54.

Singleton JL, Supalla S, Litchfield S, Schley S. From sign to word: Considering modality constraints in ASL/ English bilingual education. *Top Lang Disord* 1998; 18:16–29.

Treiman R, Hirsh-Pasek K. Silent reading: insights from second-generation deaf readers. *Cogn Psychol* 1983;15:39–65.

Yurkowski P, Ewoldt C. A case for the semantic processing of the deaf reader. *Am Ann Deaf* 1986;131:243–247.

Appendix 12B

Psychosocial Development of Children in Deafness

Nancy K. Mellon

Deafness offers a natural paradigm for examining the role that language plays in cognitive, social, and emotional development in children. Language links children to their parents and society, and it enables cognitive, social, and emotional development. When children share a common language with their parents, socialization and language acquisition occur naturally during development, but when parent and child lack a common mode for expressing themselves through language, the disconnect presents developmental challenges that are not easily overcome. Consequently, deaf children of hearing parents are more likely to have problems in acquiring language, which may lead to problems in social and emotional adjustment.

Problems in acquiring language can negatively affect every aspect of development in children. There are practical problems that accompany learning through the visual mode in a world in which so much of what children learn comes through listening (Switzer and Williams, 1967). The deaf child cannot simultaneously listen to his mother and focus on an activity because inputs must be processed visually; sequencing of stimuli becomes an issue in learning (Wood *et al.*, 1986). The deaf children of deaf parents are advantaged in this respect, because they are likely to have been diagnosed early and because their parents are more likely to be sensitive to their visual communication needs (Vaccari and Marschark, 1997). The problem of divided attention limits experiential input to deaf children (Wood, 1991).

An often overlooked aspect of difference between deaf and hearing children is the context for development and its effect on orientation in the social world. Hearing children occupy parallel worlds arising from the integration of vision and hearing (Wood, 1991). The hearing child is constantly reminded of the outside world by sounds that infiltrate his consciousness even during solitary play. In contrast, the deaf child's world is insulated from the sounds of the outside environment and is consequently more centered on the self and the child's own activities (Urban, 1989). It is likely that a difference in how the world is experienced will have consequences for the child's development of social skills and personality.

The most frequent psychologic diagnoses for deaf children are related to behavioral disorders. Deaf children are often stereotyped as impulsive, immature, egocentric, and lacking in empathy, inner control, and self-awareness (Myklebust, 1964; Schle-

N. K. Mellon: The Johns Hopkins University, The Listening Center at Johns Hopkins, Baltimore, Maryland 21287.

singer and Meadow, 1972). Behavior disorders are three times more common in deaf than in hearing populations (Watson *et al.*, 1990). Although behavioral problems are often attributed to poor parent-child communication, psychosocial problems in deaf children of hearing parents may also be related to learning experiences rather than to any innate characteristic of deafness (Schum, 1991).

Patterns of behavior naturally reflect experience. Schum (1991) proposes a developmental model of social behavior in deaf children, which links behavior problems to experiential deficits. Children use environmental experiences to develop increasingly sophisticated notions about how the world operates. Experiential efficiency requires two elements: a common communication mode to receive information and linguistic resources with which to process, code, and manipulate information. Normally, parents can foster this development through communication, helping the child learn to interpret, think about, and generalize from their experience. Poor communication disrupts this line of transmission.

Development in the child's first 3 years often progresses normally, because it is not heavily language dependent. However, when communication is at a rudimentary, concrete level and development begins to require a sophisticated language system, developmental lags may occur. Consequently, the deaf child may behave in a manner that may be appropriate for a younger child but is inappropriate or deviant for the child's age. Many behavioral problems exhibited by deaf children can be attributed to poor relational skills lack of empathy, lack of awareness of their impact on others, or inability to read emotional cues. These relational skills are achieved at a higher level of interpersonal understanding a stage that can be delayed by communication deficits (Schum, 1991).

Similarly, greater impulsivity in deaf children may be linked to delays in developing affect regulation because of problems in early communication environments (Hind-

ley, 1997). Hearing parents of deaf children likely experience greater frustration in child rearing. Frustration may leave parents less responsive to affective cues from their children and may compromise the quality of interactions with their children (Meadow and Schlesinger, 1972). Because they lack effective linguistic methods for socializing their children, hearing parents of deaf children have been found to rely more heavily on physical punishment and removal to control child behavior. These methods discourage the development of self-monitoring and give the child little information with which to understand rules. The deaf child often has to learn rules by repeated trial and error, although parental explanation could easily provide the same information.

Quittner *et al.* (1994) examined the impact of audition on the development of visual attention in children. They compared the performance of school-age hearing children on a visual attention task to two groups of deaf children: those with cochlear implants and those without implants. Deaf children without implants performed poorly compared with their hearing peers, and deaf children with cochlear implants performed significantly better than deaf children without implants. The investigators suggest that a history of auditory experience is important to the development of visual attention. Deaf children whose visual attention is poor because of inadequate auditory experience are likely to be diagnosed with attention or behavior problems.

Studies suggest that deaf children have higher rates of attention disorders than hearing controls (Kelly *et al.*, 1993). Children with acquired deafness are more than twice as likely as children with hereditary deafness to be diagnosed with attention problems. These differences may be caused by generalized brain abnormalities associated with congenital rubella, congenital cytomegalovirus infection, and bacterial meningitis. Hindley (1997) suggests that hereditary deafness is more likely to be diagnosed early and to include deaf children of deaf parents a group more likely to have fewer communication problems.

Language enables the cultural transmission of accepted patterns of behavior (Hindley, 1997). Socialization normally occurs in the midst of the society into which the child is being acculturated. If access to social norms and behaviors are undermined by communication difficulty, developmental differences are likely to arise. From this perspective, it is not deafness that puts a child at risk for delayed development, but rather it is the lack of shared communication mode between parents and children that sets the stage for developmental problems (Bebko and McKinnon, 1990; Wood, 1991; Vernon and Rothstein, 1968).

Koester and Meadow-Orlans (1994) identified language ability, not modality, as the best predictor of interpersonal communication in children, regardless of hearing status. Hearing parents who become adept at sign language can sidestep the developmental risks associated with inadequate communication. Reliance on sign language, however, naturally limits a child's communicative partners. Cochlear implants and oral education can expand the child's social boundaries and add to the child's experiential input through access to auditory information. Cochlear implants typically provide better access to spoken language than hearing aids for children with advanced levels of cochlear defect or degeneration and can help avert developmental deficits due to inadequate experiential input.

Ideally, hearing parents can develop a repertoire of communication strategies to communicate effectively with their deaf children across developmental stages. In reality, few hearing parents acquire the fluency in sign language required to adequately nurture social skills in their deaf children. This is most likely because of the difficulty inherent in learning any new language as an adult, particularly when environmental exposure to the desired language is limited. Cochlear implants offer an avenue through which deaf children can better access the family and social environment. Any improvement in communication between parent and child is likely to positively effect child outcomes in language, social, and cognitive development.

REFERENCES

Bebko J, McKinnon E. The language experience of deaf children: its relation to spontaneous rehearsal in a memory task. *Child Dev* 1990;61:1744–1752.

Hindley P. Psychiatric aspects of hearing impairment. *J Child Psychol Psychiatry* 1997;38:101–117.

Kelly D, Kelly B, Jones M, Moulton N, Verhulst S, Bell S. Attention deficits in children and adolescents with hearing loss. *Am J Dis Child* 1993;147:737–741.

Koester L, Meadow-Orlans K. Parenting a deaf child: stress, strength and support. In: Moores DF, Meadow-Orlans KP, eds. *Educational and developmental aspects of deafness.* Washington, DC: Gallaudet University Press, 1990.

Myklebust HR. *The psychology of deafness: sensory deprivation, learning, and adjustment.* New York: Grune & Stratton, 1964.

Quittner A, Smith L, Osberger M, Mitchel T, Katz D. The impact of audition on the development of visual attention. *Psychol Sci* 1994;5:347–353.

Schlesinger HS, Meadow KP. *Sound and sign: childhood deafness and mental health.* Berkeley, CA: University of California Press, 1972.

Schum R. Communication and social growth: a developmental model of social behavior in deaf children. *Ear Hear* 1991;12:320–327.

Switzer M, Williams B. Life problems of deaf people. *Arch Environ Health* 1967;15:249–256.

Urban E. Childhood deafness: compensatory deintegration of the self. *J Anal Psychol* 1989;34:143–157.

Vaccari C, Marschark M. Communication between parents and deaf children: implications for social-emotional development. *J Child Psychol Psychiatry,* 1997;38:793–801.

Vernon M, Rothstein D. Prelingual deafness: an experiment of nature. *Arch Gen Psychiatry* 1968;19:361–369.

Watson S, Henggler S, Whelan J. Family functioning and the social adaptation of hearing-impaired youth. *J Abnorm Psychol* 1990;18:143–163.

Wood D. Communication and cognition. *Am Ann Deaf* 1991;136:247–251.

Wood D, Wood H, Griffiths A, Howarth I. *Teaching and talking with deaf children.* Chichester: John Wiley, 1986.

Cochlear Implants: Principles & Practices, edited by John K. Niparko, Karen Iler Kirk, Nancy K. Mellon, Amy McConkey Robbins, Debara L. Tucci, and Blake S. Wilson. Lippincott Williams & Wilkins, Philadelphia © 2000.

13

Rehabilitation after Cochlear Implantation

Amy McConkey Robbins

The rehabilitation of children and adults who receive cochlear implants is now regarded as an essential part of the management of these patients. Impressive results from many users suggest that implants may change the trajectory of specialized learning for this population (Osberger *et al.*, 1996; Waltzman *et al.*, 1992; Gantz *et al.*, 1994). Surgical placement and appropriate fitting of a cochlear implant are necessary but insufficient prerequisites to achieving meaningful auditory integration and communicative competence. Postsurgical rehabilitation is recognized as a critical ingredient in the formula for successful cochlear implant use, particularly for implant recipients who lost their hearing before the establishment of spoken language (Geers and Moog, 1994; Nevins and Chute, 1996).

This chapter covers the topic of rehabilitation after cochlear implantation, considering rehabilitative needs in the context of preexisting linguistic skills. The first section addresses cochlear implant rehabilitation related to the prelingually deaf child and discusses speech perception, language, and speech production. The second section deals with issues of educational placement and support unique to children with cochlear implants. The third and fourth sections discuss rehabilitation issues for patients implanted in adolescence and adulthood, respectively.

THE PRELINGUALLY DEAF CHILD WITH A COCHLEAR IMPLANT

Childhood candidacy, rehabilitation need, and potential benefits of cochlear implants should be considered in the context of prelingual versus postlingual onset of deafness. The postlingually deafened child, having experienced profound hearing loss after the acquisition of language, typically shows rapid and dramatic benefit from the device. From a rehabilitation standpoint, postlingually deafened children are often characterized as more like the postlingually deafened adult than the prelingually deaf child (Fig. 13.1). Rehabilitation with the postlingually deafened child is often short term, with emphasis on communication strategies and on mapping the new percepts from the implant onto an existing linguistic code. In contrast, the prelingually deaf child with a cochlear im-

A. M. Robbins: Communication Consulting Services, Indianapolis, Indiana 46260.

Pre vs. post-lingual onset of deafness

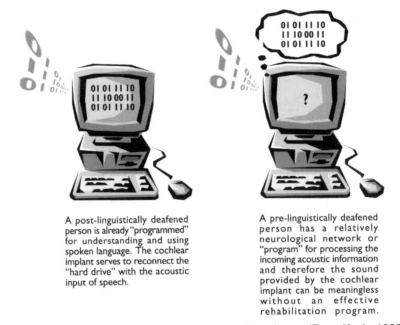

A post-linguistically deafened person is already "programmed" for understanding and using spoken language. The cochlear implant serves to reconnect the "hard drive" with the acoustic input of speech.

A pre-linguistically deafened person has a relatively neurological network or "program" for processing the incoming acoustic information and therefore the sound provided by the cochlear implant can be meaningless without an effective rehabilitation program.

FIG. 13.1. Prelingual versus postlingual onset of deafness. (From Koch, 1999.)

plant must use information from the implant to develop such a code de novo (Fig. 13.2).

For ease of reading, separate treatment is given to auditory, speech, and language skills, the three principal domains of cochlear implant rehabilitation for prelingually deaf children. Rehabilitative strategies should seek to achieve overall communicative competence, not to teach specific, isolated auditory, speech, or language subskills. These are simply means to a end. Programs that emphasize meaningful auditory integration are most effective when they take an integrated approach to therapy. The various aspects of communicative competence, listening, speaking, language, and pragmatics are interwoven in rehabilitation (Fig. 13.3). Artificially breaking down these components may lead to splintered skills and does not make the most efficient use of the limited instructional time that is available. Moreover, it is

Four components of therapy

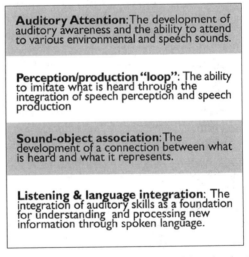

Auditory Attention: The development of auditory awareness and the ability to attend to various environmental and speech sounds.

Perception/production "loop": The ability to imitate what is heard through the integration of speech perception and speech production

Sound-object association: The development of a connection between what is heard and what it represents.

Listening & language integration: The integration of auditory skills as a foundation for understanding and processing new information through spoken language.

FIG. 13.2. Four components of cochlear implant rehabilitation therapy. (Koch, 1999, and Pollack, 1997).

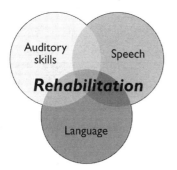

FIG. 13.3. Components of an integrated approach to cochlear implant rehabilitation.

possible to overtrain one aspect of communication to the detriment of other communicative skills. This phenomenon, referred to as *greenhousing* (Robbins, 1994a), may lead to disorders in communicative development when different subskills of communication fail to progress in synchrony. Warning signs for children whose skills have been greenhoused are addressed later in this chapter.

SPEECH PERCEPTION AFTER COCHLEAR IMPLANTATION

Auditory Capacity Versus Auditory Performance

Boothroyd *et al.* (1991) identified two measures of the auditory status of hearing-impaired listeners. The first, *auditory capacity*, refers to the ability to perceive significant contrasts among acoustic speech patterns. Auditory capacity is determined by the degree of the hearing loss, the dynamic range from threshold to uncomfortable loudness, and frequency discriminability. Boothroyd cautions that describing an individual's capacity only imperfectly predicts *auditory performance*, because auditory capacity translates to auditory performance only with appropriate amplification, experience, and conditions within the listening environment.

Similarly, a child's auditory capacity with a cochlear implant may be described by pa-

rameters such as threshold, electrical dynamic range, pitch perception, and sense of temporal aspects of speech (*e.g.*, duration, sequence). As with the hearing-aided patient, these parameters imperfectly predict how much benefit an implant patient will receive in real-world situations. Other factors, such as environmental support for audition, family commitment, educational emphasis, expectations, and quality of the rehabilitation program, are viewed as essential determinants of the child's auditory performance with a cochlear implant.

Similarities and Differences between Hearing-Aided and Cochlear-Implanted Children

Clinicians who work with deaf children wearing hearing aids often speculate on whether the same rehabilitation principles apply to children wearing cochlear implants. The answer is a resounding "yes and no." Effective principles used in working with a hearing-aided child are applicable to children wearing cochlear implants to the extent that shifts in threshold, dynamic range and pitch perception occur for both. Some of the similarities between the two groups are outlined in Table 13.1. Both groups of listeners follow the same sequence of auditory development, beginning with detection and progressing to more complex skills. For both groups, vowels tend to be perceived more accurately than consonants. When discriminating consonants from one another, the place of articulation feature (*e.g.*, *t* versus *k*) is the most

TABLE 13.1. *Similarities between hearing-aided and cochlear-implanted listeners*

Same sequence of auditory learning; *e.g.* begin with detection
Vowel perception superior to consonants
Consonant place cues most difficult
Wide individual differences
Background noise problematic
Many factors outside our control

difficult to identify. A broad range of perfor-mance is seen in both groups, highlighting the need for an individualized approach to treatment. Background noise causes signifi-cant decrements in performance for hearing-aided and cochlear-implanted listeners. In addition to masking effects on phoneme per-ception, filtering employed by the device can further compromise dynamic range. Chil-dren wearing either sensory aid present with many factors that are out of the clinician's control. These factors include the tempera-ment and intelligence of the child; the cause of deafness and condition of the surviving auditory system; and the overall personality characteristics that are known to affect learn-ing, including self-confidence, extroversion, and willingness to take risks (Head, 1983).

Clinicians may rest assured that the knowl-edge base they have developed regarding therapy with hearing-aided children will, in most cases, serve them well when working with implanted children. Nevertheless, im-portant differences exist between the two groups of children and professionals and par-ents must be cognizant of them in the ap-proach used with the child. Table 13.2 lists differences between the two groups of listen-ers. Although the sequence of auditory learning is similar for children with hearing aids and cochlear implants, the time course of learning for listening development often differs substantially. For example, implanted children are often able to demonstrate reli-able detection skills within hours or days of initial stimulation, in contrast to many pro-foundly deaf children with hearing aids who require months of training before demon-strating reliable detection responses. High-

frequency consonants are typically audible through the cochlear implant, whereas many profoundly deaf children wearing traditional amplification cannot perceive these sounds because of the electroacoustic limitations of traditional hearing aids (Fig. 13.4). However, the limited dynamic range available by means of electrically evoked hearing may present problems to cochlear implant listen-ers. The discrepancy in performance that of-ten exists between a child's performance in structured or natural settings may be even more pronounced in children early in their cochlear implant experience.

Cochlear implants provide the potential for incidental learning through natural con-sequences in the environment to a degree that may not be possible with hearing aids. Helping implanted children realize this po-tential, however, is one of the greatest chal-lenges facing clinicians. Of the differences outlined in Table 13.2, the last one is the most pivotal and may account for the rapid progress seen by many children after implan-tation and for the disappointing performance observed in others. Incidental learning ac-counts for the vast potential the child has to acquire language in a timely and efficient manner.

Teaching Curricula for Auditory Rehabilitation

Based on similarities between hearing-aided and cochlear-implanted children, clinicians find value in many existing auditory training programs. For example, Erber (1982) pro-posed a model for auditory rehabilitation that is widely implemented with cochlear im-plant children. This model posits a hierarchy of listening skills, beginning with simple de-tection of sound, discrimination, identifica-tion, and comprehension of meaningful audi-tory information (Fig. 13.5). The difficulty of stimuli at each level of the hierarchy may be adjusted by altering their linguistic complex-ity from simple (nonsense syllable) to com-

TABLE 13.2. *Differences between hearing-aided and cochlear-implanted children*

Time course of learning altered
Detection easier with cochlear implant
High-frequency sounds more salient with cochlear im-plant
Incidental learning potential

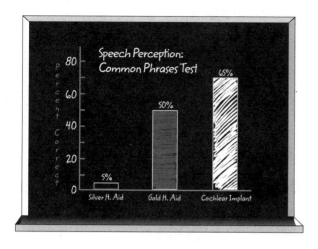

FIG. 13.4. Average open-set sentence recognition of children wearing the Clarion cochlear implant ($n = 22$; x̄ pure tone average [PTA] = 108 dB) compared with users of the Silver Hearing Aid ($n = 13$; x̄ PTA = 104 dB) and the Gold Hearing Aid ($n = 17$; x̄ PTA = 92 dB). The implant children's skills exceeded those of the hearing aid users despite an advantage in duration of device use by those using the Hearing Aid (x̄ Silver = 6.3 years; x̄ Gold = 5.2 years) compared with the cochlear implant (x̄ = 1.5 years). (Hearing aid data from Miyamoto *et al.*, 1995; implant data obtained during the U.S. clinical trial of Clarion.)

plex (paragraph-length material). Children with cochlear implants progress along this hierarchy in an order similar to that of hearing-aided children. However, the time and effort spent at various levels often needs to be adjusted to the child's learning curve. Erber's model remains a useful one for planning auditory work with implanted children.

Northcott's (1978) curriculum guide for hearing-impaired children from birth to 3 years of age describes a teaching program that has been validated over time as effective in developing oral communication (OC) skills. It is appropriate for early-implanted children for several reasons:

1. Its primary focus is on the parents and the development of communication in the home.
2. Language acquisition is viewed as the goal of training, so that auditory skill development is always set within a linguistic context.
3. Schedules of development are provided for motor, auditory, receptive language and expressive language skills, suggesting a holistic view of the developing implanted child.

This program is particularly useful in light of the increasing numbers of deaf children receiving cochlear implants before the age of 3 years. These children require a curriculum that is less structured and more parent cen-

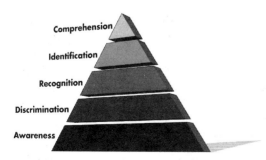

FIG. 13.5. Model of listening skill development. (Adapted from Erber, 1982.)

Essential Communication Habits

Present auditory **first!** If a child gets information visually, there will be little motivation to listen.

Signal **"listen"**... to" *push in the clutch"* & "shift" from *looking to listening.*

Provide **"uncluttered" listening "space"**... Sound cannot be sorted out against a "busy" acoustic background

Provide **"acoustic highlighting"** Emphasize key words.

Use **visual** clarifiers... Make a *direct connection* between a word & what it represents.

Speak **slowly**... Speech is comprised of very discrete bits of acoustic information presented at a very rapid rate.

Allow **processing time**... Understanding speech is a complex, multi-step cognitive process.

FIG. 13.6. Essential communication habits. (Koch, 1991.)

tered because of their young age and limited communication (Fig. 13.6). Training programs designed for older implanted children are inappropriate for this group, because such programs are less likely to employ a developmental approach to communication therapy.

Correspondence materials from the John Tracy Clinic are highly recommended for parents of young children with implants. Even those involved in other therapy programs can benefit from these materials, which are available in 26 languages and are provided free of charge. They provide an excellent supplemental resource and emphasize the parent-child relationship that is so vital in communication development.

Sindrey's *Listening Games for Littles* (1997) is an example of interleaving of language, speech, and auditory skills in a curriculum for preschool children. This program is an alternative to overly structured and analytic listening training programs, and Sindrey's lessons can capture the interest and imagination of children and therapists. Sindrey's approach is based in the auditory-verbal method that is well suited to cochlear implant children because of its emphasis on maximizing hearing for language develop-

ment. Auditory-verbal materials from Pollack (1997) and Estabrooks (1994) also have been extremely useful for implanted children.

Several other auditory programs are in widespread use with implanted children, including *Speech Perception Instructional Curriculum and Evaluation* (SPICE) (Moog *et al.*, 1995), *Miami Cochlear Implant Auditory and Tactile Skills Curriculum* (CHATS) (Vergara and Miskel, 1994), and *Developmental Approach to Successful Listening II* (DASL) (Stout and Windle, 1992).

A seven-part video training program with an extensive manual was developed at The Listening Center at Johns Hopkins. *Bringing Sound to Life: Principles and Practices of Cochlear Implant Rehabilitation* (Koch, 1999) provides professionals and parents with practical foundations and strategies for developing a rehabilitation program and integrating goals into home and classroom (Fig. 13.7). Koch provides abundant examples and explains therapy principles in ways that readers can understand and generalize. For example, Koch uses a "3-D therapy" rule to remind clinicians that cochlear implant rehabilitation has three dimensions: diagnostics, development, and demonstration (Fig. 13.8). Koch also outlines factors affecting test performance in children (Fig. 13.9). Many therapists find that an eclectic approach, combining information from several training sources, best meets the individual needs of each implanted child.

The Risk of Greenhousing

The nature of auditory therapy, in which one aspect of sound is focused on and intensely drilled, poses a risk for the development of a counterproductive pattern known as greenhousing. Robbins (1994a) used this term to describe therapy approaches that emphasize isolated, structured listening behaviors to the exclusion of other communication skills. This approach may lead to an asynchrony between auditory development

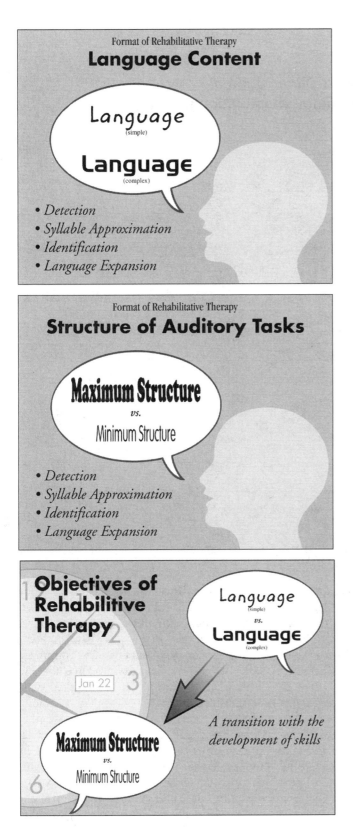

FIG. 13.7. Formats and objectives of auditory rehabilitation. (From Koch, 1999.)

The 3-Dimensions of
Cochlear Implant Rehabilitation therapy

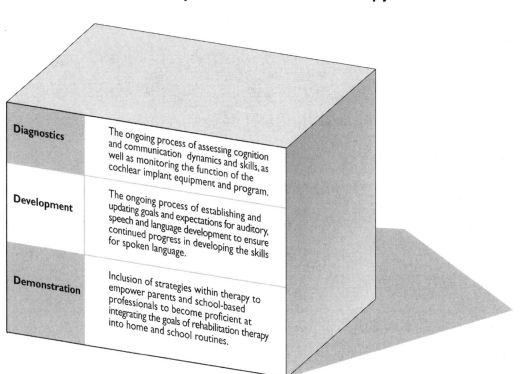

Diagnostics	The ongoing process of assessing cognition and communication dynamics and skills, as well as monitoring the function of the cochlear implant equipment and program.
Development	The ongoing process of establishing and updating goals and expectations for auditory, speech and language development to ensure continued progress in developing the skills for spoken language.
Demonstration	Inclusion of strategies within therapy to empower parents and school-based professionals to become proficient at integrating the goals of rehabilitation therapy into home and school routines.

FIG. 13.8. Three-dimensional therapy. (From Koch, 1999.)

and overall communicative competence. There are a number of "red flags" used to identify children whose auditory development is following this counterproductive pattern. First, these children may be able to engage in auditory tasks through listening alone as long as they are not required to interpret what they hear in a meaningful way. This includes the child who can make fine distinctions between pairs of nonsense syllables (*e.g.*, dop versus gop) but fails to make similar distinctions when real words are used. Second, these children may be able to perform listening tasks for rehearsed material but are unsuccessful when the same information is presented in a novel, unrehearsed situation. Third, children with greenhoused skills may rely heavily on rote or elicited imitation during communication, even after considerable practice with the language structures used. These children's successful auditory performance may depend on routinized tasks, suggesting that the skills have not generalized. For example, a school-aged child demonstrating this behavior may be able to answer the question, "What is the weather outside today?", through listening alone if asked during calendar time each morning by the teacher in a rehearsed format. If the same question occurred in the course of daily conversation, the child may fail to comprehend the identical phrase. These observations indicate the need for incidental learning emphasis at home and school.

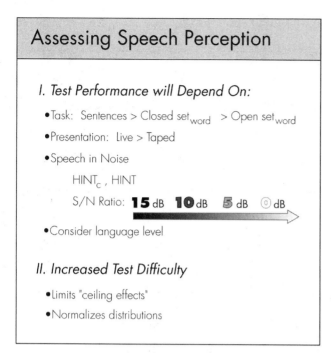

Assessing Speech Perception

I. Test Performance will Depend On:

- Task: Sentences > Closed set$_{word}$ > Open set$_{word}$
- Presentation: Live > Taped
- Speech in Noise

  HINT$_c$, HINT

  S/N Ratio: **15** dB **10** dB **5** dB ⊙ dB

  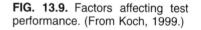

- Consider language level

II. Increased Test Difficulty

- Limits "ceiling effects"
- Normalizes distributions

FIG. 13.9. Factors affecting test performance. (From Koch, 1999.)

To reduce the risk of developing green-housed listening skills in implanted children, several strategies are suggested:

1. Alternate global and discrete listening activities in therapy. Global listening tasks rely on suprasegmental cues and the gestalt of the message, whereas discrete listening tasks require an analytic approach to recognizing fine details in the message. Both are important, but a balance is required. Traditional auditory teaching relied too heavily on many repetitions of discrete listening tasks, such as minimally different word pairs. The teacher must make certain that structured, discrete listening tasks account for no more than one-half of a child's auditory activities during therapy. Music, nursery rhymes, recognition of emotion in the voice, and listening walks can be motivating global tasks.

2. Establish listening routines, and then change the routine in a controlled, monitored fashion. Young children need routines in their schedule, and teachers of the hearing-impaired can make effective use of routines. However, overusing routines can mask the ability to judge the child's auditory understanding. By sabotaging a child's routine, teachers are able to separate situational from auditory comprehension. If a teacher greets the implanted child every morning with, "Go hang up your coat," and the child hangs up his coat, it is impossible to judge whether the child understands the command or predicts it from the context. The teacher should alternate this command with several others, such as "Put your book bag on your chair," and "Hang up a friend's coat," observing the child's response to changes in auditorily presented information.

3. Introduce open-set tasks early in rehabilitation. Do not wait for children to master

Sound-Object Association:
Connecting sound & meaning

Listening "set"	All of the possible responses to a listening task.
"Closed Set".	A clearly defined or "limited" set. All possible responses are within the specified set.
"Open Set"	A set in which the range of possible responses to a listening task is unlimited.
"Bridge Set"	A set of possible choices in which the context is clearly established, however the specific content is not defined.

FIG. 13.10. Set content affects listening performance. (From Koch, 1999.)

closed-set listening before expecting some open-set responses. Present common phrases such as "How are you?" and "Time for lunch" through listening alone. Even if the child does not understand, clarify with speechreading, and try again later. You are conveying the message that you expect the child to listen and comprehend (Fig. 13.10).

4. Make closed-set listening tasks less predictable. For example, if Sally is picking an object out of a field of four objects through listening alone, try these variations: ask for one of the objects several times, ask for an object that is not one of the choices, fail to ask for one object, call the child's name in place of an object, or present silence and observe the child's response (Fig. 13.9).

5. Set spontaneous listening goals and structured ones. Spontaneous goals can include the child responding to his name on his own, recognizing classroom auditory signals when not in a listening set, or understanding some key words in a conversation through listening alone.

6. Document instances in which the child repeats something he has overheard in conversation, uses a new word without being directly taught it, or reauditorizes by "thinking aloud" with language to solve problems.

All of these approaches suggest that the forces of generalization and incidental learning are alive and working in the child.

LANGUAGE LEARNING AFTER COCHLEAR IMPLANTATION

Research Findings

The earliest studies evaluating implant benefit in children assessed speech perception skills (see Chapter 10). Because the cochlear implant is an auditory prosthesis, assessing perception was viewed as the most direct way to evaluate device benefit. Later, speech production benefits were studied, acknowledging the close relation between speech perception and speech production. Attention has been focused on what many contend is the ultimate goal of pediatric cochlear implantation: enhancement of language development.

Early-onset profound hearing loss has devastating consequences for the development of language. During the critical period for language learning, falling between birth and about 7 years of age, children with normal hearing master almost all of the essential elements required for being a competent communicator in their language. The presence of profound hearing loss dramatically alters children's ability to extract linguistic cues from the auditory language models around them. These children are also deprived of one of the primary sources of language information; the linguistic models that are available during "overhearing" language through various sources in the environment are drastically reduced.

Children with prelingual onset of profound deafness have been shown to experience substantial delays in their mastery of all aspects of communication. Investigators have documented hearing-impaired children's deficiencies in vocabulary (Boothroyd et al., 1991, Osberger et al., 1981), grammar (Power and Quigley, 1973, Geers and Moog, 1994), concepts (Davis, 1974), and pragmatics (Kretschmer and Kretschmer, 1994) in the receptive and expressive domains. Language is the internalized, abstract knowledge system that is the basis for communication. Improvement in language has far-reaching and life-altering consequences for a deaf child, including improved reading ability (Paul, 1998), academic achievement (Goldgar and Osberger, 1986) and career attainment.

Documenting the effects of cochlear implants on language development is challenging, because the language of most unimplanted deaf children improves somewhat over time. Studies of the receptive vocabulary scores of implanted children (Dawson et al., 1995), for example, compared rate of learning with published data for normal-hearing and hearing-impaired children. The rate of language improvement increased after implantation but could not be attributed directly to implant use because such studies lacked a control group for comparison. Investigators have used various research designs to isolate maturational effects from the effects of the cochlear implant on language development. Robbins et al. (1995) used language quotients, based on a formula by Strong et al., (1994) to compare predicted language scores on the Reynell Scales (1990) with those actually achieved by children wearing the Nucleus 22-channel cochlear implant. At 15 months after implantation, observed scores were 10 months higher for receptive and 8 months higher for expressive language than the scores that had been expected based on maturation alone.

An alternative prediction method used by Robbins et al. (1997) assessed language development in cochlear-implanted children. A group of unimplanted, profoundly deaf children provided cross-sectional data that were used to generate predictive equations using the Reynell Scales. This allowed the investigators to estimate the rate of language learning in a deaf child that could be attributed to maturation. Actual language performance on the Reynell was then measured in a group of implanted children at intervals before and after implantation. These scores were then compared with those predicted on the basis of maturation. After 1 year of device use, the implanted subjects' average language scores were approximately 7 months better than those predicted from maturation. Moreover, the rate of language improvement for the implanted children was equivalent to gains seen in normal-hearing children (Fig. 13.11). Improved rate of language learning was observed for children using oral and those using total communication (TC). The subjects' absolute language levels remained considerably delayed, however, relative to hearing peers.

The subskills of linguistic development affected by cochlear implantation were studied (Robbins et al., 1997) in children with multichannel implants using various measures of language ability. The rate of English language improvement fell in or near that of normal-hearing children in areas such as understanding and use of connected language, single-word vocabulary comprehension, and ability to provide antonyms and synonyms. The slowest rate of change for the implanted children was observed in their mastery of the grammatical aspects of English. Aspects of grammar, particularly morphology (*i.e.*, word endings such as the third person *s*, plural *s*, and past tense *ed*) have been identified as some of the most fragile subskills of language. For children using TC, these morphologic markers have been identified as the ele-

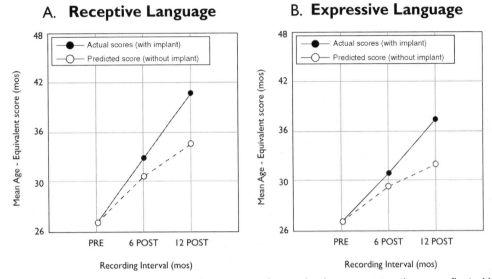

FIG. 13.11. A: Trajectory of age-equivalent scores of receptive language over time as reflected by performance on the Reynell test. Scores for 23 children with cochlear implants are plotted with the predicted scores. Predicted scores were based on observations in 89 unimplanted, profoundly deaf children who met audiologic criteria for implantation. **B:** Similar measures and comparisons for expressive language.

ments most likely to be omitted by adults who sign manually coded English (Schick and Moeller, 1992), a factor that limits the exposure TC children have to them in natural conversation.

Studies have reported language data from children implanted with the Clarion multichannel implant (Robbins *et al.*, 1999). Twenty-three children using the continuous interleaved sampling speech processing strategy were administered the Reynell Developmental Language Scales preoperatively and after 6 months of Clarion use. Significant improvements were observed in average age equivalent scores over time for receptive and expressive skills, although the absolute language levels of the implanted children remained delayed relative to their hearing peers. The children's rate of language growth in the first 6 months of implant use also was calculated. A score of 100 indicates a normal developmental rate (*i.e.*, 6 months' language growth in a 6-month period). The Clarion children, on average, progressed at a rate that exceeded that of normal-hearing chil-

dren (*i.e.*, 9 months' receptive and expressive language growth in 6 months) (Fig. 13.12). This study differed from most others of this nature in that the children's age at implant was considerably younger than that seen in other investigations. The average age at implantation of these subjects was 38 months, and more than one-half of the subjects were implanted at the age of 2 years. These findings provide further evidence in support of early implantation, a topic to be discussed later in this chapter. There was no significant difference between the language performance of children who used OC or TC.

Summary of Research Findings

The studies cited previously in this chapter provide research evidence regarding the effects of cochlear implants on language development in children. Robbins (1999) provided a summary of such evidence, which is presented in this section.

Improved speech processing strategies provide more language enhancement. The

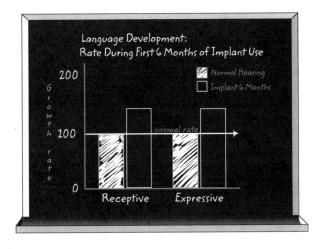

FIG. 13.12. Rates of language development in 23 prelingually deaf children wearing the Clarion implant. A language rate of 100 indicates development consistent with that of hearing children (*i.e.*, 6 months' language growth in 6 months). The Clarion children averaged 9 months' language growth in 6 months. Absolute scores for the implanted children remain delayed relative to hearing peers. (From Robbins AM, Bollard PM, Green J. Language development in children implanted with the CLARION cochlear implant. *Ann Otol Rhinol Laryngol Suppl* 1999;177:113–118.)

amount and quality of information provided by the speech processor has a measurable effect on language improvement. With each generation of speech processor technology, more improvements are observed in language outcomes. Compare, for example, the nebulous effects on language of the single-channel implant with those provided by multichannel implants with spectral peak or continuous interleaved sampling strategies.

Children with cochlear implants outperform their profoundly deaf peers who use hearing aids. In studies comparing the language performance of implanted children with that of their unimplanted, deaf peers with similar degrees of hearing loss, faster rates of language learning and higher overall language achievement levels consistently have been documented in the implant subjects. The average profoundly deaf child learns language at about one-half the rate of normal-hearing children (*i.e.*, 6 months' language in 1 year). If it is the case that a cochlear implant converts a profoundly deaf child to a severely hearing-impaired one (Boothroyd and Eran, 1994), this conversion represents a monumental leap in achievement potential, given what is known about the differences in ability of these two groups.

Cochlear implants allow deaf children to begin to learning language at a rate equivalent to that of normal-hearing children. Several studies demonstrated that the average child who receives a multichannel cochlear implant learns approximately 1 year of language in 1 year's time. This effect seems to be particularly true for those implanted before the age of 6 years.

Most deaf children remain delayed in their language skills, even after implantation. This appears to be the case because of the significant delays that already exist in children's language at the time they receive their implants. To avoid this continued delay, children must learn language at a faster than normal rate after implantation to catch up to their hearing peers, as some appear to be doing (Robbins *et al.*, 1999; Bollard, 1999), or they must receive their implants early enough to prevent an uncloseable gap from forming between language age and chronologic age.

A wide range of language benefit is observed across children. Virtually every study of the performance of implanted patients, whether adults or children, has yielded a wide range of performance outcomes. The study of language enhancement in this population is no exception. Regardless of the specific device used, some children do extremely well with their implants, performing as "stars" in the upper end of the continuum, whereas a small number of children receive limited benefit from their implants. The attempt to tease out what factors may account for this variability is ongoing. It is important to keep this large performance variance in mind, especially when reviewing data that have been averaged across subjects.

OC and TC children improve in their language skills after implantation. This finding has been reported by a variety of investigators using several different assessment procedures. It stands in contrast to the results reported for speech perception or speech production benefit in children with implants. In both these areas, children using OC have been shown consistently to outperform their counterparts who use TC (Osberger *et al.*, 1998; Osberger *et al.*, 1994; Geers and Moog, 1994). It is not clear whether the mechanisms by which language is enhanced through a cochlear implant are the same for children using OC and TC.

Earlier age at implantation provides a better chance of children receiving language enhancement from their implant. This trend for better performance in children implanted younger also has been documented in speech perception studies (Waltzman *et al.*, 1997). Many factors favor early age at implantation, including neural plasticity and the notion of critical periods. Another factor that may account for this advantage is the ability of the younger child to learn language incidentally. This topic is addressed later in this chapter.

Mechanisms by Which Cochlear Implants Improve Language in Prelingually Deaf Children

The investigations cited previously confirm that cochlear implants provide measurable language enhancement for children, particularly young children, who receive them. What is less certain is the mechanism or mechanisms by which this enhancement takes place, although some hypotheses are possible.

Access to the Spoken Language Code

For a profoundly deaf child with limited hearing aid benefit, more of the cues necessary to interpret the spoken language code are available through a multichannel cochlear implant than through hearing aids. Even the best cochlear implant users do not hear normally; the signal they receive is degraded. However, state-of-the-art cochlear implants appear to provide a rich enough signal to give "linguistic access" in many of the children who receive them. Data from group studies cited earlier and from case studies (Svirsky, 1998) confirm that some congenitally deaf children are able to learn English language through information from their cochlear implant.

An example of this increased linguistic access is the availability of morphologic marker cues that are available to a profoundly deaf listener through a cochlear implant but usually not through a hearing aid. The structure of English is such that many morphologic markers occur at the ends of words, where they are produced with a weak intensity and are marked by high-frequency consonants such as t, s, and s, which may not be auditorily salient. Rudmin (1983) reported on Pittman's findings that there were 21 linguistic functions of s and its voiced cognate z in the English language. Missing or misinterpreting just these two sounds could be extremely detrimental to morphologic acquisition by OC children. Merely detecting these sounds does not ensure that the child will have comprehension of the linguistic meanings, which is a much longer and fundamentally different learning process. Nevertheless, a person cannot learn to interpret auditory phenomenon if she or he does not hear them. The cochlear implant, although not replicating the spoken code perfectly, provides more pieces of the language puzzle.

In the case of children using TC, morphologic markers have been identified as the elements most likely to be omitted by adults who sign manually coded English (Schick and Moeller, 1992). This finding limits the exposure that TC users have to morphologic information during signed conversation. Children using TC gain auditory access to these markers through their cochlear im-

Emergence of Spontaneous Language with Cochlear Implants in Children

Rates of language development were tested in 23 prelingually deaf children wearing the Clarion implant. A language rate of 100 indicates development consistent with that of hearing children (*i.e.*, 6 months' growth in 6 months). The Clarion children averaged 9 months' language growth in 6 months. The absolute scores of the implanted children remain delayed relative to normal-hearing peers.

Because the ultimate goal of implantation is to facilitate comprehension and expression of spoken language, there is a clear need to evaluate the strategies adopted by children to communicate spontaneously after implantation (Schopmeyer *et al.*, 1999). Information through spontaneous language involves the conversion of thought into speech. This conversion relies on mental representations of lexical, phonologic, and syntactic structure (Jackendoff, 1994).

Children with cochlear implants were videotaped during play sessions to obtain 20-minute language samples. Subjects were 1 year 4 months to 9 years 11 months of age. An age-matched group of unimplanted candidates was used to establish the effects of normal maturation on vocabulary development. Children were engaged to play in the presence of the parents and a clinician. Tapes were analyzed for lexical items produced by the child in seven semantic categories.

The semantic categories analyzed were based on those previously described (Laughton and Hasentstab, 1986.) Categories included AGENT (person or actor), ACTION, OBJECT (*i.e.*, what is acted on), LOCATION, POSSESSION, MODIFIERS (*i.e.*, adjectives or adverbs); and SOCIAL CONVENTIONS (*e.g.*, hi, please, yes). Words were counted by different lexical items only; if a word was used more than once, it was counted only one time.

The study of implanted children revealed an increase in the mean number of lexical items produced from 15 preoperatively to 27 at 6 months after implant activation. The mean number of lexical items produced by age-matched subjects without and with cochlear implants were 13 and 28, respectively. Although these comparisons reach only marginal statistical significance, the trend is a positive one.

When broken into individual semantic categories, the participants demonstrated similarities to normally hearing children: use of items within every category and heavy representation of AGENT, ACTION, and OBJECT. The high number of MODIFIERS used appears to be related to a preponderance of color labels. The low incidence of POSSESSION may be more likely to arise.

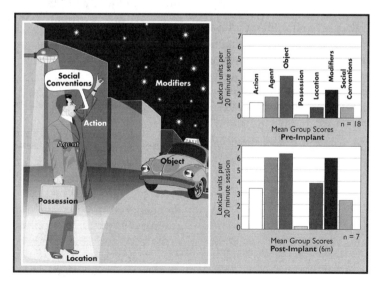

plants and may therefore learn them auditorially.

Cochlear Implants Increase Visual Attention

It is possible that cochlear implants have a global, multisensory effect on language learning, a hypothesis supported by the findings of Quittner *et al.* (1994). These researchers reported increases in selective visual attention in children after cochlear implantation and posited that attention may be viewed as a behavior of the whole organism. They also suggested that improvements in selective visual attention should precede gains in auditory word recognition in children with cochlear implant. Increases in visual attention translate into more vigilance and less distractibility, both of which create a positive environment for language learning. Most profoundly deaf children do not have adequate residual hearing to use audition as a way of monitoring their environment. This means they must periodically look up from the task at hand to monitor their surroundings. For a student in a classroom, this means that his attention to the book in front of him or the mathematical problem being written on the board is constantly being interrupted as he looks around and then returns to the task at hand. If the cochlear implant allowed the child to develop a listening mechanism for monitoring his environment, the child could concentrate on his work while processing auditory signals around him (*i.e.*, "That's the sound of the water fountain at the back of the room; that's the sound of someone throwing paper in the trashcan. I can ignore those.").

Ability to Cue into a Speaker

Hearing-impaired children who rely on lip-reading often miss the first parts of sentences spoken by others in conversation. This occurs because they are not visually cued into the speaker as he or she begins to talk. Anecdotal reports suggest that the cochlear implant ameliorates this problem because listeners are immediately aware when someone is speaking and can direct visual attention to that speaker. This means that, rather than processing only the second half of a message, the cochlear implant user has full access to the whole conversation, even if the user relies heavily on lip-reading for language comprehension.

Potential for Incidental Language Learning

The potential for incidental language learning is perhaps the most compelling hypothesis to explain language enhancement from cochlear implants. Incidental language learning is the avenue by which children with normal hearing learn language. This avenue usually is unavailable to deaf children, who must be directly taught every language skill they know.

Traditionally, auditory development in profoundly hearing-impaired children was viewed as a process of auditory training. This implied that the child required didactic training to achieve each of the listening skills along a hierarchy of auditory development, and there were virtually hundreds of these skills. The assumption was the child learned only what was directly taught. This was not an unreasonable assumption before the advent of multichannel cochlear implants, given that many profoundly deaf children were able to recognize only patterns of auditory information rather than to discriminate the fine temporal and spectral structure of speech. Listeners who lack precision in these percepts are considered "pattern perceivers." Boothroyd (1984) demonstrated that children who perceived only patterns of auditory information could still use sound to make a remarkable number of discriminations of the speech signal. However, these pattern perceivers did not access enough of the auditory code to use listening as their primary source of language learning. For these children to learn spoken language, a direct, systematic approach to training was required. The children were, in large part, unable to make use of incidental learning, as a means of acquiring language. This incidental language learning is the means by which normal-hearing children learn language. It is the most efficient and perhaps the only way to truly master a spoken language code.

Incidental learning takes place when a child acquires knowledge or skills through naturally occurring events. The ability to generalize is central to an incidental learning model because such a model assumes that the developing child's cognitive system is able to make use of similarities and differences within situations to generalize across them. For example, a child who is hurt by touching the burner on his mother's gas stove probably will not attempt to touch the burner on his grandmother's electric range. He has generalized information from one context to another. Rather than having to be individually taught not to touch every heat source in the home, he eventually realizes that other hot items, such as a curling iron, boiling tea kettle, or casserole that just came out of the oven, also cause pain. One of the reasons the child can make these generalizations is that his sensory system—in this case, his sense of touch—is intact. If the child did not feel pain normally, it is unlikely that he would be able to generalize this information and would need to be shown every source of dangerous heat separately. This is analogous to the case of the profoundly deaf child with little residual hearing. Because his sensory input system—in this case his sense of hearing—is so limited, the chances of using incidental learning for generalization are substantially reduced (Boothroyd, 1985).

Cochlear implants provide the potential for deaf children to make use of generalization and incidental learning to an unprecedented degree. However, the signal provided by the implant is not complete; even implant recipients using state-of-the-art speech processing technology receive a degraded auditory signal. Children often receive a cochlear implant after several years of auditory deprivation, during which they have learned to process information visually. Even with the improved auditory signal provided by the cochlear implant, these youngsters need systematic and intensive training to reach their auditory potential.

Didactic Versus Generalization Approaches to Language Rehabilitation

Teaching methodologies in deaf education must change to accommodate the increased generalization ability of deaf children with cochlear implants. If clinicians continue to assume that a child's learning completely depends on didactic instruction, opportunities for incidental learning will be lost. Because didactic therapy lessons are designed to address specific skills, clinicians working with an implanted child should also identify real-world situations in which these same skills may be applied and generalized by the child. Failure to adopt an emphasis on incidental learning lessens the effectiveness of parents to use "teachable moments" at home to foster their child's auditory progress (Fig. 13.13).

Given the improved auditory learning potential with cochlear implants, the goal is not to teach the child every skill he will ever need to know but to select teaching targets that can be generalized to other targets, which can be generalized to other targets, and so on (Fig. 13.14). This approach promotes independent learning skills and helps the child become a responsible communicator.

Age at Implant Is a Critical Factor

A child's potential for incidental learning and generalization is greatest in the early

Preparing for incidental learning through didactic activities

Didactic therapy activity	Incidental learning application
Dolly dress-up	Getting dressed
Teddy bear tea party	Setting table, language at meals, doing the dishes
"Cooking" with "Playdo"	Baking cookies, preparing dinner
Category games	Grocery shopping, sorting toys, doing laundry
"Simon Says"	Following directions, body parts
"I Spy"	Descriptions, associations, functions of objects

FIG. 13.13. Preparing for incidental learning through didactic activities. (From Koch, 1999.)

years and slowly decreases with age. All implanted children require a combination of didactic instruction and opportunities for incidental learning. Typically, children who receive an implant at an earlier age require less didactic instruction and benefit more from incidental learning. Although children who are older at the time of implantation may still benefit from incidental learning, it is likely that their curriculum will need to be heavily weighted with didactic instruction if they are to acquire useful skills (Fig. 13.15).

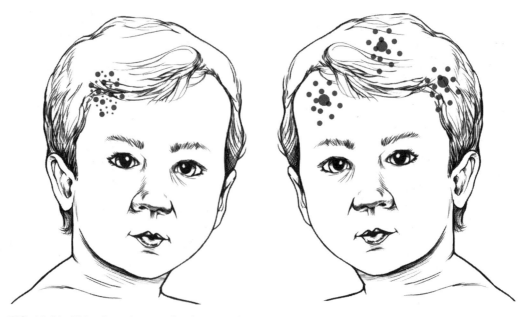

FIG. 13.14. Didactic and generalized approaches to communicative competence. The didactic model *(left)* attempts to target the behaviors needed for communicative competence by teaching every skill needed. To foster incidental learning *(right)*, therapy goals are selected that can be generalized to other skills, gradually producing a competent communicator.

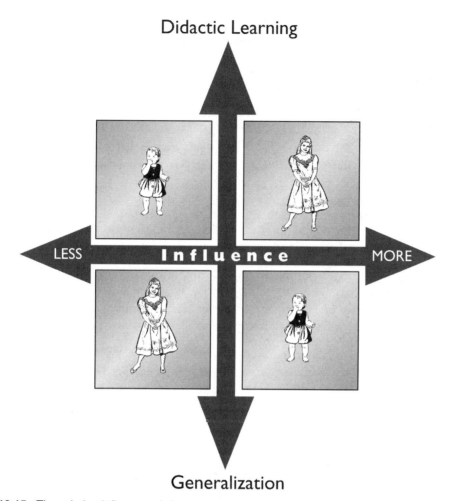

FIG. 13.15. The relative influence of didactic learning versus generalization for younger and older children. A child implanted at a young age requires less emphasis on didactic instruction, instead relying heavily on the innate ability to generalize. A child implanted later typically depends more on didactic instruction, and generalization has less influence. All implanted children need a combination of both types of learning to maximize device benefit.

This phenomenon, along with other evidence (Waltzman *et al.*, 1994; Brackett *et al.*, 1997; Fryauf-Bertschy *et al.*, 1997), argues for early implantation of children.

SPEECH TRAINING AFTER COCHLEAR IMPLANTATION

Speech is a system of oral movements that generate sounds (Fig. 13.16). These sounds may be used as the medium by which individuals communicate linguistically coded thoughts. The process of speech development requires that the child learn the intimate connection that exists between the sounds of speech and the oral movements that create those sounds (Boothroyd, 1982). Even in the earliest weeks and months of infancy, normal-hearing children begin to make this connection with the reflexive behaviors of crying, sneezing, and gurgling. This connection is reinforced and elaborated with each stage of speech acquisition, including babbling, jargoning, and the beginning of

	Voiced	Unvoiced
Fricative	v, TH, zh, z	f, th, sh, s, h, wh
Plosive	b, d, g	p, t, k
Nasal	m, n, ng	---
Affricate	j	ch
Resonant	l, r, w, y	---

FIG. 13.16. Summary of the features of speech and English phonemes.

real word use, a phenomenon that generally occurs around the first birthday. In normal-hearing children, speech development begins at birth and is virtually complete by the time the child begins school. Throughout the early years, it is the child's hearing that directs the development and control of speech acquisition. In later childhood, children rely more on how sounds should *feel* during speech, but early speech development is mediated by *hearing* (Fig. 13.17).

Profound hearing loss is a major impediment to speech development because it interferes with two essential processes: the child's ability to perceive the speech signal (Fig. 13.18) and the ability of the child to monitor his own speech (Calvert and Silverman, 1983). Both these processes are essential for accurate speech development. These two problems then create secondary difficulties for the deaf child. One such difficulty is that, because OC does not emerge during its critical period, an asynchrony develops between cognitive and communication skills. The greater the length of time that elapses between the emergence of developmental readiness and the mastery of subskills to fulfill that readiness, the more difficult it becomes for development to follow its intended course (Boothroyd, 1982).

Because of these difficulties, children with profound hearing loss generally do not develop intelligible speech without a substantial amount of systematic and intensive training. Even with this training, the intelligibility of many profoundly deaf children has been disappointingly low (Monsen, 1978; Osberger and McGarr, 1982; Carney, 1986),

largely because the electroacoustic limitations of traditional hearing aids did not allow enough of the segmental elements of speech to be conveyed to the listener. Improvement in speech skills is one of the objectives most often cited by parents seeking a cochlear implant for their child.

Research Findings

Speech production improvements after cochlear implantation have been documented using a variety of procedures. Serry and Blamey (1999) and Tye-Murray *et al.* (1995) examined speech improvements as a function of percentage of phonemes or words correctly produced. Other investigators have calculated a ratio of changes in meaningful or nonmeaningful speech attempts (Tobey *et al.*, 1994) or as a percentage of words spoken by the child that are recognizable to a naive listener (Osberger *et al.*, 1994). Taken together, these results suggest that cochlear implants enhance speech production abilities to a degree that was not possible with conventional hearing aids (Fig. 13.19). Serry and Blamey (1999) further analyzed speech production benefit from the cochlear implant by calculating the rate of phoneme improvement over time. Results suggested that implanted children took an average of 15 months from the time a speech sound was recognizable in their phonetic repertoire to the time the sound was correctly produced at least one-half of the time. A wide range of performance has been documented in studies of speech production enhancement, suggesting that multiple factors such as age at onset of deafness, time of

Phoneme Perception & Production:
Building Blocks of Listening

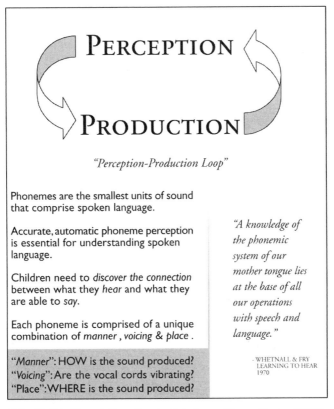

PERCEPTION

PRODUCTION

"Perception-Production Loop"

Phonemes are the smallest units of sound that comprise spoken language.

Accurate, automatic phoneme perception is essential for understanding spoken language.

Children need to *discover the connection* between what they *hear* and what they are able to *say*.

Each phoneme is comprised of a unique combination of *manner* , *voicing* & *place* .

"*Manner*": HOW is the sound produced?
"*Voicing*": Are the vocal cords vibrating?
"*Place*": WHERE is the sound produced?

"A knowledge of the phonemic system of our mother tongue lies at the base of all our operations with speech and language."

- WHETNALL & FRY
LEARNING TO HEAR
1970

FIG. 13.17. Perception–Production loop. (From Koch, 1999.)

implantation, communication methodology and rehabilitation may affect production and receptive outcomes.

Speech Training Procedures

The speech training method proposed by Ling (1976, 1989) is widely used with children wearing cochlear implants. This method uses a developmental approach to spoken communication, beginning with syllables, and recommends an order of teaching for speech sounds in English. Emphasis is placed on audition as the modality of choice for developing spoken language, whenever possible, and on the transfer of speech skills from drills to meaningful use. Although this method

was written before cochlear implants were available for deaf children, Ling's suggested teaching techniques remain highly compatible with the needs of most implanted children.

Word Associations for Syllable Perception (W*A*S*P*) (Koch, 1999) provides a tool to systematically develop a child's phoneme perception and production. Using simple pictures and toys representing increasingly complex phoneme combinations, the program is useful for developing a child's perception-production feedback loop and for monitoring the function of the cochlear implant (Figs. 13.20 through 13.22).

Robbins (1994) outlined six guidelines for speech training programs for children with

Audition of Speech Sounds

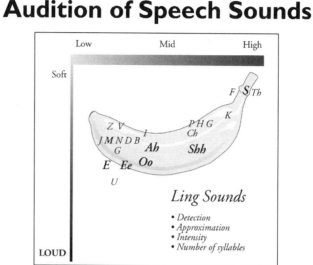

FIG. 13.18. Audibility of speech sounds. (From Koch, 1999.)

cochlear implants (Table 13.3). These guidelines may be used as principles for developing speech skills in implanted children, regardless of the specific speech training curriculum chosen:

1. Integrate perception and production goals. Therapy tasks should contain a listening and speaking component whenever possible. This allows the clinician to cover considerably more training in

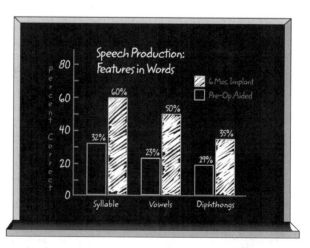

FIG. 13.19. Speech production results are shown for 24 prelingually deaf children preoperatively with hearing aids (x̄ pure tone average = 112 dB) and 6 months postoperatively with their Clarion implants. Significant improvement (*p* < .01) was documented in the production of syllables, vowels and diphthongs. Average age at time of implant was 3.6 years. (From Brown , McDowall. *Ann Otol Rhinol Laryngol* 1999;108[Suppl 177, Pt 2]:110–112.)

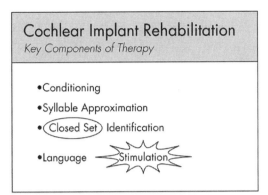

FIG. 13.20. Components of cochlear implant therapy. (From Koch, 1999.)

each session, without extra preparation of materials. By interweaving perception and production goals into the same activities, the connection between listening and speaking is made more salient to the child.

2. Develop a dialogue rather than tutorial therapy style. A dialogue format approaches communication lessons in a way that more closely replicates the give and take of real-world communication (Blank and Marquis, 1987). Rather than the teacher serving as the dominant conversational partner (as in a tutorial format), the dialogue format emphasizes turn-taking and switching of roles by child and clinician. When the child takes the role of teacher, he or she asks the questions and gains practice on the production of target stimuli.

3. Emphasize generalization of speech skills to real-world situations. Spoken language skills have a greater chance of being put to use in the real world if they have been developed through purposeful, result-producing experiences than if developed solely through rote exercise. One way to encourage generalization is through the use of bridging activities that maintain the essential purpose of a therapy task but include modifications to more closely approximate natural communication. These

modifications include creating a time delay between the explanation of the task and the opportunity for the child to use the speech target, setting up communication interaction in which the child must use a particular speech target when not expecting to do so, or constructing a situation in which the child's judgment is required in making communication choices. Another time-honored way to emphasize carryover is to use vocabulary in speech training sessions that are essential to the child's functioning in his daily life. For example, if the child adores soccer, the vocabulary chosen should include many words from this sport.

4. Use communication sabotage. First described by Lucas-Arwood (1980) in the child language literature, communication

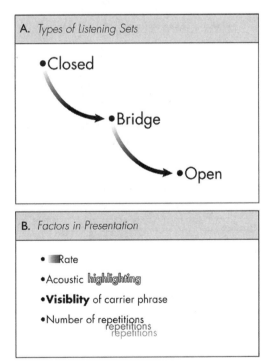

FIG. 13.21. A: Types of listening tasks classified by the level of context and cued information that accompany speech presentations. B: Factors in presentation to be considered in implant rehabilitation.

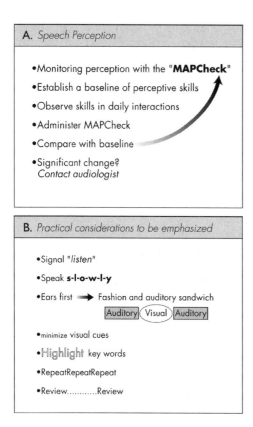

A. *Speech Perception*

- Monitoring perception with the **"MAPCheck"**
- Establish a baseline of perceptive skills
- Observe skills in daily interactions
- Administer MAPCheck
- Compare with baseline
- Significant change?
  Contact audiologist

B. *Practical considerations to be emphasized*

- Signal "*listen*"
- Speak **s-l-o-w-l-y**
- Ears first ➡ Fashion and auditory sandwich
  [Auditory] (Visual) [Auditory]
- minimize visual cues
- Highlight key words
- RepeatRepeatRepeat
- Review...........Review

FIG. 13.22. A: Ongoing monitoring of implant-mediated perceptions is a fundamental aspect of auditory rehabilitation. **B:** Effective auditory rehabilitation requires emphasis on key factors in the presentation of speech sounds.

sabotage is used as a component of speech training and assessment. As a training tool, the purpose of sabotage is to teach the child that he must be prepared for the unexpected and that listening is unpredictable. As an assessment tool, sabotage allows the clinician to observe whether

TABLE 13.3. *Principles for developing oral communication skills in implanted children*

Integrate perception and production goals
Develop a dialogue rather than a tutorial therapy style.
Emphasize generalization to real-world situations.
Use communication sabotage.
Use contrasts as stimuli in listening and speaking tasks.
Make communicative competence the goal.

true mastery of speech skills has occurred or the skills are tentative.

5. Use contrasts as stimuli in listening and speaking tasks. The use of speech contrasts, described by Ling (1976), Elbert and Gierut (1986), and Hodson and Paden (1991), involves juxtaposing contrasted sounds during speech training. When targets are contrasted with one another, the child is able to more clearly discern the distinguishing speech feature or features. The use of contrasts has also been suggested by Lindamood and Lindamood (1997), who incorporate this technique into their phonologic training programs. These researchers contend, for example, that if a child is trained what is "not r," she or he can more easily recognize what "is r." This technique is particularly well

suited for children with multichannel cochlear implants because both members of the contrasted pair are audible through their device, allowing the children auditory feedback about their productions and those of the teacher. Pictured material useful for developing contrasts include Contrastive Word Pairs (Kiernan and Zentz, 1990) and Language Approach to Open Syllables (Young, 1981). As the clinician develops speech sounds from isolation and syllables into real words, phrases, and running conversation, an Expansion-Reduction approach may be very helpful (Fig. 13.23). This approach may be visualized as a ladder for speech training. The clinician drills skills at the level appropriate to the child, moving up the ladder (expanding demands) when the child is successful with a speech target and stepping down the ladder (reducing demands) if the child is unsuccessful. For example, a

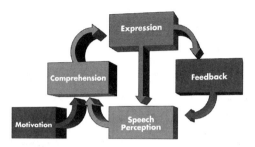

FIG. 13.24. Components of communicative competence.

child might be working on single-syllable words that begin with the alveolar sound /t/ (top; toes; tape). If the child successfully produces the words at this level, the clinician immediately moves up the ladder, putting the words in short phrases (a top; my toes; the tape). If the child is unsuccessful at producing the single words, the clinician steps down the ladder, reducing the production demand to a consonant-vowel syllable (to; toe; tae). Drills continue at this level until the child is successful, and the clinician steps up the ladder again. At any given time in therapy, a child typically is working on various speech targets at different rungs of the ladder.

6. Make communicative competence the goal. Speech skills are not meant to develop in isolation, but rather in synchrony with other communication abilities. Intelligible speech is only useful if a child has something to communicate to others and has the underlying language skills to do so. Goals for speech development must fit in with the child's overall communicative abilities (Fig. 13.24).

Effect of Communication Mode on Speech Production Skills of Implanted Children

Several studies have examined the effect of communication mode on the speech intelligibility of children with cochlear implants. The results of these studies have confirmed that,

Expansion - Reduction Method
Ladder of Speech Training Skills

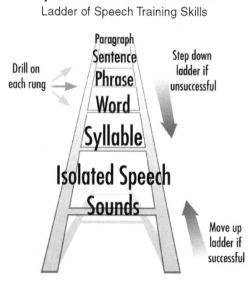

FIG. 13.23. The ladder of speech training skills used in the expansion-reduction method. The clinician quickly raises or lowers task difficulty during speech lessons to accommodate the child's level of success.

among implanted children, those who use OC demonstrate higher levels of speech intelligibility than those who use TC (Osberger, *et al.*, 1993; Osberger, *et al.*, 1994; Geers *et al.*, 1998., Osberger *et al.*, 1998). Many factors may account for this advantage, including the fact that children with less residual hearing tend to be placed in TC programs. However, this factor was carefully controlled for in the Osberger *et al.* (1994) study. An impressive advantage in speech intelligibility still was demonstrated by OC children, even when their TC counterparts were matched for preimplantation hearing levels. This may be related to the amount of time spent on speech training in OC or TC programs, to better teacher training in the area of speech, to levels of expectations set by parents and teachers, to the speech models of classroom peers, or to a combination of these factors. Osberger *et al.* concluded that, "Even if the amount of speech training, teacher preparation and parental expectations for the use of speech can be improved in total communication, the development of intelligible speech may still occur more often in children who use only speech to communicate than in children who use signs plus speech for communication. If signs are the more salient aspect of communication, auditory and speech information will receive secondary attention. It may be that children who use total communication do not reach their potential in speech development because of problems inherent in their method of communication."

The reader should keep in mind that this advantage in performance of OC over TC children has not been maintained when language skills are evaluated in implanted children. Whereas OC children outperform TC children in their speech production skills, both communication groups show similar language benefits from the cochlear implant. However, that several independent studies have confirmed a speech production advantage for OC children warrants serious consideration. TC continues to be the preferred option for a certain percentage of implanted children, but the family and school must be cognizant of the likelihood of reduced speech intelligibility in these youngsters.

EDUCATIONAL PLACEMENT AND SUPPORT OF IMPLANTED CHILDREN

The academic achievement levels of hearing-impaired children in the United States have historically been substantially lower than those of their normal-hearing peers. The reading achievement of hearing-impaired students, as measured on standardized tests, is disappointingly poor. For example, Holt's data from the SAT-8s showed a median reading grade equivalent of fourth grade in a large group of 17-year-old students with hearing loss. Cochlear implants have positive effects on educational achievement (Boothroyd *et al.*, 1998) but depend heavily on the ability of the system to adapt to the changing needs and skill levels of the implanted child.

Schools play a pivotal role in furthering the language and academic development of implanted children. The school's role in serving the child with a cochlear implant is threefold. The primary role of the school is to serve the academic needs of the child—to teach reading, mathematics, and the other essential academic subjects so that the implanted child functions at a level commensurate with normal-hearing peers. The school's second role is to create an environment that reinforces and expands the child's abilities with his cochlear implant. This means providing the child with many opportunities to listen and speak within daily classroom routines and to provide augmentative therapy directed at developing specific skills related to the cochlear implant. The school's role includes serving as a member of the cochlear implant team, giving feedback to the team regarding the benefit the child receives from the device and input regarding the child's progress in language, academic, and other

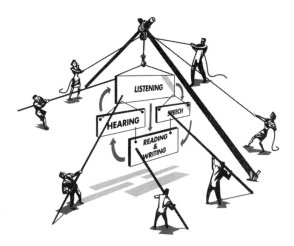

FIG. 13.25. The acquisition of communication skills is multifaceted. A team effort is required to build and support a child's communication mastery with the cochlear implant.

developmental skills. School personnel are in a unique position to provide such input, because the hospital-based team members, including the physician, audiologist, and speech pathologist, see the child only occasionally. In contrast, teachers have daily contact with the child, more familiarity with the child's unique characteristics of personality and temperament, and the perspective of viewing how the child learns and performs differentially across situations.

Importance of the Individualized Educational Plan

For all the technologic benefits afforded by cochlear implants, clinical experience suggests that these benefits are only fully realized if the child's educational program provides a high level of support to the child. One of the most important steps in ensuring such support is the writing of the child's individualized educational plan (IEP). In many ways, the IEP should be viewed as a partner to the cochlear implant because, as Flexer (1994) observes, "The IEP is the only ticket into the system of resource allocation that allows a child to receive any special technology, services, or strategies in school." The highest level audiologic, therapy, or interpreter recommendations cannot and usually

will not be implemented by the school unless these recommendations are written into the IEP. Even when a school recognizes that an implant child needs a special type of assistance or intervention, unless the parent is knowledgeable enough about the needs of the child to request the service and write it into the IEP, the school is under no obligation to offer this assistance or intervention. For this reason, the parents and implant center personnel must be prepared to formulate concise, measurable goals related to the child's cochlear implant that may be included in the IEP.

Relationship between the Cochlear Implant Center and the School

Another factor that influences implant success in children is the degree of partnership that exists between the cochlear implant center and the child's school. Each is critically important to the other. Both possess information about the implant child that can help in serving his or her needs. The degree to which that information is shared is one of the determinants of how the child progresses with his device (Fig. 13.26).

Nevins and Chute (1996) outlined a model of the relationship between the cochlear implant center and the child's school. They em-

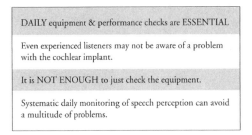

DAILY equipment & performance checks are ESSENTIAL

Even experienced listeners may not be aware of a problem with the cochlear implant.

It is NOT ENOUGH to just check the equipment.

Systematic daily monitoring of speech perception can avoid a multitude of problems.

FIG. 13.26. Key considerations in troubleshooting the device and monitoring speech perception.

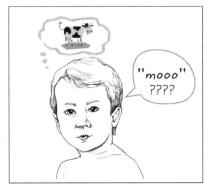

A child may be "familiar" with a word, but have never "heard it.

"mooo" ????

FIG. 13.27. Familiarity with vocabulary influences all aspects of listening, and it is common for a child born with a profound hearing loss to have significant gaps in vocabulary. It is important that the professional be aware of the child's familiarity with the vocabulary contained within a listening set and that the parent and professional recognize the difference between linguistic familiarity (*e.g.*, through a visual system, sign, lip-reading, print) and auditory familiarity. A child may be familiar with the sign representing *cow* but have no familiarity with the spoken word. If the vocabulary is new or only recently introduced, the child is unable to match the stimulus with an "image" of the word filed in the auditory memory. It takes time, repetition, and review before a child with a cochlear implant can develop an auditory memory with sufficient vocabulary to perform even simple identification tasks. (From Koch, 1999.)

phasize the importance of a preimplantation school visit made by a cochlear implantation team member. Nevins and Chute state that the single most important goal of the preimplantation visit is the establishment of a trusting relationship between the school and the cochlear implant center. In addition to establishing this working trust, other objectives of the visit before implantation are to evaluate the educational environment and observe the child as she or he functions within that environment and to share information about the cochlear implant and discuss reasonable expectations for device benefit for that child.

The preimplantation visit and other interactions should be viewed as a two-way exchange of information between the two agencies. Information is shared from center to school regarding the functioning of the cochlear implant, the child's performance on tests, and other details (Fig. 13.27). Information shared by the school to the center gives insights about the child that may be used to better manage the child and his or her family. Nevins and Chute recommend postimplantation interactions, including an additional school visit, training for care and maintenance of the implant, and assistance with the writing of appropriate auditory goals.

Because the implant center and school are sometimes far away from one another, teams must sometimes find alternative and creative ways to exchange information about the im-

planted child (Table 13.4):

1. Use videotapes as the medium to exchange information. School personnel can videotape sessions with the child and send these to the implant center, allowing the

TABLE 13.4. *Exchanging information between the cochlear implant center and the school*

Send copies of a videotaped session.
School personnel should accompany the child to an appointment at the implant center.
Suggest workshops that school staff may attend.
Share helpful resources and curricula.
Arrange periodic conference calls.

implant staff a view of the child in his or her educational environment. After a diagnostic session at the implant center, the feedback session with the parents can be videotaped and sent to the school. In this way, the school is privy to the same information as the parents regarding the child's test results and implications for educational management.

2. Invite school personnel to accompany the child during a visit to the cochlear implant center, where they can observe or participate in programming or rehabilitation sessions.

3. Provide the school staff with information about regional workshops and meetings related to implants specifically or management of hearing-impaired children in general.

4. Exchange lists of printed resources, curricula, and books that are helpful in managing children with implants, and update this information regularly.

5. Arrange conference calls in which several professionals (and perhaps the parents) can be on the line at the same time to "meet" about issues related to the implanted child.

Using the Child's Curriculum for Auditory Skill Development

Auditory work carried out with the implanted child should be integrated as much as possible with other communicative skills. For this reason, it is helpful to use material from school curricula as stimuli during auditory sessions. For example, vocabulary words or spelling list words may be used as stimuli during closed-set listening activities; newspaper articles from social studies class may be used for an open-set discussion of fact versus opinion; or a novel being read in class may be used for speech tracking practice. Suggestions for incorporating academic material into listening training may be found in Firszt

and Reeder (1996) and Nevins and Chute (1996).

Educational Placement Decisions for Implanted Children

Least Restrictive Environment

The legal guidelines for determining appropriate educational placement for hearing-impaired children, as dictated by Public Laws 94-142 and 101-476, are the same as for other handicapped children. Central to these guidelines is the notion of placing the child in "the least restrictive environment" in which he may succeed educationally. The law also stipulates that each child's unique needs and educational goals must be outlined in an IEP, which serves as a contract between the school and family and is rewritten each academic year. The importance of a least restrictive environment is balanced by "most appropriate placement." A child should be in an environment in which she or he has "full access to curricular information." The benefits of educational inclusion (formerly referred to as "the mainstream") for an implanted child cannot be overemphasized. These benefits include a higher standard of educational performance in regular classrooms (Ross, 1982), better communication models provided by normal-hearing peers, and improved speech intelligibility (Jensema et al., 1978).

Although these benefits are powerful and persuasive, they are only enjoyed by those who have the prerequisite skills to learn in the regular educational environment. In other words, the goal is not to place cochlear implant children in regular classrooms at all costs, but to choose that environment because the child has the skills to succeed there while expanding their cognitive and linguistic repertoire. Harrington (1974) asserts that hearing-impaired children have a unique linguistic problem that can severely restrict their ability to profit from an unplanned language presentation in the regular classroom.

Unless the language levels of deaf children are within 1 or 2 years of the levels of those in the regular class in which they are placed, they are virtually cut off from the entire verbal input process that is basic to educational experiences. An implanted child who is ill prepared for the regular classroom because of language and academic deficits may fall even further behind his or her peers in that environment if an accelerated rate of learning cannot be maintained.

The sense of failure and loss of confidence that comes from performing poorly are not risks to be taken lightly. Matkin (1988), for example, cautioned against a "failure-based" model of educational placement for hearing-impaired students in which they were placed in regular classrooms until they failed, reassigned to more restricted placements, and then given the support services they should have received all along. The key to successful educational inclusion for any child with hearing loss, including the implanted child, is to ensure that he or she is adequately prepared for placement in the regular classroom through early intervention, use of audition, and a concentrated rehabilitation program of language and communication development (Bess and McConnell, 1981). Longitudinal studies of children with cochlear implants in inclusive educational placements are imperative for evaluating how these children succeed in this environment.

Several evaluation tools can help make decisions about educational placement for a child with hearing loss, including those wearing cochlear implants. Two useful screening measures are the Screening Inventory for Educational Risk (SIFTER) (Anderson, 1989) for school-aged children and the Preschool SIFTER (Anderson and Matkin, 1996) for preschool children. Teachers complete questionnaires that sample the child's skills in academics, attention, communication, class participation, and school behavior relative to normal-hearing children. These straightforward tools are not diagnostic measures but rather are screening instruments used to identify children who merit further observation and testing. Although the SIFTER and Preschool SIFTER were not specifically designed for use with implanted children, they have proven useful for this population (Wray et al., 1997).

The Educational Resource Matrix (ERM) (Koch et al., 1997) is a tool with which to assess the resource use in placement of children with cochlear implants in educational programs. The educational placement is examined along a continuum from a full mainstream setting to placement in a residential school for the deaf. Support services such as speech therapy, interpreter services, and academic tutoring are also plotted along a continuum from no services at all to more than 6 hours of services per day. Using the ERM, the educational resource use can be examined over time for an individual child and for the population of implanted children as a whole. The ERM can also be useful in examining cost-effectiveness of the cochlear implant in children.

Koch et al. (1997) tracked patterns of use of educational and rehabilitative resources for 42 children with cochlear implants. Their initial cost-benefit projections based on observed advancement toward educational independence in the educational resource matrix indicated an extremely favorable net current value of the implant (i.e., cost savings minus cost). Further studies of this aspect of pediatric cochlear implantation are ongoing.

These data suggest that implanted children are able to make the transition to less restrictive environments after experience with their device. For children who have successfully transferred from more to less restrictive placements, continued monitoring of academic performance is warranted. Difficulties may arise when the child experiences educational transitions, such as moving from elementary to middle school or middle school to high school. These transitions may require changes in the support services offered. Professional guidance at these times it critical.

TABLE 13.5. *Educational modifications for children with cochlear implants*

Individualized education plan goals should reflect increased auditory potential.

The child is expected to demonstrate his newly acquired auditory skills at school.

Staff expectations should increase for speech, language, auditory skills; expectations should be put into practice.

A total communication child should be moved as far down the auditory continuum as possible.

The role of the interpreter is altered.

Generalization emphasis seeks to enhance opportunities for incidental learning, replacing strictly didactic approach.

After a child receives his cochlear implant, a variety of modifications are normally required in his educational program. For some children, particularly those in TC programs, these modifications may be fairly radical, as the educational setting seeks to take advantage of the child's new-found listening skills. Some modifications that are typically required are listed in Table 13.5.

Special Needs of the Implanted Child Using Total Communication

Children using TC make up a substantial proportion of the pediatric implant population. Some have questioned whether a TC approach is compatible with a cochlear implant. The answer to this question deserves a review of the historical development of TC.

The philosophy of TC evolved in the early 1970s. Before that time, deaf educators were divided into two primary camps: oralists, who advocated the use of speech and lip-reading without signs, and manualists, who advocated the use of sign language. The TC approach was originally intended to promote the use of any method of communication that was needed to develop language competence in the child. This included OC, signing, oral-signed communication, audition, fingerspelling, speechreading, and cued speech. It was also recognized that, depending on the situation, children might require different methods or combinations of methods. Hypothetically, a TC child would use speech alone with hearing people in a store or restaurant, simultaneous speech and sign with a hearing-impaired classmate, or signing alone with a deaf adult. Implied in this definition of TC is the notion that a person would use any method needed and not use what was not needed.

If this interpretation of TC is accepted, the method seems compatible with cochlear implants. A persons would use sign to augment spoken communication when it was needed and not use sign if it were not needed. Over time, however, the definition of TC has become synonymous with simultaneous communication (*i.e.*, the combined use of speech and sign in all situations) (Strong and Charlson, 1987). The insistence on full-time simultaneous communication was a concerned response to what many saw as a bastardization of TC: teachers who spoke and used an occasional sign or teachers who signed silently and used an occasional spoken word. The insistence on simultaneous communication at all times was meant to ensure that the child had full access to ongoing language models at all times, a critically important component of incidental learning capabilities. Cochlear implants have altered the notion of full language access and the need for every TC child to have sign and speech in all situations. Many TC children who successfully use their cochlear implants can communicate orally with complete effectiveness at home or in social settings, but they cannot do so at school because of the heavy informational and linguistic load inherent in academic content material. For such children, signing is a necessary aid to full communication access but not in every situation or with all people.

To make use of the auditory in formation conveyed by a cochlear implant, the child, whether using TC or not, must have considerable auditory practice, experience, and reinforcement for listening. Because of the

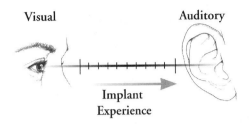

FIG. 13.28. The auditory-visual continuum for language learning. Therapy should be directed at moving each implanted child as far toward the auditory end of the continuum as possible.

heavy emphasis placed on visual learning within a TC program, the TC child typically receives less of this type of practice, experience, and reinforcement than does an OC child (Fig. 13.28).

Recommendations for Total Communication Children with Cochlear Implants

Several recommendations have been offered for TC children with cochlear implants:

1. Begin a frank discussion about these issues with home and school before surgery. The team must determine if there is enough flexibility in these environments to accommodate and reinforce the child's new sensory avenue for learning (*i.e.*, audition).
2. Adopt the philosophy that the child will move along the continuum to become as auditory as is possible for him or her (Fig. 13.29). Many TC children are exclusively visual learners at the time of implantation. How far each child moves depends on many factors. However, clinical experience suggests that a visual learner enrolled in a TC program that does not reinforce real-word consequences for listening and speaking will remain a visual learner despite the cochlear implant.
3. Resolve that adults will provide to the TC child whatever modality is needed to communicate successfully—but only what is needed. As situations arise in which the child is successful orally, as he begins to understand some phrases by listening

alone and as he acquires an intelligible spoken vocabulary, his auditory and oral skills will be respected, and signs will not be used in those situations. Over time, we hope to see the repertoire of such situations expand. During rehabilitation tasks, present information first through listening, provide visual clarifiers, and then finish with auditory information. This creates an "auditory sandwich" (Koch, 1999) for the child (Fig. 13.30).

4. Explain to the child that at different times his teachers and family members may sign to him, may just talk to him, may emphasize lip-reading, or may emphasize listening and that they will help him learn to make use of all this information from the cochlear implant. Avoid conveying any value judgments about modes of communication. Comments such as, "We don't want you to depend on sign language" imply an inferiority of one system over another when it is a positive rather than a negative thing that the child is developing fluency in several different communication modalities.

REHABILITATION FOR THE ADOLESCENT RECEIVING A COCHLEAR IMPLANT

Some unique issues exist regarding adolescents receiving cochlear implants. Assuming the adolescent is prelingually deaf, these issues revolve around making modifications in three specific areas: modifying the counseling techniques used during the selection pro-

Recipe for an Auditory Sandwich

• Present the auditory information first – repeat as many times as is necessary to make an "auditory impression" (The first "slice of bread" in the sandwich.)

• Provide a *visual* clarifier (the contents of the sandwich), such as the object or picture, a sign or Cue.

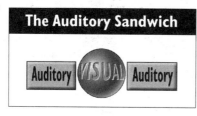

• Finish the sandwich by restating the auditory information.

Utilizing this strategy should become automatic throughout the day. Language within daily routines such as preparing lunch, going out to the grocery store and getting ready for bed should be presented auditorally first. Saying "time to go!" *before* making a move toward the door will be more valuable than saying it, for the first time, at the door.

This "auditory sandwich" technique effectively reduces dependence on signs or lipreading. If the child responds after being given the auditory information- there is little reason to provide the visual support. Thus the child becomes the best indicator of when it is time to drop a sign or Cue.

FIG. 13.29. The auditory sandwich. Using this strategy should become automatic throughout the day. Language within daily routines such as preparing lunch, going to to the grocery store, and getting ready for bed should be presented auditorally first. Saying "time to go!" *before* making a move toward the door is more valuable than saying it, for the first time, at the door. This auditory sandwich technique effectively reduces dependence on signs or lip-reading. If the child responds after being given the auditory information, there is little reason to provide the visual support. In this way, the child becomes the best indicator of when it is time to drop a sign or cue. (From Koch, 1999.)

cess, modifying the expectations for the benefits received from the implant, and modifying rehabilitation activities so they are relevant and motivating to those in this age group.

Modifying Preimplantation Counseling Procedures

When the consideration for cochlear implantation involves an adolescent, it is imperative that he or she be directly involved in the decision-making process. Although parents are recognized as having the authority to make decisions in the best interest of their children, experience teaches that the adolescent's wishes must be considered and respected when determining implant candidacy. Because adolescence is a time when youngsters increasingly assert their independence from their parents, forcing a teenager against her or his wishes to have a cochlear implant or to wear it is difficult at best. That is not to say that every objection made by the adolescent candidate is a valid one, but every objection does deserve an informed response from members of the cochlear implant team.

To be fully part of the counseling process, the adolescent must have access to all the information presented to the family about the cochlear implant. In the case of an adolescent who uses sign language, it is critical that a team member who is a fluent user of sign language interact with the family. In the event that no member of the implant team is fluent enough to communicate fully with the adolescent, an interpreter should be employed during family counseling sessions. It is not advisable for the parents to serve as interpreter for the teenager during these sessions, because they are busy processing a considerable amount of new information. The youth should receive information from an objective source.

Modifying Expectations for Cochlear Implant Benefit

When families consider an implant for an adolescent child, they should be shown data gathered from other users implanted at later ages. Allowing families to see the markedly poorer speech perception results of older-implanted compared with younger-implanted children (Fryauf-Bertschy et al., 1997) may help shape more realistic expectations of benefit. After seeing such results, families may decide against the cochlear implant as an option for their teenager. In either case, the family has made a well-informed decision that is based on fact. Large group studies that include many younger children are an inappropriate comparison group when predicting benefit in adolescents and may cause the family to develop unrealistic expectations for the child implanted at an older age.

Prelingually deaf adolescents who present for cochlear implantation may be appropriate candidates if they meet the following criteria: consistent use of amplification during childhood, a history of good oral and auditory training, communication skills adequate to understand the benefits and limitations of a cochlear implant, willingness to participate in postoperative rehabilitation, and a strong desire to have a cochlear implant. The speech recognition benefits derived by some prelingually deafened children implanted later in childhood, including at early adolescence, have been documented by Osberger et al. (1998) (Fig. 13.30). The subjects in their study showed faster rates of learning and higher levels of speech recognition than they had previously achieved with hearing aids. An important finding, however, was that subjects who used OC achieved significantly higher scores on four of the five outcome measures compared with subjects who used TC. The TC subjects, as a group, were deafer than the oral subjects. However, even controlling for preimplantation hearing levels, the investigators concluded that older, prelingually deafened children who use OC have the potential to derive significant benefit from current cochlear implant technology. Implant benefit is more limited, however, in children with a long duration of deafness who use TC.

Modifying Rehabilitation for the Adolescent

The focus of rehabilitation for an adolescent shifts considerably from that applied to younger children. Above all, rehabilitation activities must be meaningful and motivating for the adolescent's age and interest level. Books and therapy materials designed for young children are boring and even insulting to a teenager. One guideline is to use as

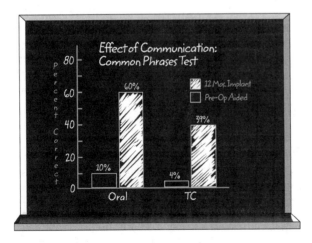

FIG. 13.30. Children implanted with CLARION after the age of 5 years in oral communication (OC; $n = 26$) and total communication (TC; $n = 13$) programs demonstrated increased benefit in open-set sentence recognition compared with preoperative performance with hearing aids ($\bar{x}$ pure tone average: OC = 107 dB; TC = 111 dB). Postoperatively, Clarion children who use OC outperform children who use TC, despite similar age at implantation (OC = 8.9 years; TC = 9.9 years).

therapy materials stimuli that are part of the teenager's life. Motivating stimuli may include rap or rock music, video games, or useful environmental sounds such as recognizing the microwave timer. A teenager fascinated with cars may be motivated to learn to discriminate the sound of a well-tuned engine from an engine that runs roughly. Improved competence with the telephone is a goal of virtually every teenager with a cochlear implant. A telephone training course, such as Castle's (1984), can promote telephone proficiency, even in implant users who have limited or no open-set speech recognition ability, by teaching the patient to use a verbal code.

Speech therapy with adolescent implant users tends to be directed more at improving the intelligibility of specific words, phrases, and sentences that are functionally important to the adolescent, rather than training the entire phonetic inventory. Likewise, a good portion of therapy time may be spent on improving social language skills, conversational pragmatics, and even social etiquette. Many aspects of politeness and deference are conveyed through changes in the suprasegmental patterns of a spoken message. Adolescents who have not had access to such cues are unaware of the subtle shadings in meaning inherent in these cues. This often leads to poor socialization with hearing peers and teachers. Improving these social language skills has been reported by adolescent implant users as one of the most beneficial aspects of receiving the device.

Academic content material is an excellent source of postimplantation rehabilitation stimuli for teenagers. Many of these students are struggling to maintain an adequate academic standing. When rehabilitation focuses on listening or speaking skills and uses the vocabulary and concepts contained in current assignments, the clinician "kills two birds with one stone." The teenager's compliance also increases as a result of the combined motivations, such as to improve listening skills and get a better grade in social studies, for attending therapy.

The adolescent implant user is expected to take on a greater sense of personal responsibility in his or her approach to rehabilitation. Contracts that spell out specific commitments to therapy homework, follow-through, or attendance may be effective when set up between clinician and adolescent. This is often more successfully done without direct parental involvement because there may be an ongoing power struggle between parent and child at this age.

Nevins and Chute (1996) outline practical therapy lessons for the adolescent implant user in the auditory, speech, and speechreading domains. Tye-Murray's (1997) curriculum for older teenagers also offers helpful suggestions.

REHABILITATION FOR THE ADULT IMPLANT USER

As with children, we deal separately with the rehabilitation issues pertaining to prelingually and postlingually deaf adults. These groups present very different pictures clinically.

Postlingually Deaf Adults

Most adults receiving cochlear implants experienced postlingual onset of profound deafness. Edgerton (1985) outlined several factors that determine the degree to which postlingually deaf adults benefited from single-channel cochlear implants, and these factors remain relevant today with multichannel patients: amount of open-set speech understanding obtained through the implant, auditory and spoken language competence before receiving the cochlear implant, personality and motivation, preimplantation patient expectations, social-vocational history and status, visual processing capabilities, family attitudes, general health, the presence of other mental or physical disabilities in addition to deafness, suitability of specific rehabilitation approaches, and the degree of professionalism and completeness with which approaches are implemented. Many of these factors are beyond the clinician's control, but the choice of rehabilitation approaches and the way these approaches are implemented have a decisive impact on the patient's success with the device.

The goals for rehabilitation with postlingually deaf adults are to optimize the communication benefits received from the cochlear implant and to improve the communication relationships adversely affected by deafness. The rehabilitation process in postlingual adults typically is made up of two types of activities, *auditory training* and *communication strategy procedures.* Most adult patients require a rehabilitation program that consists of a mixture of these activities, although the proportion of time spent in each one varies greatly across patients.

Auditory training procedures consist of "guided listening" tasks or special listening practice to improve auditory perceptual skills (Erber, 1993). These procedures fit in the hierarchy of listening behaviors mentioned earlier in this chapter, beginning with detection and progressing through open-set speech understanding. Auditory training procedures may address *analytic listening skills,* with which the patient listens for fine differences between sounds, or *synthetic listening skills,* with which the patient interprets for the gestalt of a message.

Communication strategy procedures address issues related to conversational technique, repair strategies, assertiveness training, interpersonal skills, and coping mechanisms. They focus on how the patient "puts it all together" when communicating with others. During these procedures, the therapist and patient consider the effects of typical situations, environments, topics, and conversational goals on the fluency of communication. Communication strategies are developed to help adults overcome many of the complex conversational difficulties that result from an acquired hearing loss. Attention is drawn to the speech and language habits of frequent communication partners. Building on the strong language foundation of postlingual patients, the adult implant user may climb the ladder back to successful com-

munication with the help of clinicians and family members (Fig. 13.31).

Clinical judgment is used to determine the proportion of time a patient spends on auditory training and communication strategies during postimplantation rehabilitation. Because of advances in speech processing technology, many postlingually deaf adults enjoy very high levels of open-set speech understanding within a short time after initial stimulation. These adults may be able to use the telephone with little difficulty and understand conversation without lip-reading. Other adult patients may receive less speech understanding and require more analytic training to develop these skills. Experience suggests that patients with the following characteristics may need more rehabilitation time spent on auditory training: those who were deaf for many years before implantation, those with reduced open-set speech understanding, and those requiring longer periods to adjust to the new speech code conveyed by their device.

Rehabilitation Resources for Postlingually Deaf Adults

Most adult patients can benefit from keeping a daily listening journal. Patients are asked to make entries in the journal describing what they hear with their implant, recording memorable experiences related to their newfound listening skills, any problems and solutions they experience with their equipment, and communication interactions that take place with others. For example, a patient with 1 month of implant experience may write about an incident at a shoe store when he could not understand the clerk. The goals for making entries in the journal are to record what occurred and adopt a problem-solving perspective to assess what could be done the next time to improve the situation. Initially, most patients do much recording and little problem solving because the many new auditory experiences and sensations take center stage. As time goes on, the patient increases the amount of problem solv-

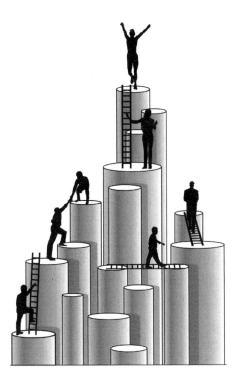

FIG. 13.31. Building on the strong language foundation of postlingual patients, the adult implant user may climb the ladder back to successful communication with the help of clinicians and family members.

ing that takes place on paper. In the case of the shoe salesman, such solutions may include an entry such as "The next time that happens, I need to be more direct about my hearing loss and tell the clerk up front that I'm having trouble understanding him. If need be, I may request a salesperson I can understand better."

In the first days and weeks after initial stimulation, patients may be asked to write a journal entry every day, particularly if their skills are changing rapidly. As time passes, the entries are limited to three or four times per week and then left to the patient's discretion. Constructing a written record of any behavior is an effective way to monitor it, because it draws attention to the behavior and heightens internal awareness. This has the effect of examining the behavior more closely. Such heightened perceptual awareness is one of the benefits of keeping a listening journal. Another benefit is that the journal serves as a longitudinal record of the

progress experienced by the patient. This is often helpful during periods when the patient is discouraged about having reached a plateau or is experiencing some other difficulty. The journal can be immensely insightful to others who read it, provided the patient is comfortable sharing it. Clinicians may learn much about what cochlear implants are from a first-person perspective, a view they do not get otherwise. Prospective implant patients and their families have benefitted from reading another implant recipient's journal as a way of preparing for the challenges and rewards that lie ahead.

Learning to Hear Again with a Cochlear Implant (Wayner and Abrahamson, 1998) is an auditory rehabilitation curriculum guide for hearing-impaired adults wearing cochlear implants. Sections of the guide deal with topics of major importance in rehabilitation, such as speechreading, communication strategies (Trychin and Boone, 1987), and coping behaviors. The program is user-friendly for the clinician who may carry out the activities with an individual patient or in small group settings. The researchers state that "deafness cannot be rehabilitated by cochlear implants alone" and emphasize the importance of family involvement. The chances of an implant patient's success are greatly increased when communication partners are involved in rehabilitation. Frank discussion is sometimes required to modify expectations that the cochlear implant can solve all a family's communication difficulties. The guide provides many suggestions for encouraging family members in their communication interactions with a hearing-impared relative. It also contains several excellent self-assessments for cochlear implant users to complete. These evaluate the extent of difficulty imposed by the hearing loss from the patient's own viewpoint.

One self-assessment scale in the guide is the "Communication Performance Assessment." It contains statements that are scored by the patient on a 5-point scale of from 1 (never) to 5 (always). Sample questions from the scale include: "Listening to conversation requires a lot of concentration and effort for me"; "I have difficulty understanding if I cannot see the speaker's face"; "I don't hear important sounds around me like a doorbell or the phone"; "I feel self-conscious when asking others to repeat what they've said." Results from this and other scales in the guide may help chart progress over time and provide an assessment of the patient's functioning in real-world situations.

The investigators also spend considerable time focusing on coping strategies for the implanted patient. They characterize coping as involving a positive, problem-solving attitude, not being synonymous with mastery, requiring effort that may or may not succeed, and involving learning from difficult situations. Coping mechanisms are divided into those that are emotion focused (*i.e.*, designed to make a person feel better), such as thoughts, realistic expectations, or avoidance behaviors, and those that are problem focused and designed to solve the difficulty.

Among the latter, training is suggested for anticipatory strategies (*e.g.*, plan questions to ask, anticipate environmental problems such as excessive background noise, decide how to narrow and specify questions beforehand) and for repair strategies that are used after conversational breakdown occurs (rephrase, ask for repetition of a specific word or phrase, write a brief message). The guide provides practical suggestions for clinicians to focus on these behaviors with clients in one-on-one or small-group sessions.

A second helpful resource for postlingually deaf adults is *Communication and Adult Hearing Loss* (Erber, 1993), a guide to improving conversational interaction skills. This book offers a self-help approach to communication training, providing suggestions and information directly to the adult with a hearing loss. This helpful guide is not written specifically for patients wearing a cochlear implant, but it is highly appropriate for such individuals, many of whom have experienced longstanding hearing loss and have developed counterproductive conversational behaviors.

Erber's suggestions for improving conversational skills are based on the shared assumptions of people who enter into conversations: conversation is not a monologue; people change conversational roles as necessary according to the circumstances; people expect differences of opinion to be negotiated; communicators do not expect tedious precision in a spoken message; and communicators expect you to be sensitive to their overt verbal or subtle nonverbal expressions of puzzlement when they do not understand. These assumptions are frequently violated by persons with hearing loss, including those who have received cochlear implants. Much of Erber's text is directed at suggestions for practicing appropriate conversational conventions. Families of adult cochlear implant users will also find this book to be of value.

The Prelingual Adult

Many prelingually deafened adults (those deafened before the development of speech and language skills) are not candidates for a cochlear implant, primarily because of the long duration of deafness and resulting atrophy of neural elements. Deaf adults whose communication is based exclusively on sign language have not been shown to use a cochlear implant effectively, because their world is organized almost entirely without sound. Most of these adults are members of the Deaf culture, a culture rich in tradition and unified through American sign language (ASL). ASL is not a manual translation of English but a unique language with its own syntax, morphology, and vocabulary. Because ASL has no written or spoken correlate, it cannot be used simultaneously with spoken English.

Some prelingually deaf adults are good candidates for cochlear implantation and have been shown to use the device effectively. These adults typically have a history of consistent hearing aid use, providing stimulation to the auditory nerve, received auditory and speech training in childhood, and have good oral language proficiency.

Tye-Murray (1997) wrote a communication training program that is highly appropriate for prelingually deaf adults. *Communication Training for Older Teenagers and Adults: Listening, Speechreading, and Using Conversational Strategies* contains many lessons for analytic listening and global conversational skills. The extensive speechreading component of this program also suits the rehabilitation needs of many prelingually deaf adults.

As with any subgroup of patients, candidacy for cochlear implantation of prelingually deaf adults must always be made on an individual basis. An implant team's experience with similar patients may bias them when judging new candidates, but each patient presents with a unique situation that merits consideration by the implant center staff. Compelling reports in the literature (Golan, 1997) document the fact that even some adults with very long-standing deafness have benefited greatly from receiving a cochlear implant. Each candidate deserves to

be evaluated on his or her own merit. Group performance data reveal how statistically likely or unlikely it is that a potential candidate will perform well on test measures but can never predict perfectly what quality of life benefits an individual may enjoy from the cochlear implant.

REFERENCES

Bess F, McConnell F. *Audiology, education and the hearing-impaired child.* St. Louis: CV Mosby, 1981.
Bollard PM, Chute PM, Popp A, Parisier SC. Specific language growth in young children using the CLARION cochlear implant. *Ann Otol Rhinol Laryngol Suppl* 1999 177:119–23.
Boothroyd A. Auditory perception of speech contrasts by subjects with sensorineural hearing loss. *J Speech Hear Res* 1984;27:134–144.
Boothroyd A. Residual hearing and the problem of carry-over in the speech of the deaf. *American Speech-Language-Hearing Association (ASHA) Rep* 1985;15:8–14.
Boothroyd A, Eran O. Auditory speech perception capacity of child implant users expressed as equivalent hearing loss. *Volta Rev* 1994;96:151–168.
Boothroyd A, Geers A, Moog J. Practical implications of cochlear implants in children. *Ear Hear* 1991; 12:81S–89S.
Boothroyd-Turner D, Boothroyd A. Characteristics and attainment of congenitally deaf children with cochlear implants. Paper presented at the Alexander Graham Bell International Convention; Little Rock, AR, June 30, 1998.
Brackett D, Zara C. Communication outcomes related to early implantation. *Otolaryngol Head Neck Surg (in press).*
Calvert D, Silverman R. Speech and deafness. Washington, DC: AG Bell, 1983.
Castle D. *Telephone training course.* Rochester, NY: National Technical Institute for the Deaf (NTID), 1994.
Dawson PW, Blamey PJ, Dettman SJ, Barker EJ, Clark GM. A clinical report on receptive vocabulary skills in cochlear implant users. *Ear Hear* 1995;13:288–294.
Elbert M, Dinnsen DA, Powell TW. On the prediction of phonologic generalization learning patterns. *J Speech Hear Disord* 1984;49:309–317.
Edgerton B. Rehabilitation and training of postlingually deaf adult cochlear implant patients. *Semin Hear* 1985;6:65–88.
Erber N. *Auditory training.* Washington, DC: AG Bell Publications, 1982.
Erber N. *Communication and adult hearing loss.* Abbotsford, Australia: Clavis Publishing, 1993.
Estabrooks W. *Auditory-verbal therapy for parents and professionals.* Washington, DC: AG Bell, 1994.
Firszt J, Reeder R. *GOALS: guidelines for optimizing auditory learning skills.* Washington, DC: AG Bell, 1996.

Flexer C. *Facilitating hearing and listening in young children.* San Diego: Singular Publishing, 1994.

Fryauf-Bertschy H, Tyler RS, Kelsay DM, Gantz BJ, Woodworth GG. Cochlear implant use by prelingually deafened children: the influences of age at implant and length of device use. *J Speech Hear Res* 1997;40:183–199.

Gantz B, Tyler R, Woodworth G, Tye-Murray N, Fryauf-Bertschy H. Results of multichannel cochlear implants in congenital and acquired prelingual deafness in children: five-year follow up. *Am J Otol* 1994;15:1–8.

Geers A, Moog J. Spoken language results: vocabulary, syntax, and communication. *Volta Rev* 1994;96:131–148.

Golan L. Going against the odds: getting a cochlear implant after 55 years of total deafness. *Volta Voices* 1997;4:29–32.

Harrington JD. The integration of deaf children and youth through educational strategies: highlights. *Q Bull NY League Hard Hear* 1974;53:6–8.

Head J. Skills + knowledge + x-factors = effective speech teaching. In: Hochberg I, Levitt H, Osberger MJ, eds. *Speech of the hearing impaired.* Baltimore: University Park Press, 1983.

Hodson BW, Paden EP. Targeting intelligible speech, 2nd ed. Austin, TX: Pro-Ed, 1991.

Jackendoff R. *Patterns in the mind: language and human nature.* New York: Basic Books, 1994:53–56.

Kiernan, Zentz. *Contrastive word pairs.* Baltimore: KZ Associates, 1990.

Laughton J, Hasentab M. *The language learning process: implications for management of disorders.* Rockville, MD: Aspen, 1986.

Lindamood P, Lindamood P. *Lindamood phoneme sequencing for reading, spelling and speech (LiPS).* San Luis Obispo: Gander Educational Publishing, 1997.

Ling D. Speech and the hearing-impaired child. Washington, DC: AG Bell, 1976.

Ling D. Foundations of spoken language for hearing-impaired children. Washington, DC: AG Bell, 1989.

Kretschmer R, Kretschmer L. Discourse and hearing impairment. In: Ripich D, Creaghead N, eds. *School discourse problems.* San Diego: Singular Publishing, 1994:263–296.

Koch M. *Bringing sound to life.* Baltimore: York Publishing, 1999.

Moog J, Biedenstein J, and Davidson L. *Speech perception instructional curriculum and evaluation (SPICE).* St. Louis: Central Institute for the Deaf, 1995.

Nevins ME, Chute PM. *Children with cochlear implants in educational settings.* San Diego: Singular Press, 1996.

Northcott W. *Curriculum guide—hearing-impaired children 0 to 3 years and their parents.* Washington, DC: AG Bell, 1978.

Osberger MJ, Moeller MP, Eccarius M, McConkey A, Johnson D. Expressive language skills. In: Osberger MJ, ed. *Language and learning skills of hearing-impaired students.* ASHA monograph no 23. 1981:54–65.

Osberger MJ, Robbins AM, Todd SL, Riley AI. Speech intelligibility of children with cochlear implants. *Volta Rev* 1994;96:169–180.

Osberger MJ, Robbins AJ, Todd SL, Riley A, Kirk KI,

Carney AE. Cochlear Implants and tactile aids for children with profound hearing impairment. In: Bess F, Gravel J, Tharpe AM, eds. *Amplification for children with auditory deficits.* Nashville: Bill Wilkerson Press, 1996.

Osberger MJ, Fisher L, Phillips SZ, Geier L, Barker MJ. Speech recognition performance of older children with cochlear implants. *Am J Otol* 1998;19:152–157.

Pollack D. *Educational audiology for the limited-hearing infant and preschooler.* Springfield, IL: Charles C Thomas, 1997.

Power DJ, Quigley SP. Deaf children's acquisition of the passive voice. *J Speech Hear Res* 1973;16:5–11.

Reynell JK, Gruber CP. *Reynell developmental language scales.* Los Angeles: Western Psychological Services, 1990.

Robbins AM. A critical evaluation of rehabilitation techniques. Presented at the 5th Symposium on Cochlear Implants in Children; New York, NY, 1994a.

Robbins AM. Guidelines for developing oral communication skills in children with cochlear implants. *Volta Rev* 1994b;96:75–82.

Robbins AM. Language Development. In: Waltzman S, Cohen N, eds. *Cochlear implants.* New York: Thieme, 1999.

Robbins AM, Bollard PM, Green J. Language development in children implanted with the CLARION cochlear implant. *Ann Otol Rhinol Laryngol Suppl* 1999;177:113–118.

Robbins AM, Kirk KI. Speech perception assessment and performance in pediatric cochlear implant users. *Semin Hear* 1996;17:353–369.

Robbins AM, Osberger MJ, Miyamoto RT, Kessler KS. Language development in children with cochlear implants. 1995.

Robbins AM, Svirsky MA, Kirk KI. Children with implants can speak, but can they communicate? *Otolaryngol Head Neck Surg* 1997;117:155–160.

Robbins AM, Svirsky MA, Miyamoto RT. Aspects of linguistic development affected by cochlear implants. Presented at the International Symposium on Cochlear Implants; New York, NY, May 1997. (To appear in Waltzman S, Cohen, eds. *Cochlear implants.* New York: Thieme.)

Rudmin F. The why and how of hearing /s/. *Volta Rev* 1983;85:263–269.

Serry TA, Blamey PJ. A 4-year investigation into phonetic inventory development in young cochlear implant users. *J Speech Hear Res* 1999;42:141–154.

Schopmeyer B, Mellon N, Dobaj H, Niparko J. Emergence of expressive vocabulary in children with cochlear implants. In: Waltzman S, eds. *Proceedings of the Vth International Cochlear Implant Conference.* New York: Thieme *(in press).*

Schick B, Moeller MP. What is learnable in manually coded English sign systems? *Appl Psycholing* 1992;13:313–340.

Stout GG, Windle JV. *Developmental approach to successful listening, II.* Englewood, CO: Resource Point, 1992.

Strong CJ, Clark TC, Walden BE. The relationship of hearing-loss severity to demographic, age, treatment, and intervention-effectiveness variables. *Ear Hear* 1994;15:126–137.

Tobey E, Geers A, Brenner C. Speech production

results: speech feature acquisition. *Volta Rev* 1994; 96:109–129.

Trychin S, Boone M. *Communication rules for hard of hearing people: manual.* Bethesda, MD: SHHH Publications, 1987.

Tye-Murray N. *Communication training for older teenagers and adults: listening, speechreading and using conversational strategies.* Washington, DC: AG Bell, 1997.

Tye-Murray N, Spencer L, Woodworth GG. Acquisition of speech by children who have prolonged cochlear implant experience. *J Speech Hear Res* 1995;38: 327–337.

Vergara K, Miskiel L. *The Miami cochlear implant auditory and tactile skills curriculum (CHATS).* Miami, FL: Intelligent Hearing Systems, 1994.

Waltzman S, Cohen N, Shapiro W. Use of a multichannel cochlear implant in the congenitally and prelingually deaf population. *Laryngoscope* 1992; 102:395–399.

Waltzman SB, Cohen NL, Gomolin RH, Shapiro WH, Ozdamar SR, Hoffman RA. Long-term results of early cochlear implantation in congenitally and prelingually deafened children. *Am J Otol* 1994;15 [Suppl]:9–13.

Wayner D, Abrahamson J. *Learning to hear again with a cochlear implant.* Austin: Hear Again, 1988.

Wray D, Flexer C, Saunders . Classroom performance of children who are deaf and hard of hearing learning spoken communication using an auditory-verbal approach. *Volta Rev (in press).*

Young EC. *Language approach to open syllables.* Tucson: Communication Skill Builders, 1981.

Appendix 13A

Rehabilitation for the Hearing Impaired:
A Historical Perspective

Mark Ross

Clinical models of cochlear implant rehabilitation are reminiscent of past efforts to improve on the communication benefits provided by hearing aids. Aural rehabilitation (AR) for the hearing-impaired is not a new topic or concern on the clinical scene. In the United States, the first formal AR organization, the New York League for the Hard of Hearing, was established more than 85 years ago as a self-help effort by several hard of hearing individuals. The self-help aspects were soon augmented by a paid professional staff. Before World War II, several Leagues for the Hard of Hearing were organized around the country. Soon after World War II, these groups banded together as the American Hearing Society. A number of centers still exist with origins from this period.

The major AR procedure initially offered at the time was lip-reading, later called *speechreading* to reflect a focus on the total

communicative setting rather than just the lip movements. Facial expressions, the experiential situation, linguistic and contextual cues, and the use of residual hearing are all subsumed under the concept of speechreading. Prosthetic devices (mostly hearing aids), although primitive by today's standards, offered some assistance to a limited group of people with hearing loss. Speechreading classes, in addition to their own intrinsic contribution, became a kind of camouflaged medium through which the social and self-help aspects of the program could be provided. Attending lip-reading "classes" was deemed acceptable; implying that a person needed some kind of "therapy" (AR) was not.

AR gained impetus during World War II. Many young men sustained hearing losses as a result of noise exposure, and it was the responsibility of U.S. government to rehabilitate them. The armed services organized hearing testing and AR programs for their active-duty personnel, calling on the talents of professionals from various fields, mainly

M. Ross: Professor Emeritus, The University of Connecticut, Storrs, Connecticut 06268.

specialists in speech correction or remediation (the later terminology was *speech-language pathology*), educators of the deaf, psychologists, otolaryngologists, and electronic engineers. Later, as these young men were discharged from the service, the responsibility for providing AR was shared by the Veterans Administration.

From the beginning, a dual emphasis could be seen in the activities of those who concentrated on the nonmedical management of hearing loss. On one track, the focus was placed on diagnostic tests for hearing. This included the creation of new diagnostic devices and procedures, including those for selecting specific hearing aids (which soon profited by major advances in electroacoustics). For many years, this track constituted the bulk of research efforts by the newly emerging audiologic profession, with data-based research publications the primary avenue for professional advancement.

AR constituted a second track. The major emphasis was on lip-reading classes, supplemented by "auditory training" lessons designed to help patients benefit from the novel auditory sensations they received; this followed rather crude efforts at "selective amplification" (*i.e.*, attempting to determine the most appropriate amplification pattern for people with different degrees and types of hearing losses). Instruction in lip-reading usually began with an explanation of the lip movements necessary to articulate the various classes of "sounds." Clients were instructed in concepts such as homopheneous sounds (*i.e.*, those that look alike on the lips), the necessity for lip focus, and modifications due to sound blending. Later, the analytic focus gave way to a more synthetic approach, in which difficulty-graded lip-reading lessons were administered under various listening conditions (*i.e.*, with and without voice and background noises and linguistic or contextual clues). The psychosocial impact of the hearing loss, hearing tactics, and other coping strategies were not included as formal material. However, because the AR programs lasted 1 to 3 months and servicemen

were quartered in the same barracks, many informal interactions naturally occurred that, in retrospect, may have been the most valuable aspect of the entire program.

After World War II, many of the personnel who provided clinical services in Army and Navy hospital joined academia (where many also completed their doctorates), primarily in departments of speech, and began to develop an audiologic curriculum based on their clinical activities and perceived future professional needs. As a new profession striving to be recognized as a unique entity, the content emphasized the fundamentals of hearing science, audiometric testing, auditory perception, and differential diagnostic procedures. Soon after audiology entered academia, it became clear that AR was being relegated to a secondary position in the hierarchy of the audiologic profession. Research in AR was and remains notoriously difficult to implement; we still have difficulty relating any component of AR therapy procedure to improvement in communication skills, although we are doing better when it comes to psychosocial self-perception. It was probably more satisfying to conduct research related to the factors and variables (*e.g.*, definable auditory stimuli) that could be precisely controlled and in which the results could unambiguously be related to the stimulus conditions.

The history of AR related to hearing aid use should be remembered when considering the field of cochlear implant rehabilitation. More and more patients will be receiving these devices, and no matter how sophisticated they become, it is unlikely that they will ever produce auditory sensations identical to those occurring in a normal auditory system. Persons using implants will always experience a somewhat novel auditory sensation that they will have to learn to interpret and integrate with speechreading cues.

AR conducted with cochlear implant patients provides the profession of audiology an opportunity to revisit its roots by improving communication abilities through AR therapeutic strategies. Because of advances in materials and training procedures, the previously uncontrolled AR efforts for hearing aid wearers can be improved and applied to implant users. Quantifying the positive impact of AR for cochlear implant patients is a necessity, not just to convince colleagues and clients of its value, but to support lobbying efforts for service-delivery models by which AR can be supported by third parties. AR for cochlear implant users must be seen as an integral and supportable component of the total rehabilitation process.

Appendix 13B

Motor Skills in Childhood Deafness

Betty Schopmeyer

Auditory and visual inputs work together in the normally developing infant to provide information about the environment. Audition informs the individual about location and the physical characteristics of objects (Savelsbergh *et al.*, 1991). The infant's earliest responses to auditory stimuli include visual-motor behavior as he moves his eyes or head to localize sound. The synergy between auditory, visual, and motor development suggests that the lack of early auditory input contributes to motor delays in the deaf.

Studies of motor skills in deaf children report deficits in balance and other motor areas, especially those tasks requiring fast or complex movement execution (Wiegersma and Van Der Velde, 1983; Savelsbergh *et al.*, 1991). Studies of reaction time and speed of movement response in deaf children cite clear differences in both areas between deaf and hearing subjects. Possible explanations of the observed deficits are described by Wiergersma and Van Der Velde (1983) in four categories:

1. *Organic factors.* Vestibular defects, often associated with deafness, have a pervasive influence on motor performance in the areas of balance and in eye-hand and total-body coordination. Neurologic deficits may be associated with the specific cause of an individual's hearing impairment.

2. *Sensory deprivation.* Infants and young children practice movements that produce sound, which helps them achieve motor control. This practice behavior includes vocal play and babbling. In daily life, hearing individuals are able to use the sound effects generated by actions to acquire knowledge of their own performance and to help them automatize target motor behaviors. Sound supplements visual, tactile, and proprioceptive information about spatial orientation, speed, pressure, and sequential movement. Auditory deprivation may impede motor development and adaptive movement learning.

3. *Language (verbal) deprivation.* A hearing child has a firm connection between movement or skill learning and verbal representation of the motor components of the skill. By means of language, internal or external, it is possible to bring about changes in the motor behavior of the child by referencing movement experiences the child has had in the past. The deaf child, who often is seriously deficient in language knowledge, is unable to use this verbal encoding with the same efficacy. In learning any new complex movement, there is a cognitive stage during which

verbal-conceptual strategies support execution. Many people use some form of verbal rehearsal before activities are automatized. The lack of inner language for encoding this self-regulatory rehearsal affects the motor learning of deaf individuals.

4. *Emotional factors.* Parents of deaf children may experience frustration about communication barriers that may lead to overprotection, neglect, or other maladaptive parenting behaviors. The self-concept of the deaf child may be affected, resulting in shyness and low self-confidence. These characteristics may cause the deaf child to be less willing to explore his environment and to enter into novel situations that challenge his motor abilities to progress.

The literature concerning motor development in the deaf implies concomitant effects on speech motor skills. Motor learning for speech production and the development of oral-verbal praxis depend on intact sensory receptor mechanisms and the subsequent integration of acoustic information with visual, proprioceptive, and kinesthetic feedback (Hodge, 1994). *Praxis* may be defined as the smooth, rapid, automatic retrieval and execution of movement patterns (Broesterhuizen, 1997). Young children begin to acquire neural connections between auditory and motor events at a very young age: the period between 3 and 12 months of age may be the most sensitive period for the eventual acquisition of speech motor control in terms of establishing and automatizing the fundamental movement routines for speech (Netsell, 1981; Hodge, 1994). During this period, many deaf children remain undiagnosed. They do not have the auditory-communicative motivation to practice the integration sound with motor skill, limiting their ability to organize appropriate combinations of motor signals that produce desired phonetic targets. It has been suggested that the acoustic patterns of speech contain a code for the motor actions required to generate these patterns, enabling the young child to develop neural connections coding spatial-temporal plans for speech production (Hodge, 1994). Later, when provided with auditory information through cochlear implantation, deaf children struggle with the effects of their limited experience with the phonetic-acoustic and other sensorimotor consequences of vocalizing, including a small repertoire of sound-movement patterns to choose from when trying to produce speech. There is also some evidence that children experiencing delays in speech-motor skills learn word-specific motor programs that cannot be separated into component parts (*i.e.,* syllables and phonemes) to be reassembled into other programs, limiting their flexibility and exacerbating the gap between chronologic-cognitive age and speech ability.

A child receiving a cochlear implant at a young age is provided with auditory stimulation, but the residual effects of deafness on his motor system for speech may still be operating. Deaf individuals may vary in their innate praxis abilities, thereby accounting for the differences in oral language skills often seen between two deaf people with apparently identical profiles in terms of the commonly cited factors of age, onset, cause, degree, and intervention. Broesterhuizen (1997) describes a prognostic test battery incorporating fine motor, memory for rhythm, and successive memory tasks (eupraxia battery) that accurately predicts success in oral language acquisition when administered to preschool deaf children.

Clinicians working with deaf children intuitively recognize speech-motor difficulties as speech emerges. Given the importance of the integration of visual, auditory, and sensory-motor integration in speech acquisition, it appears that further investigation of motor and particularly speech-motor skills is critical for understanding of speech production in the deaf and in deaf individuals receiving cochlear implants. There are significant implications for modifying intervention programs to include more emphasis on motor skill and sensory-motor integration.

REFERENCES

1. Broesterhuizen MLHM. Psychological assessment of deaf children. *Scand Audiol Suppl* 1997;26[Suppl 46]:43–49.
2. Hodge MM. Assessment of children with developmental apraxia of speech: a rationale. *Clin Commun Disord* 1994;4:91–101.
3. Netsell R. The acquisition of speech motor control: a perspective with directions for research. In: Stark R, ed. *Language behavior in early infancy and childhood.* New York: Elsevier/North Holland, 1981:127–156.
4. Savelsbergh GJP, Netelenbos JB, Whiting HTA. Auditory perception and the control of spatially coordinated action of deaf and hearing children. *J Child Psychol Psychiatry* 1991;32:489–500.
5. Wiegersma PH, Van Der Velde A. Motor development of deaf children. *J Child Psychol Psychiatry* 1983;24:103–111.

Cochlear Implants: Principles & Practices, edited by John K. Niparko, Karen Iler Kirk, Nancy K. Mellon, Amy McConkey Robbins, Debara L. Tucci, and Blake S. Wilson. Lippincott Williams & Wilkins, Philadelphia © 2000.

SECTION VII

Cultural Aspects of Cochlear Implantation

14

Culture and
Cochlear Implants

John K. Niparko

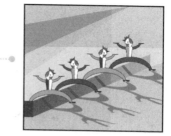

In the long-standing controversy over the best way to raise a deaf child, the cochlear implant is another cultural divide. A contentious and often emotional debate has surrounded the practice of cochlear implantation since its inception. Rival arguments are well recognized in lay publications (Barry, 1991; Dolnick, 1993; Solomon, 1994; Bassis *et al.*, 1980; Arana-Ward, 1997), among advocacy (National Association of the Deaf, 1993; Lane, 1994; World Federation of the Deaf, 1996) and professional organizations (Cohen, 1994; Balkany *et al.*, 1996), and by the legal profession (Brusky, 1995).

A number of concerns arise in discussions of the ethics of cochlear implantation, from the deeply personal to those of society at large. Although discussions of the ethics of cochlear implantation are often broad in their cultural implications, they can have explicit impacts. Objective analysis of specific concerns is a practical matter in candidacy considerations and in sustaining use of a cochlear implant, particularly among those deafened before acquiring language. This chapter examines several themes that underlie discussions of the ethical principles related to cochlear implantation.

In discussions of the ethics of cochlear implantation, a writer's background is key to a reader's understanding of the perspectives offered. By way of disclosure, I am a hearing otolaryngologist with interests in clinical and basic science research related to congenital deafness and to cochlear implants. It has been asserted that such an orientation may prevent a full understanding of cultural arguments against cochlear implantation (Gentry, 1988). Moreover, with regard to religious affiliation, I am not Amish. I have also been told personally that this aspect of my background prevents understanding the opposition to cochlear implantation held by some Amish communities. I defer to such judgments. My intent is to familiarize the reader to prior written work on cultural dynamics and the disparate viewpoints regarding cochlear implantation. Final judgments are left to personal motivations and to the wisest teachers of all, time and experience.

J. K. Niparko: Department of Otolaryngology—Head and Neck Surgery, The Listening Center at Johns Hopkins, The Johns Hopkins University, Baltimore, Maryland 21205-1809.

CULTURAL DYNAMICS

Definitions and Background

Culture is defined as the total way of life of a group of people and provides the defining features of every society (Bassis *et al.*, 1980). A society consists of people who interact within socially structured relationships and share a common culture. Cultural practices as they relate to educational approach, socialization, and parental and cultural authority are themes woven into arguments marshaled for and against cochlear implantation. An understanding of the basic principles that underlie cultural dynamics can provide useful background information in considering cross-cultural conflicts.

A people's culture provides what Kluckhohn (1949) described as a design for living. Such designs endow humans with learning opportunities that are unavailable to other animals. Although animals can learn, their needs are met principally by genetically programmed patterns of instinctual behavior. Instinct enables the early acquisition of behaviors needed for survival. Needed periods of learning are relatively brief, promoting behaviors that are key to survival despite relatively short periods of nurturing.

Human infants, in contrast, are born with only the few reflexes required for respiration, feeding, and simple withdrawal from danger. An overall biologic program for living is lacking. When instilled with cultural teachings, a child begins to assimilate the products of group life that serve as a guide for living.

Human culture is passed from generation to generation and is acquired through learning. Generations pass a slightly modified version of a culture onto the next. No generation begins building a way of life from scratch, and the experience of past generations can serve as a foundation for the next. The legacy is manmade and represents the collective wisdom and motivation of a people's ancestry. It is a social rather than a cultural heredity (Lutton, 1945).

All cultures are composed of material and nonmaterial elements. Material culture refers to the tangible substance that people use to meet their needs. Nonmaterial culture consists in intangible elements that guide a people's outlook and behavior. Because cultures are transmitted from one generation to the next, material and nonmaterial elements are subject to evolutionary pressures from a natural selection of ideas and new developments.

Material elements represent those that often come to mind when thinking of foreign cultures manner of dress, books, music, food, architecture, tools, and transport. Technologic advancement has a strong impact on the material elements of a culture. The effect of this impact is increasingly pervasive in industrialized cultures today.

Technologies are described as systems of knowledge that have practical, material application. The level of technology within a culture is greatly influenced by nonmaterial cultural elements. That is, beliefs, customs, and norms can strongly influence technologic development within a culture. A culture's adoption of technology can influence patterns of interpersonal communication and how a culture relates to its environment. Technology can influence cultures to use environment resources in often dramatically different ways. For example, hunting-gathering, housing, division of labor, transportation, and communication are cultural elements that have been markedly altered throughout history by a culture's embrace of or resistance to technologic advances.

Nonmaterial culture consists in intangible elements that guide a people's outlook and behavior; values, norms, and sanctions are the cultural constructs that serve as guidelines of what is right, desirable, and worthy of respect. The degree to which behaviors are shaped by these guidelines depends on a culture's level of emotional commitment. Some norms are sacred and violations of them unconscionable.

Language is a unique element within the framework of material and nonmaterial cultural elements. Language makes it possible to acquire, sustain, or modify cultural designs for living. The nonmaterial elements that reflect the meaning that people attach to actions can be expressed effectively only through language. The ability to transmit insight learning is crucial to the cohesion of society. Language serves as the vehicle through which this information is transmitted.

Language also exerts a pervasive effect on perspective, as examined brilliantly by Sapir (1921) and Whorf (1956). The Sapir-Whorf hypothesis holds that the language of a people channels their thoughts and perceptions. Different languages channel disparate patterns of thinking into stereotypical patterns and can influence the way the world is viewed.

A corollary of the Sapir-Whorf hypothesis is that unless a culture has a word or expression for something within the repertoire of their language, they cannot conceive of it. An often quoted example of this relates to the Eskimo concept of snow. Although white flakes that fall from the sky in winter are encompassed in a single word in simple English, the Eskimo vocabulary characterizes snow in more than 20 different words that represent different forms of snow. The expanded linguistic repertoire enhances perception of subtle variation in snow's texture, weight, saturation, and dispersal—attributes not perceived routinely in a selective way by non-Eskimos.

The Study of Cultural Differences

Judgments offered as part of the cochlear implant controversy tend to have an either/or quality. Attributes of the practice of implantation tend to be classified as right or wrong, good or bad, success or failure. This approach often leads to absolute positions. Accepting one principle leads to rejecting the opposite. Arguments that involve values shaped by our cultural prospective, however, are filled with complexity and intricacy.

The study of differences in judgments that reflect cultural background represents an important dimension of anthropologic study.

Cultural differences are common between foreign lands but are also experienced by members of subcultures within larger societies. When immersed in an unfamiliar cultural setting, cultural differences often yield a sense of disorientation and stress known as cultural shock. Cultural shock occurs because we have learned to live much of our daily life according to cultural patterns that are established early in life, and often so thoroughly that they become habit. Symptoms of cultural shock also include feelings of incompetence and isolation. Familiar behavioral cues are absent and replaced by patterns that can seem to be baseless. Everyday life can become unpredictable.

Ethnocentrism is the tendency to evaluate other cultures in terms of one's own. Ethnocentric judgments often yield the conclusion that an unfamiliar culture is inferior. The origin of ethnocentric viewpoints is a lack of familiarity with material and nonmaterial elements of a culture. The lack of access to a culture's language could be expected to motivate an ethnocentric viewpoint.

Cultural relativism offers an alternative approach to studying cultural contrasts. Cultural relativism stems from the view that cultural beliefs and practices must be understood within the context of that culture's setting and on its own terms. If we are to understand a culture from a relative viewpoint, its merits must be judged with sensitivity to its native values and norms.

CULTURAL VIEWS OF DEAFNESS

Cultural dynamics are highly evident in ethical discussions of cochlear implantation. Cultural dynamics of culture transfer, technology, and most notably language are relevant to these views. The cultural minority composed of users of American sign language (ASL) is commonly referred to as the Deaf culture or Deaf World. The upper case D is significant and is used to succinctly express identity with a shared culture, rather than individuals grouped by a medical condition.

A well-publicized reaction to cochlear implantation occurred when Deaf culture advocates reacted to a story aired on the CBS news magazine "60 Minutes" in the fall of 1992. Reporter Tom Bradley commented that he had never been more captivated than by the story's featured implant recipient. This 7-year-old girl with postmeningitic deafness demonstrated scholastic success, music ability, and impressive receptive and productive speech skills.

In response, Deaf activists offered scathing editorial comment that later aired on the program. It was stated that the piece reflected child abuse and genocide. Such views have been amplified in published commentary (Lane, 1993; Dolnick, 1993; National Association of the Deaf, 1993; Lane and Bahan, 1998). In a reprise of this documentary with an update in 1999, Mr. Bradley observed that the positions held by the National Association of the Deaf toward implantation were under reconsideration.

A shared language, it is held, makes for a shared identity (Dolnick, 1993). Cultural linguists recognize that signed languages are full-fledged natural languages (Lane and Bahan, 1998). These languages exert a broad impact on those who are fluent users. Distinct patterns of social organization are observed within communities that employ signed languages, and there are aspects of membership in Deaf communities that are unique and unfamiliar to hearing individuals.

To understand this concept better, deafness should be distinguished from intermediate levels of hearing loss (Dolnick, 1993). Whereas most members of hearing society are familiar with hearing limitations under challenging listening conditions, deafness extends beyond limited speech recognition. Deafness, particularly when early in onset, confers a life experience that is radically different because of a systematically different language base not shared by the majority hearing culture. Even incidental communications can be restricted to others who sign. Most early-deafened children are born to hearing parents and do not share a basic mode of communication with their parents.

Deaf children who employ ASL typically acquire a sense of cultural identity primarily through visual language and primarily through peers rather than their parents.

Although it has been observed that ASL represents a highly expressive language with grammatical complexity, ASL presents communicative limitations (Dolnick, 1993). ASL does not exist in written form, and in literate societies, written words serve to increase vastly the efficiency with which culture in transmitted. This is not to suggest that people who do not write cannot transmit their culture from one generation to the next, but writing is an enormous asset and a necessity in complex, advanced cultures (DeBlij, 1982). It may be possible to create poetry in ASL, but such works cannot be disseminated with the facility provided by the written word. Although digital technology may impact on this aspect of ASL, functional illiteracy often observed in educational settings that employ ASL (Holt, 1993) constrains access to important conduits of information provided by writing.

Differences in cultural values between users of ASL and speakers of English appear to lie at the heart of controversies of cochlear implantation. Lane and Bahan (1998) assert that Deaf values lead to a very different assessment of pediatric cochlear implant surgery from that held by most within the mainstream (hearing) culture. Arguments against cochlear implantation center largely on congenitally deaf children as candidates and often concern the impact of the device on these children as implant recipients and the impact of the device on Deaf culture. These concerns are examined here.

Failure of Cochlear Implants to Foster Language Acquisition in Children Born Deaf

Lane (1993) and Lane and Bahan (1998) assert that, although the literature on cochlear implantation is poorly established, the literature that is available reflects poor performance in several domains. These investigators have assembled data sets from reports in children deafened before the age of 3 years who received cochlear implants. Tests of open-set speech recognition are isolated for analysis because they are held by these researchers as the tests of speech perception that are most generalizable to everyday communication, and these data suggest the following:

- Mean scores overstate speech perception capabilities.
- Children born deaf score zero or close to zero.
- The few subjects revealing exceptionally high speech perception scores are without proper controls, because these children may derive more benefit from circumstances surrounding implantation (*e.g.* rehabilitation) than from the implant itself.

Based on this analysis, Lane and Bahan assert that cochlear implants are of unproven benefit and innovative and therefore ethically problematic when applied to children. The investigators extend their inferences to explain patterns of nonuse of cochlear implants. Children from schools for the deaf who are nonusers are often those who incurred their deafness before the age of 3 years and demonstrate poor levels of speech recognition (Rose *et al.*, 1996).

There are, however, several aspects of Lane's and Bahan's (1998) interpretation of the implant literature that should be examined to permit a fuller understanding of the impact of implants on young children. The previous analysis evaluates only early published results, examines only the most stringent of auditory-only testing conditions, reviews studies in cohorts of children with an average age of implantation that exceeded five years of age (far higher than current practices), and reviews limited periods of cochlear implant use (a weighted average of approximately 2.5 years).

Their interpretation also deemphasizes a critical influence on performance levels with a cochlear implant: duration of use. The Lane and Bahan (1998) data sets support prior

findings (Miyamoto *et al.*, 1994) that open-set word recognition improves with longer implant experience. Scores on tests of open-set word recognition were substantially greater when the mean length of use of the device exceeded 3 years. Granted, myriad variables also influence results with in any one child, but longer duration of use correlates the most strongly with improved scores of speech reception.

Lane and Bahan (1998) conclude that not a single case has been reported of a child acquiring language because of an implant. This assertion is not sustainable in view of more recently published data. Robbins *et al.* (1998) documented accelerated acquisition of receptive and expressive language in implanted children with more than 3 years of implant experience. Similarly, enhanced spontaneous use of language (Schopmeyer, 1999) and development of prelinguistic behaviors (Tait and Lutman, 1994) have been reported in congenitally deaf children with implants.

As a corollary, Lane (1993) and Lane and Bahan (1998) take issue with prior reports (California Department of Vocational Rehabilitation), indicating that deaf individuals demonstrate severe vocational limitations. The investigators assert that there is no evidence that implanted children will have a better outcome. Later reports suggest that implanted children evidence scholastic gains, documenting greater movement toward educationally independent settings relative to age-matched aided children with similar levels of baseline hearing (Francis *et al.*, 1999). Although observational tracking incorporates a range of incompletely controlled variables, the assertion that no documented scholastic gains exist for implanted children is inaccurate.

Cochlear Implantation and Conflict in Cross-cultural Values

Opinions from the National Association of the Deaf (1993) and the World Federation of the Deaf (1996) are well-recognized examples of Deaf cultural expression of values relevant to cochlear implantation. For Deaf individuals who rely on visual language for communication, primary reliance on vision is held as a nonmaterial cultural variant and not an impairment. The Deaf culture perspective offers that deafness is not a disease that fits within an infirmity model and renders meaningless the notion that treatment is needed. Children who are merely Deaf are perfectly healthy, and it is unethical to operate on healthy children (Lane and Bahan, 1998). Because hearing culture views hearing loss as an impairment, parents and doctors feel an ethical obligation to alleviate that impairment. The inability of the Deaf culture to embrace this position is characterized as a cross-culture conflict of values. Lane and Bahan (1998) hold that this conflict is without a resolution that is morally valid.

The ethical dilemma that arises from these opposing positions is indicative of an argument mired in ethnocentric perspectives. The dilemma is rooted in discrepancies of basic values. One approach to the dilemma is to attempt to define the factors that are critical in ascribing cultural membership.

The position that early-onset deafness is critical to cultural assignment isolates deafness as the sole human characteristic that should dictate cultural identification when a child is unfortunately born deaf. This position ignores other physical characteristics that are usually intact, including those within the hearing pathway. The neural tracts and synaptic stations of the central auditory pathway are formed, often remarkably intact, and reveal connectional integrity even in congenitally profoundly deaf individuals. Growth and development of the neural tracts and organs that enable voicing and articulation and the behaviors for oral language competence are ignored by mandating visual language for the congenitally deaf. The notion that hair cell degeneration should be the sole phenotypic manifestation of the parentally derived genetic blueprint (the human genotype consists of more than 80,000 genes) to dictate cultural assignment seems arbitrary,

particularly in view of the option of providing physiologically similar inputs to these systems through cochlear implantation.

Lane and Bahan (1998) argue that, if implant teams maintain as their sole responsibility their perceived health of a child patient (as from a hearing society perspective) and if most hearing parents select to pursue implantation for their deaf children, it would be virtually impossible to ensure survival of Deaf culture without subjugating parental authority to a lesser priority. These investigators assert that the development and provision of cochlear implantation undermines survival of the Deaf culture, an outcome that is disquieting to the Deaf World.

Lane and Bahan (1998) provide support for the notion that society has an interest in preserving minority cultures and offer an analogy related to American Indian culture. They cite congressional enactment of the Indian Child Welfare Act of 1978 as evidence. The act was designed to limit transracial adoption of children out of American Indian cultures. The enactment states that "it is the policy of this nation to protect the best interests of Indian children and to promote the stability and security of Indian tribes." Supreme Court decisions have similarly ruled that Native-American tribal interests and the best interests of the child should be considered in cases of potential transracial adoption.

An alternate interpretation of these enactments, however, can lead lead to a different conclusion. Limiting transracial adoption in effect promotes acculturation according to parental origins.

Another point of departure from this analogy relates to forced choice. Implanting deaf children of deaf parents is rarely sought or offered. Even attempts to pressure hearing parents with deaf children into implantation is fraught with troublesome clinical and legal implications. Although Lane and Bahan (1998) admit that surgical programs that implant deaf children do not ostensibly have as their intent the destruction of Deaf culture, they posit that "a general intent to commit genocide can be established, in the absence of a specific intent, from proof of reasonable foreseeability."

PARENTAL AUTHORITY

One of the most compelling lines of discussion relevant to controversies surrounding cochlear implantation is related to parental authority. Deaf activists argue that hearing people, solely by virtue of not being deaf, are incompetent to make decisions in the best interests of deaf children. Consequently, hearing parents decisions to implant deaf children are often ill-founded and ill-fated (Fleisher, 1993). In America, there is firm legal foundation that establishes parental authority as paramount.

A cogent discussion of the legal findings relevant to implant controversies has been provided in a legal comment by Brusky (1995). She applied legal opinion to explore the issue of whether parents possess the right to decide whether a minor child should receive a cochlear implant. Her comment recognizes conflicting interests among the available decision makers. She observes that hearing parents, solely by virtue of having hearing, may have an inherent conflict of interest with their deaf child's best interests. The Deaf community may offer relevant input into the decision whether to implant a deaf child. However, the comment cites shortcomings of the legal recognition of the deaf community's interests in such a personal, family decision.

Parents, more than any other potential party, should appropriately assume the principal decision-making responsibility about whether to implant their child. Brusky (1995) cites more than 10 U.S. or State Supreme Court decisions that recognize parents fundamental liberty interest in the care, custody, and management of their children, including the right to make medical treatment decisions for minor children. This position stems from combined considerations of legal support of parental autonomy, a child's individual choice, and the human bonds entailed by the parent-child relationship. The right of a parent to choose whether their child should receive an implant is, however, limited when a child is sufficiently mature and capable of giving informed consent.

Beyond precedents that establish support for the primacy of parental authority is the notion that the best interests of a deaf child deserve special consideration. Brusky's Comment (1995) asserts that such decisions are highly subjective. Hearing parents and the Deaf community may disagree about whether a child should receive a cochlear implant, but both undoubtedly have the best interests of the child at heart. Because of the subjective nature of this decision, legal safeguards should be emphasized. The existing legal framework resolves much of the conflict surrounding childhood implantation provided that the decision-making process is reflective, deliberate, and exercised truly with the best interests of the child in mind.

Because hearing parents may lack detailed understanding of cultural alternatives, full disclosure of available information is crucial. Providers of implants have the duty to ensure that all patients or their parents fully comprehend the implant procedure, including its risks and benefits. Similarly, parents should be made aware of the existence of a widely accepted and fulfilling cultural alternative. Implant providers should use a thorough and deliberate process of candidate selection and carefully compare a candidate's potential with expectations. These duties are essential to fully informed consent, a fundamental concept that recognizes a patient's values and preferences. Advocates of Deaf World culture also carry a responsibility to provide accurate information to parents of deaf children.

CONCLUSIONS

Arguments over the role of cochlear implantation can serve a useful purpose in informing decisions by those affected by congenital deafness. The visceral nature of cultural arguments places a bright light of scrutiny on the validity of evidence presented on both sides of the issue. A true argument presents evidence for or against a proposition, and is capable of being objectively tested by means that are agreed on. This requires common ground.

A more fruitful discussion of cochlear implantation can be achieved if both sides of the cultural debate can acknowledge that there is no perfect solution to the language problem that ensues when deaf children are born to hearing parents. Despite a perception that the medical community is pitted against the Deaf World, it is the parents that seek out cochlear implants for their deaf children. Ultimately, the decision to implant a deaf child rests with her or his parents.

Both sides of the cultural divide wish to improve the quality of life of deaf children. Parents have an understandable desire to transmit their cultural heritage to their children through their natural language. With proper support, cochlear implantation can facilitate this process in deaf children of hearing parents. Advocates of Deaf World also believe they have something to offer deaf children, a culture based on shared identity derived by virtue of their deafness. Their desire to embrace deaf children is certainly compelling.

At the root of the cultural debate is language. Selecting a communication mode for a child's first language entails making a cultural choice. Achieving mastery of ASL, or of spoken language through cochlear implantation, prepares a child for membership in very different cultures. Each culture has its strengths and limitations, and each choice therefore entails tradeoffs. Such decisions must be highly individualized and made only after careful consideration of the child's abilities and the available options for education, socialization and support.

Selecting a cochlear implant for a deaf child entails extended commitment by family, teachers, therapists, implant teams, and the child. Immersion in ASL entails similar challenges. Hearing parents are typically unprepared to mentor sign skills in their chil-

dren, and must learn ASL themselves to do so. Because ASL is the language of a minority culture, choosing ASL demarcates boundaries in a child's ability to communicate with mainstream society.

Both sides of this cultural debate share a common challenge. Language delays consequent to late diagnosis may imperil language acquisition in either modality. This issue constitutes fertile ground for collaboration, as each side can surely agree that achieving language competence is an overarching priority for deaf children. Although bilingual education has intuitive appeal, it remains a theoretical rather than a practical option. Deaf children of hearing parents experience difficulty acquiring a first language in spoken language or ASL. The former requires functional hearing, and the latter appropriate models. Both language modalities require early exposure. Given these conditions, acquiring the necessary subskills in two different modalities presents a daunting challenge. The impact of language choice on quality of life must be objectively compared using measures of outcome that have cross-cultural relevance. All interests share in the responsibility of developing such measures.

REFERENCES

Arana-Ward M. As technology advances: a bitter debate divides the deaf. *Washington Post* 1997;May 11:1–3.
Balkany T, Hodges A, Goodman K. Ethics of cochlear implantation in young children. *Otolaryngol Head Neck Surg* 1996;114:748–755.
Barry J. Silence is golden? *Miami Herald* 1991;Sept 22.
Bassis M, Gelles R, Levine A. Culture. In: *Sociology: an introduction.* New York: Random House, 1980:63–93.
Brusky AE. Making decisions for deaf children regarding cochlear implants: the legal ramifications of recognizing deafness as a culture rather than a disability. *Wisc Law Rev* 1995:235–270.
California Vocational Rehabilitation report.
Cohen N. The ethics of cochlear implants in young children. *Am J Otol* 1994;15:1–2.
DeBlij H. *Human geography: culture, society, and space.* New York: John Wiley & Sons, 1982:217–235.
Dolnick E. Deafness as culture. *Atlantic Month* 1993; 272:37–51.
Fleisher L. Whose child is this? *Hear Health* 1993:21–23.
Francis HW, Koch ME, Wyatt JR, Niparko JK. Trends in educational placement and cost-benefit consider-

ation in children with cochlear implants. *Arch Otolagyngol Head Neck Surg (in press)*.

Gentry R. Why we won at Gallaudet. *Gallaudet Today* 1988;May-June: .

Holt J. Stanford achievement test, 8th edition. *Am Ann Deaf* 1993;138:172–175.

Lane H. *The mask of benevolence.* New York: Vintage Books, 1993.

Lane H, Bahan B. Ethics of cochlear implantation in young children: a review and reply from a Deaf-World perspective. *Otolaryngol Head Neck Surg* 1998; 119:297–313.

Mitsakos ML. *Earth's geography and environment.* Evanston, IL: McDougal, Littell & Co, 1991.

Kluckhohn C. *Mirror for man.* New York: McGraw-Hill, 1949.

Lane H. The cochlear implant controversy. *World Fed Deaf News* 1994;3:22–28.

Miyamoto R, Osberger M, Cunningham L, *et al.* Single-channel to multichannel conversions in pediatric cochlear implant recipients. *Am J Otol* 1994;15:40–45.

Rose D, Vernon M, Pool A. Cochlear implants in prelingually deaf children. *Am Ann Deaf* 1996;141:258–262.

Sapir E. *Language.* New York: Harcourt Brace, 1921.

Schopmeyer B, Mellon NK, Dobaj H, Grant GD, Niparko JK. Use of Fast ForWord® to enhance language development in children with cochlear implants. *Ann Otol Laryngol Rhinol,* in press.

Solomon. Deafness is beautiful. *New York Times Sunday Magazine,* August 28, 1994:40–45, 65–68.

Tait M, Lutman M. Comparison of early communicative behavior in young children with cochlear implants and with hearing aids. *Ear Hear* 1994;15:352–361.

National Association of the Deaf. Cochlear implants in children: a position paper. 5th National Association of the Deaf, April, 1993.

Whorf B. *Language, thought, and reality.* New York: John Wiley & Sons, 1956.

World Federation of the Deaf. *Proceedings of the XII World Congress of the World Federation of the Deaf.* Vienna: The Federation, 1996.

Appendix 14A

The Implications of Parental Choice of Communication Mode:
Understanding the Options

Nancy K. Mellon

Realistic appraisals of the impact of all options are needed to guide parents in acting in a child's best interests. Nowhere is this more apparent than with the concept of cochlear implantation of a young deaf child. Too much optimism invariably leads to disappointment, and even implant teams readily admit that implants are not a panacea for deafness. Although a cochlear implant may not be a viable option for every child, expectations of ASL should be realistic as well. ASL may be acquired naturally by deaf children and presents important opportunities for cognitive development. However, acquisition of language competence in ASL is also subject to constraints. Parents must balance the strengths and limitations of each communication mode when selecting a methodology for educating their children.

Challenges in acquiring ASL are related to factors involving parents and the child. If hearing parents are to mentor their children's language acquisition they must develop linguistic competence in ASL themselves. Many adults experience significant difficulty learning a second language whether spoken or signed (Marschark, 1997). Most hearing parents fail to learn sign; those who do often demonstrate limited competence (Vaccari and Marschark, 1997). The child's parents may fail to provide a fully fluent, sophisticated model for language. They can, however, provide a fully fluent model in spoken language, and improving the child's ability to access that language is a worthy goal.

The effects of achieving linguistic competence in ASL or in spoken language cannot

N. K. Mellon: The Johns Hopkins University, Listening Center, Baltimore, Maryland 21287.

be compared directly. Each carries very different cultural, educational, and social implications. Linguistic competence in ASL requires receptive and expressive use of sign and mastery of the complex grammar that governs its use. It does not, however, require mastery of reading and writing, because ASL has no written form. Moreover, its grammar differs significantly in terms of syntax and morphology from English grammar and is expressed through visuospatial rather than sequential auditory parameters (Crystal, 1997). ASL uses a complex system of simultaneous sign modulations similar in function to the sequential inflections of spoken morphology. Transferring language skills based in simultaneous processing to a language system organized temporally and sequentially is likely to be problematic. Linguistic skills in ASL do not transfer readily to spoken language and the subsequent development of reading and writing.

Hearing children base their reading and writing skills on a foundation developed through listening and speaking (Bench, 1992). Because they can hear speech, children with implants can bring a familiarity with the language to the process of reading and writing. This is an important consideration for many hearing parents as literacy provides the underpinnings for academic achievement and communication through the Internet, telecommunications, and the print media.

Communication in ASL is conducted by face to face interactions. This fact necessarily limits a signer's access to others. Interpreters and telecommunications relays may extend the range of potential communication partners. Unfortunately, they also place an intermediary in the communication process, changing the nature of what would otherwise be a one to one exchange. Intermediary communication devices often require use of a language vehicle other than ASL. Practical constraints may limit the individual's use of ASL in extending social boundaries and engaging in individual interactions.

Although ASL is considered a full and complex language in its own right, some 15% of all manual vocabulary in signed discourse is finger-spelled (Padden and Ramsey, 1998). Semantic possibilities in sign language are limited in some ways. Whereas roughly 4,000 signs have been recorded in ASL (Crystal, 1997), the average American high school graduate knows approximately 45,000 words, and the average 6 year old commands a vocabulary composed of an estimated 13,000 words (Pinker, 1994).

Advocates of a bilingual approach with deaf children believe that all deaf children should learn sign language as a first language (Singelton *et al.*, 1998). Acknowledging that hearing parents lack the ability to sign fluently, they assign the role of first language mentors to the schools. The ASL-first approach fails to address the time constraints on first language acquisition and research that clearly links *early* exposure and linguistic competence (Mayberry, 1993).

Although children with implants may acquire less than perfect speech, they may have the potential to show improved literacy. Implants may also provide children access to a wider array of communication partners. Dependence on ASL is natural and fully functional within the deaf community but can limit the child's facility in communicating within a hearing family, the community, and the society of their birth. Because most vocational opportunities for the developing child probably exist in mainstream society, development of spoken language skills may ultimately prove more adaptive for the child's future.

Parents carry a heavy responsibility in selecting a communication strategy for their child. Parents who choose to educate their deaf children using ASL only are making a cultural choice, foreclosing the child's options with regard to hearing culture. The deaf child is likely to benefit optimally from oral education only if residual hearing can be exploited to its fullest at the earliest possible opportunity, because language outcomes in deaf children improve with earlier detection and intervention (Yoshinaga-Itano *et al.*, 1998).

Theoretically, the goal of raising bicultural-bilingual deaf children is a good one. However, given parental limitations in terms of providing appropriate language models, the persistent delays in diagnosing hearing loss, and the less than perfect auditory inputs delivered by hearing aids and cochlear implants, deaf children are likely to continue to demonstrate difficulty in developing linguistic competence. As technology and programs of early detection and intervention improve, so too should language outcomes for hearing-impaired children.

REFERENCES

Bench R. *Communication skills in hearing-impaired children.* San Diego: Singular Publishing Group, 1992.

Crystal D. *The Cambridge encyclopedia of language,* 2nd ed. Cambridge: Cambridge University Press, 1997.

Marschark M. *Raising and educating a deaf child: a comprehensive guide to the choices, controversies, and decisions faced by parents and educators.* Oxford: Oxford University Press, 1997.

Mayberry R. First-language acquisition after childhood differs from second-language acquisition: the case of American Sign Language. *J Speech Hear Res* 1993;36:1258–1270.

Padden C, Ramsey C. Reading ability in signing deaf children. *Top Lang Disord* 1988;18:16–29.

Pinker S. *The language instinct.* New York: William Morrow, 1994:150–151.

Singleton J, Supalla S, Litchfield S, Schley S. From sign to word: considering modality constraints in ASL/English bilingual education. *Top Lang Disord* 1998;18:16–29.

Vaccari C, Marschark M. Communication between parents and deaf children: implications of socio-emotional development. *J Child Psychol Psychiatry* 1997;38:793–801.

Yoshinaga-Itano C, Sedey A, Coulter D, Mehl A. Language of early- and later-identified children with hearing loss. *Pediatrics* 1998;102:1161–1171.

Cochlear Implants: Principles & Practices, edited by John K. Niparko, Karen Iler Kirk, Nancy K. Mellon, Amy McConkey Robbins, Debara L. Tucci, and Blake S. Wilson. Lippincott Williams & Wilkins, Philadelphia © 2000.

Subject Index

A

ACE (advanced combination encoder) speech processors, 141, 161, 162

Acoustic environment, CIS processors and, 147

Acoustic signals, and information technology, 3

Acoustic trauma, 69–70

Advanced Bionics Corporation, Inc., 114, 149, 237–240 (*see also* Clarion cochlear implants)

AGC (automatic gain control), *144*, 145, 149

Aging

brain plasticity in, decline of, 48–49, 52–53

hearing loss in (*see* Presbycusis)

AIED (autoimmune inner ear disease), 82–83

Alport's disease, 64

American sign language (ASL), 301

Deaf culture and use of, 373–376

grammar of, 305–306

parental choice and use of, 379–381

used by prelingually deaf adults, 361

Aminoglycosides, ototoxic effects of, 70–72

Amplitude spectra, 10, *11*

and discharge rates of auditory neurons, 17

Anatomy, of ear

inner, *12,* 13–14, *110* (*see also* Inner ear)

middle, 11, *12,* 13 (*see also* Middle ear)

outer, 11, *12* (*see also* Outer ear)

Anteroventral cochlear nucleus (AVCN), 19

basic synaptic configurations of, 19–20, *21*

cells types within, 19–21

neural response types in, *21*

Aplasia

cochlear, 210

Michel's, 64

Mondini's, 64, *65, 66*

Approval process (*see* Food and Drug Administration)

Arthro-ophthalmopathy, hereditary, 63

Ascending auditory pathway, 22–25 (*see also* Central auditory system)

auditory cortical fields in, 24–25

cochlear nucleus and information processing in, 18–22

inferior colliculus in, 22

lateral superior olive in, 22–23

medial geniculate body in, 23–24

medial superior olive in, 22–23

nuclei in, major, 19–22, *20*

ASL (*see* American sign language)

Assessment(s)

of implant candidacy, 173–181, *179*

auditory skills, 178–179

developmental pediatric, 180–181

educational placement evaluation in, 180

general health and psychologic, 177, 180

hearing, 173–175, 178

language, 179–180

neurologic, 180–181

occupational therapy in, 180

ophthalmologic, 180

otologic and medical, 175–177, 178

of speech perception (*see* Outcomes; Speech perception)

for surgery

etiologic, 191

medical and otologic, 189–191

radiologic, 191–193

Auditory brain stem implants, 211

speech perception outcomes in adults with, 242–243

Auditory capacity, 325

Auditory cortex, 24–25

fields on superior temporal gyrus of brain, *24*

plasticity of, 46

primary (A1), *47*

Auditory experience, of language development, 36–37

fetal environment in, 294

infant-directed talk (IDT) in, 294–295

infant preferences in, 295–296

innate perception in, 292–294

intermodal, 300

six month perception of, 296–299

six to nine month perception of, 299

word learning in, 300

Auditory nerve, 14–18

Auditory neurons, 3, 14–18 (*see also* Central auditory system)

aging of, 68–69 (*see also* Presbycusis)

amplitude spectra and discharge rates of, 17

in ascending auditory pathway, 22 (*see also* Ascending auditory pathway)

best frequencies of, 15

brain input and, 14–18 (*see also* Central auditory system)

in cochlea, 18–22

hearing loss and effect on, 93–96

injury and effects on, 57–59

synaptic configurations of, 19–20

in cortex, 24–25

differentiation of, 33–34

behavioral development and, 34–37

environmental influence on, 34, 41

electrical stimulation and biological effect on, 98–99

hair cells and, synaptic contact between, 15 (*see also* Auditory receptor cells)

Auditory neurons (*contd.*)
  hearing loss and effects on histology of, *94,* 94–95, *95*
  hearing loss and effects on size of, 93–96
  loss of, 57–63
    with age, 58
    with cochlear implantation, 60, 62–63
    normal, 58
  myelination of, 48–49
  noise and effects on, 69–70
  normal, *110*
  ototoxic effects of medications on, 70–72
  pathology of, 57–63 (*see also* Spiral ganglion cells)
    autoimmune disease and, 82–83
    genetic, 63–68
    infection and, 72–76
    Meniere's disease and, 81
  patterns of connection of, establishing, 33–34
  rate-level functions of, 15, *16*
  rate response of, 15–18, *16*
  responses of, *22*
    classification of, 18
    types of, *21*
  size of, hearing loss and, 93–96
  speech and necessary, 59–62
  spontaneous activity and sound conduction in, *17,* 18
  survival of, 57–63
  two-tone suppression of, 15
  type I and type II, basic response properties of, 14–15, *16*
Auditory perception (*see* Perception, auditory)
Auditory performance, 325
Auditory physiology (*see* Physiology, auditory)
Auditory receptor cells, *12,* 13
  location, structure and function of, 14
  synaptic contact between auditory neurons and, 15
Auditory sandwich, 355
Auditory scene analysis, 27
Autoimmune injury, mechanism of, 83
Autoimmune inner ear disease (AIED), 82–83
  treatment of, 83
Automatic gain control (AGC), *144,* 145, 149
AVCN (*see* Anteroventral cochlear nucleus)

B

Background noise, in sensorineural hearing loss, 27–28
Bacterial meningitis, 74
Bandpass channels, 134–135
Basilar membrane, of inner ear, *12,* 13–14
Batteries, 115
Behavioral development (*see also* Brain plasticity)
  auditory experience and, 34–37
  differentiation of neurons and, 33–34
Behind-the-ear (BTE) housing, 110
Benefit determinations, factors included in, 271
Best frequency (BF), 15
Binaural analysis, lateral superior olive in, 23
Brachial-otologic-renal syndrome, 63
Brain plasticity, 33–53
  adult, 45–49
    auditory cortex and, 46–47
    nature of, 45–46
    other brain areas and, 47–48
    sensory deprivation and, 45–48
    training effect and, 48
  in animal models of deafness, 42–44
  behavioral plasticity and, 37–39
  cochlear implants and, 49–53
  decline of, in aging, 48–49, 52–53
  early experiences and, 41–42 (*see also* Language development)
  genetic factors in, 41
  learning and memory in, 53
  monocular deprivation and visual cortex development, 37–38, *38*
  mouse vibrissae damage and cortical development, 38–39, *40*
  and neural compensation, in humans, 44–45
  pleuripotency of cortex in, 39–41
Bringing Sounds to Life (Koch), 328
BTE (behind-the-ear) housing, 110
Bushy cells, 19–20, 22
  low and high spontaneous rate, *22*

C

C124M cochlear implants, 116–117, *117,* 161
CA (compressed analog) speech processors, 149–152
  CIS speech processors compared with, 152–155
  stimuli produced by, *151*
Candidacy, cochlear implant, 173–181, *179*
  auditory skills assessment in, 178–179
  developmental pediatric assessment in, 180–181
  educational placement assessment in, 180
  general health and psychologic assessment in, 177, 180
  hearing assessment in, 173–175, 178
  language assessment in, 179–180
  neurologic assessment in, 180–181
  occupational therapy assessment in, 180
  ophthalmologic assessment in, 180
  otologic and medical assessment in, 175–177, 178
Central auditory system, *20,* 22–25 (*see also* Auditory neurons)
  auditory cortical fields in, 24–25
  cochlear implantation and effects on, 96
    animal studies of, 97–100
  cochlear nucleus and information processing in, 18–22
  electrical stimulation of auditory neurons and effect on, 98–99
  hearing loss and effects on, 93–96
    histologic staining pattern changes in, *94,* 94–95, *95*
  inferior colliculus in, 22
    convergent input into, 23
  lateral superior olive in, 22–23
  medial geniculate body in, 23–24
  medial superior olive in, 22–23
  nuclei in, major, 19–22, *20, 23*
  pathologic changes in, 93
Central Institute for the Deaf (CID)
  speech perception categories of, 230t

speech perception test batteries of, 230–231, 231t
studies of speech performance after child cochlear implantation by, 248
Cerebral cortex
areas associated with language development in, *307*
language development and, 310–312
left hemisphere in, 309–310
right hemisphere in, 307–308
language mode and hemispheric specialization of, 310–312
neurons of, 24–25 (*see also* Central auditory system)
pleuripotency of, 39–41
Channel vocoders, 133–135, *134*
Chopper(s)
sustained (ChS), *22*
transient (ChT), *22*
Chopper responses, 21, *21, 22*
Chopper units, 21
CID (*see* Central Institute for the Deaf)
Ciliary tufts, 13
CIS-Link processor, 160
CIS speech processors, 129, 141
CA speech processors compared with, 152–155
in Clarion cochlear implants, 240
design strategies for, 145–149, *146*
evaluation of, 148–149, *149*
in Med El cochlear implants, 240–241
SPEAK speech processors compared with, 160–161
Cisplatin, ototoxic effects of, 72
City University of New York Sentences, 229
Clarion cochlear implants, *238–239*
adult speech perception after implantation of, 237–240
child speech perception after implantation of, 245–246
progenitor of, *114*
speech processor design for, 149–152, *238*
CIS, 240
SAS, 163–164, 240
Classic conditioning, 48
Clinical device studies, 122
CNC (Constant–Nucleus–Consonant) word lists, 229

Cochlea
aging and effects on, 68–69 (*see also* Presbycusis)
anatomy of, *12*, 13–14, *110*
radiographic, *176*
auditory neurons of, 14–18
damage to, 57–63 (*see also* Sensorineural hearing loss)
auditory receptor cells of, 13–14 (*see also* Auditory receptor cells)
autosomal dominant structural malformations of, 64
basal turn of, photomicrograph of, *62*
conduction of sound waves in, 13–14
conduction of sound waves to, 11
endolymphatic hydrops in, 79, *80*
frequency-specific areas of, *58*
hair cells of, 13–14 (*see also* Auditory receptor cells)
stimulus frequencies and, 14
histologic section of normal, *59–60*
impedance matching system of, 13
implanted system in, 112, *114*
injury to, 57 (*see also* Sensorineural hearing loss)
bacterial meningitis and, 74–76
measles and, 74
medications and, 70–72
Meniere's disease and, 79–82, *80, 81*
mumps and, 72, 74
otitis interna and, *75, 76*
otitis media and, *75, 76*
rubella and, 72, *73*
syphilis and, 76
ionic pumps of, specialized, 13
link of auditory brain stem and, 23
noise and effects on, 69–70
normal
histologic section of, *59–60*
radiographic image of, *176*
nucleus of, 18–22
hearing loss and pathologic effect on, 93–96
major subdivisions of, 19
neurons within, 19–22, 22–25 (*see also* Ascending auditory pathway)

response effects on, *22*
response types of, *21*
synaptic configurations within, 19–20
otosclerotic invasion of, *78,* 78–79
ototoxic effects of medications on, 70–72
radiographic image of normal, *176*
removal in animals, effects of, 42–44
spiral ganglion cells of, 14 (*see also* Spiral ganglion cells)
Cochlear Corporation, 234–237 (*see also* Nucleus cochlear implants)
Cochlear hair cells, 3 (*see also* Auditory receptor cells)
Cochlear implant system(s), 1–2, 49–51, 109–127 (*see also* Implantation, cochlear)
C124M, 116–117, *117* (*see also* C124M cochlear implant)
candidacy for, 173–177 (*see also* Candidacy)
channel, 106 (*see also* Channel vocoders)
Clarion, *114,* 149–152 (*see also* Clarion cochlear implants)
COMBI 40, 112, *112* (*see also* COMBI 40/COMBI 40+ cochlear implants)
components of, 109–113, *111, 112*
cultural impact of, 5–6 (*see also* Cultural impact)
design of, 113, *114,* 115t, 118 (*see also* Design)
electrodes of, 109, 110, 117–118
partial insertion of, 112, *114*
reference, 110
fitting, 165–166
Food and Drug Administration approval of, 3–4, 122–127 (*see also* Food and Drug Administration)
future trends in, 167–168
history of, 103–106
information processing by, 136–137 (*see also* Speech processors)
Med El, 112, *112, 113* (*see also* COMBI 40/COMBI 40+ cochlear implants)
microcircuitry of, 119–121, *120* (*see also* Microcircuitry)
microphone of, 109, 113–115

Cochlear implant system(s) (*contd.*)
  Nucleus, 141–145 (*see also* Nucleus cochlear implants)
  patient variables and, 166–167
  signal processing by, 27–28
  speech processor of, 109, 110, 115–116, *120* (*see also* Speech processors)
  speech representation by, 129–168 (*see also* Speech representation)
  technologic development of, 119–121
  transmission link of, 109, *111,* 116–117
  trends in, 167–168
Cochlear implantation (*see* Implantation, cochlear)
  linguistic implications of, 5–6 (*see also* Rehabilitation)
Cochlear Ltd., 112, 143, 156 (*see also* C124M cochlear implants)
Cochlear malformation, implantation in, 208–210
Cogan's syndrome, 82
Coils, transmitting and receiving, 109, 110
COMBI 40/COMBI 40+ cochlear implants, 112, *112, 113,* 161, 162–163
  adult speech perception after implantation of, 240–241
  child speech perception after implantation of, 246
  electrode arrays of, 118
Communication
  methods of, in hearing loss, 182 (*see also* Language development; Signed language)
  parental, with deaf children, 183–186, 316 (*see also under* Cultural impact)
Communication and Adult Hearing Loss (Erber), 360
Communication Training for Older Teenagers and Adults (Tye-Murray), 361
Competing noise, in outcome testing, 228
Complex sound representation, 15, 17, *17*
Compressed analog (CA) speech processors, 149–152
  CIS speech processors compared with, 152–155

stimuli produced by, *151*
Consensus Conferences, 4
Consonant sounds, classification of, 131–132, 131t
Continuous interleaved sampling (CIS), 129, 147, *148* (*see also* CIS speech processors)
Contrastive Word Pairs (Kiernan and Zentz), 347
Cortex (*see* Cerebral cortex)
Cortical neurons, 24–25 (*see also* Central auditory system)
Cost-benefit ratio, 270 (*see also under* Outcomes)
Cost-effectiveness, assessment instruments of, 271
Cost-effectiveness ratio, 270 (*see also under* Outcomes)
Cost-utility ratio, 270 (*see also under* Outcomes)
Cost-utility yield, determination of, 271–272
Critical period, and brain plasticity, 51
Critical period hypothesis, 2, 34–37
Cultural impact, of cochlear implantation, 5–6, 372
  background and definitions, 372–373
  Deaf culture and, 373–378
  ethnocentric perspectives in, 376
  implantation failure in deaf children, 374–375
  parental authority and, 377
Cytochrome oxidase measurement, of neuronal activity, 98

D
dB SPL, 10
DCN (dorsal cochlear nucleus), 19
Deaf culture, 373–378
Deafness (*see* Hearing loss)
Deformity, common cavity, 210
Delayed-onset hearing loss, autosomal dominant, 64
Design
  cochlear implant, 113, *114,* 118
  fitting in, 165–166
  options and considerations in, 115t
  patient variable in, 166–167
  problems of, 137

speech processor, 138–139, 164–165
  compressed analog (CA), 149–152
  continuous interleaved sampling (CIS), 145–149
  F0/F1/F2, *141,* 141–143, *142*
  feature extraction and multipeak, 141–145
  implementation of, 166
  interleaved pulses (IP), 138–141
  MPEAK, 143–145, *144*
  n-of-m, 161–163
  simultaneous analog stimulation (SAS), 163–164
  SPEAK, 156–157, *158*
  spectral maxima sound processor (SMSP), 155–156
  successful, 165–167
  trends in, 167–168
Developmental Approach to Successful Listening, DASL, (Stout and Windle), 328
Device approval process, 3 (*see also* Food and Drug Administration)
DFNB1 locus mutations and, 68
Digital signal processing (DSP) chips, 115–116, *120*
Djourno, A, and Eyries, C, 103, 105
Dorsal cochlear nucleus (DCN), 19
Doyle, 106
Drugs (*see* Medications)
DSP chips, 115–116, *120*

E
Ear
  inner, *12,* 13–14, *110* (*see also* Inner ear)
  middle, 11, *12,* 13 (*see also* Middle ear)
  outer, 11, *12* (*see also* Outer ear)
Ear drum, 13
Educational placement, of implanted children, 278–279, 280, 349
  curriculum and skill development in, 351–355
  individualized plans in, 349
  relationship between implant center and school in, 349–352
  trends in, 281–283

Educational Resource Matrix (ERM), 278–280, 352
Electrodes, of cochlear implants, 109, 110, 117–118
  partial insertion of, 112, *114*
  reference, 110
Endbulb of Held, 19–20, 23
  function of, 43
  synapses of, in normal and deaf cats, *44*
Endolymphatic hydrops, 79, *80*
ERM (*see* Educational Resource Matrix)
ERPs (*see* Evoked response potentials)
Evoked potentials
  in assessment of implant candidacy, 173–175, *174*
  intracochlear, 116–117, *117*
Evoked response potentials (ERPs), in speech perception, 308–309
Expressive language, *334*

F
F0/F1/F2 speech processors, *141,* 141–143, *142*
  in Nucleus cochlear implant systems, 235, 244–245
F0/F2 speech processors, 142–143
Feature extraction and multipeak processors, 141–145
Filters
  preemphasis, 145–146, *146*
  transfer function of vocal cords as, 130
Fitting, of cochlear implant systems, 165–166
Fluoride, and arrest of otosclerosis, 79
Food and Drug Administration (FDA), 122–127
  approval process of, 3–4, 123–126
    standard sequence of, 122
  classification of otolaryngologic implants by, 123
  definitions approved by, 122
  investigational device exemption (IDE) regulation of, 123–126
  Modernization Act of 1997, 126–127
  presentation of premarket approval application to, 126
Formant frequencies, 11
Formant peaks, 10, 130

Formant vocoders, 135–136, *136*
F0/F1/F2 speech processors, *141,* 141–143, *142*
Frequencies, of sound waves, 9–10, *11*

G
GASP (Glendonald Auditory Screening Procedure), 246, 251
Genetic origins, of sensorineural hearing loss, 63–68
  Alport's disease, 64
  arthro-ophthalmopathy, hereditary, 63
  brachial-otologic-renal syndrome, 63
  delayed-onset hearing loss, autosomal dominant, 64
  DFNB1 locus mutations and, 68
  Hunter's syndrome, 66
  Hurler's disease, 66
  Jervell and Lange-Neilsen syndrome, 66, 67
  Klippel-Feil syndrome, 66
  large vestibular aqueduct syndrome (LVAS), 65–66
  Marshall-Stickler syndrome, 63
  Melnick-Fraser syndrome, 63
  Michel's aplasia, 64
  Mondini's aplasia, 64, *65, 66*
  neurofibromatosis, 64
  Norrie's syndrome, 68
  Pendred's syndrome, 66, 67
  Refsum's disease, 66
  Stickler's syndrome, 63
  Usher's syndrome, 66, 67
  von Recklinghausen's disease, 64
  Waardenburg's syndrome, 63
  Wildervaank's syndrome, 68
Glendonald Auditory Screening Procedure (GASP), 246, 251
Grammatic language development, 304–305
Greenhousing, 325
  avoiding risk of, 328–331

H
Haemophilus influenzae, 74
Hair cells (*see* Auditory receptor cells)

Head-level unit, 109, 110
Hearing
  brain mechanisms of (*see* Brain plasticity; Cochlea)
  physiology of, 2, 14–30 (*see also* Physiology, auditory)
Hearing aid use, recruitment and, 28–30
Hearing loss
  adjustment to, parental, 181–186
  adult (*see* Rehabilitation; Speech perception)
  animal models of, brain plasticity in, 42–44
  assessment of (*see* Assessment)
  brain plasticity and, 42–44, 49–51
  changes associated with
    central auditory system and, 93–96
    origin of, 43–44
  childhood, 181–186
    language development in (*see* Language development; Rehabilitation; Speech perception)
    motor skills in, 365–367
    psychosocial development in, 319–321
  cochlear implants for, 49–51 (*see also* Cochlear implant systems)
    performance of, 51–53
  congenital, treatment of, 51
  diagnosis of, 173–177 (*see also* Assessment)
    parental response to, 181–183
  electrical stimulation of auditory neurons and reversal of, 98–100
  epidemiology of, 88–91
  genetic pathology of, 63–68 (*see also* Genetic origins)
  language development in (*see* Language development)
  neuronal damage/loss in, *110*
  parental adjustment to, child outcomes and, 183–186
  parental response to diagnosis of, 181–183
  prevalence of
    in adults, 90–91
    in children, 88–90
  psychosocial development of children with, 319–321

Hearing loss (*contd.*)
    reading development and, 315
        (*see also* Language devel-
        opment)
    assessment methods in,
        317–318
    educational programs in, 318
    home environment in, 317
    inferential and metacognitive
        factors in, 316–317
    parent-child communication
        in, 316
    school environment in, 317
    sound and symbol correspon-
        dence in, 315–316
    vocabulary and syntax in,
        316
    sensorineural (*see* Sensorineu-
        ral hearing loss)
    severe to profound, 57 (*see
        also* Sensorineural hearing
        loss)
    synaptic changes in, 52
    treatment of, 51–52 (*see also*
        Implantation, cochlear,
        technique of)
    brain plasticity and, 49–51
    cochlear implants in, 49–51
    performance of, 51–53
Hemispheric specialization, lan-
    guage and, 307–312
High resolution computerized to-
    mography (HRCT),
    191–193
Histologic otosclerosis, 77–78
History, of cochlear implants,
    103–106
House, William F, 106 (*see also*
    3M/House device)
HRCT (high resolution computer-
    ized tomography), 191–193
HUI (Health Utilities Index), On-
    tario, 273
Hunter's syndrome, 66
Hurler's disease, 66
Hypoplasia, cochlear, 210

I

IDE (Investigational device ex-
    emption) regulation, of
    FDA, 123–126
Impedance matching system, of
    cochlea, 13
Implant(s) (*see also* Cochlear im-
    plant systems)
    classification of, used in otola-
        ryngology, 123
    FDA definition of, 122

Implant team, evolution of, 5
Implantation, cochlear, 2, 49–51,
    189
    in adults, 208–210 (*see also*
        Outcomes; Rehabilitation)
    assessment for
        etiologic, 191
        medical and otologic,
            189–191
        radiologic, 191–193
    auditory brain stem implants,
        211
    benefits of (*see* Implantation,
        cochlear, outcomes of)
    bony growth impeding, 76
    brain plasticity and, 51–52
    in children, 200–203 (*see also*
        Outcomes; Rehabilitation)
    age and effects on, 262–265,
        318, 336, 339–341
    literature metanalysis of,
        260–265
    in cochlear malformation,
        208–210
    in cochlear ossification,
        203–208
    complications of, in adults,
        211–216
        facial nerve injury, 214–215
        incision and flap design,
            211–212
        surgical risk, 211
        tinnitus, 215–216
        vertigo, 216
        vestibular function, reduced,
            216
        wound breakdown, 215
    complications of, in children,
        216–218
        device failure, 218
        studies of, 217–218
        surgical risk, 217
    cost effectiveness of, 269–272
        (*see also* Outcomes)
        adults, 272–275
        children, 275–286
    critical periods and, 51–52
    cultural impact of, 5–6 (*see
        also* Cultural impact)
    Deaf culture arguments
        against, 373–376
    and effects on central auditory
        system, 96
    animal studies of, 97–100
    failure of, in deaf children,
        374–375
    histologic results of, 218–219
    history of, 103–106

language acquisition and, 5 (*see
        also* Language develop-
        ment; Rehabilitation)
    literature metanalysis of child,
        260–265
    in Meniere's disease, 81–82
    MRI imaging followup after,
        210–211
    music and, 266–268
    neuronal injury/loss and,
        59–63, 93–96, 109, *110*
    otosclerosis and, 78–79
    outcomes of, 4, 30, 51–53 (*see
        also* Outcomes; Rehabili-
        tation)
    procedural timing for, 51
    rehabilitation after, 5 (*see also*
        Rehabilitation)
    reimplantation surgery, 218
    research on, 226–227, 253–254
    risks of, 4 (*see also* Implanta-
        tion, cochlear, technique
        of; Outcomes)
    signal processing in, 27–28
    speech perception after,
        325–331 (*see also* Out-
        comes; Rehabilitation;
        Speech perception)
    technique of, 193–200
        facial nerve, monitoring,
            198–199
        flap design, 193
        insertion of device, 196–197
        mastoidectomy, 193, 195
        modifications with labyrin-
            thectomy, 197–198
        preoperative considerations,
            193
        radiographs, postoperative,
            199–200
        scala tympani, opening,
            195–196
    technology of, 1–2, 109–127
        (*see also* Cochlear implant
        systems)
    uniqueness of, 3
Incidental language learning,
    338–339
Incus, 13
Indiana University School of
    Medicine (IUSM)
    speech perception test batteries
        of, 230, 232t
    studies of speech performance
        after child cochlear implan-
        tation, 247
Individual variation, in speech
    perception, 233–234

Ineraid cochlear implants, 163–164 (*see also* CA speech processors)
Infant-directed talk (IDT), 294–295
Infectious diseases, and sensorineural hearing loss, 72–76 (*see also* specific disease)
  bacterial meningitis, 74
  measles, 74
  mumps, 72, 74
  rubella, 72, *73*
  syphilis, 76
Inferior colliculus (IC)
  contralateral, 22
  convergent input into, 23
Information processing
  in cochlear nucleus, 18–22
  in sensorineural hearing loss, 25–28
  by speech processors, 136–137
Inner ear, *12*, 13–14 (*see also* Cochlea)
  auditory receptor cells of, 13–14
  autosomal dominant structural malformations of, 64
  conduction of sound waves in, 13
  hair cells of, 13–14
  ionic pumps of, specialized, 13
Institutional Review Board (IRB)
  presentation of data in premarket approval application, 126
  role of, 125–126
Integrated circuit technology, 109
  of cochlear implants, 119–121
  of speech processors, 115–116, *120*
Interleaved pulses (IP), 138, *140*
Interleaved pulses (IP) processor, *138*, 138–141
  comparisons of, with other designs, 139–141
Intermittency and duration, of sound, 10
Investigational device exemption (IDE) regulation, of FDA, 123–126
Ionic pumps, of cochlea, 13
IUSM (*see* Indiana University School of Medicine)

J

Jervell and Lange-Neilsen syndrome, 66, 67

John Tracy Clinic, 328

K

Klippel-Feil syndrome, 66

L

Labyrinthitis, suppurative, *75*, 76
Labyrinthitis ossificans, 74–76
  cochlear implantation in cases of, 78–79, 203–208 (*see also* Otosclerosis)
  device choice for, 205–208
  procedure choice for, 205–208
Language, cultural significance of, 373
Language Approach to Open Syllables (Young), 347
Language development, 5, 291–292, 303–306 (*see also* Brain plasticity; Speech perception)
  after cochlear implantation, 5–6, 292, 331–341 (*see also* Rehabilitation)
  age of child and, 336, 339–341
  auditory experience of, 36–37
  fetal environment in, 294
  infant-directed talk (IDT) in, 294–295
  infant preferences in, 295–296
  innate perception in, 292–294
  intermodal, 300
  six month perception of, 296–299
  six to nine month perception of, 299
  word learning in, 300
  cerebrocortical areas associated with, 25, *307*
  grammatic, 304–305
  hemispheric specialization of, 310–312
  incidental, 338–339
  left hemisphere in, 309–310
  modality of, and hemispheric specialization, 307–312
  neurobiologic basis of, 308–309
  neurolinguistic theory of, 306–308
  parental influence on, 183–186, 294–295
  phonologic, 303–304

  pragmatic, 303
  reading and writing in, 305–306 (*see also* Reading development)
  semantic, 304
  speech production during, 300–301
  social influences in, 301–302
  vocal imitation in, 302–303
  treatment of impaired, 51–52
Large vestibular aqueduct syndrome (LVAS), 65–66
Lateral superior olive (LSO), 22–23
  tonographic organization of, 22
Learning to Hear Again with a Cochlear Implant (Wayner and Abrahamson), 359
Least restrictive environment, 351–352
Left hemisphere, in language development, 309–310
Lexical Neighborhood Test (LNT), 245, 249
Linguistic implications, of cochlear implantation, 5–6 (*see also* Rehabilitation)
Listening Games for Littles (Sindrey), 328
LNT (Lexical Neighborhood Test), 245, 249
Locke's theory, of neurolinguistics, 306–308
Loop diuretics, ototoxic effects of, 72

M

MAC (Minimal Auditory Capabilities) Battery, 229
Malformation, cochlear, implantation in, 208–210
Malleus, 13
Marshall-Stickler syndrome, 63
Maternal adjustment, and child outcomes, 183–186
Measles, 74
Measurements of mismatch negativity (MMN), 299
Med El GmbH (Medical Electronic Corporation), 112, 160, 240–241, *242–243* (*see also* COMBI 40/COMBI 40+ cochlear implants)
Medial geniculate body (MGB), 23–24
Medial nucleus of trapezoid body (MNTB), 22–23

Medial superior olive (MSO), 22–23
  histology of cells of
    in idiopathic labyrinthitis, 94
    in meningitis, 95
  tonographic organization of, 22
Medications, ototoxic effect of, 70–72
Melnick-Fraser syndrome, 63
Meniere's disease, 79–82
  cochlear implantation in, 81–82
  pathologic physiology of, 79–81
  symptoms of, 79
  type of hearing loss in, 79
Mental grammar, 292–294, 306–307
MGB (medial geniculate body), 23–24
Miami Cochlear Implant Auditory and Tactile Skills Curriculum, CHATS, (Vergara and Miskel), 328
Michel's aplasia, 64
Michelson, RP, 106
Microcircuitry, 109
  advances in, 3
  of cochlear implants, 119–121
  of speech processors, 115–116, 120
Microphone, 109, 113–115
Middle ear, 12
  conduction of sound waves in, 13
  conduction of sound waves to, 11
  dimensions of, importance of, 13
Mini Speech Processor (MSP), 143–145, 144
Minimal Auditory Capabilities (MAC) Battery, 229
Minimal Pairs Test, 245
Minimal sensorineural hearing loss (MSHL), 90
MLNT (Multisyllabic Lexical Neighborhood Test), 249
MNGIPs (myelin-associated neurite growth inhibitory proteins), 48–49, 49
MNTB (medial nucleus of trapezoid body), 22–23
Modernization Act of 1997, FDA, 126–127
Mondini's aplasia, 64, 65, 66
Morphometry, computer-assisted, 94–95
MPEAK speech processors, 143–145, 144

SPEAK speech processors compared with, 157–160, 159
used in Nucleus cochlear implants, 235, 244–245
MRI (magnetic resonance imaging)
  as adjunct to HRCT before surgery, 192–193
  contraindications for implantation with future, 191
  followup after cochlear implantation, 210–211
MSHL (minimal sensorineural hearing loss), 90
MSP (Mini Speech Processor), 143–145, 144
Multichannel cochlear implant systems, 106
  outcomes for, 137
    adult speech perception, 234–241
    child speech perception, 244–247
Multimodal speech perception, 228
Multisyllabic Lexical Neighborhood Test, 249
Mumps, 72, 74
Music, and cochlear implantation, 266–268
Myelin-associated neurite growth inhibitory proteins (MNGIPs), 48–49, 49
Myelination, of neurons, 48–49

N
n-of-m speech processors, 139, 155–156, 160
  ACE implementation of, 162
  design strategies of, 161–163
National Association of the Deaf, 375
National Center for Health Statistics (NCHS), hearing loss surveys by, 90–91
National Institutes of Health (NIH)
  Consensus Conferences of, 4
  Consensus Statement of, 129
Native language magnet (NLM) theory, 296–299
Neisseria meningitidis, 74
Nerve fibers (see Auditory neurons)
Neural compensation, in humans, 44–45 (see also Brain plasticity)

Neurobiologic basis, of language development, 308–309 (see also Brain plasticity)
Neurofibromatosis, 64
Neurolinguistic theory, of language development, 306–308
Neuronal systems, modifiable, 2 (see also Brain plasticity)
Neurons, auditory (see Auditory neurons)
Noise-induced hearing loss, 69–70, 91
Nonsignificant risk (NSR) studies, 122
Nonsimultaneous stimuli, 152
Norrie's syndrome, 68
Northcott's curriculum guide, 327
Nucleus cochlear implants, 236–237
  adult speech perception after implantation of, 234–237
  child speech perception after implantation of, 244–245
  design strategies of, 141–145
  electrode arrays of, 118
  MPEAK speech processor with, 143–145, 144
  speech processors used with, 235–237

O
Octopus cells, 22
Olivocochlear bundle, 23
Ontario HUI (Health Utilities Index), 273
Open-set and closed-set test formats, 228
Oral communication, 327
Organ of Corti, 12, 13
  aging and effects on, 68
  tonographic organization of, 19
Ossicles, middle ear, 12, 13
Otitis interna, and sensorineural hearing loss, 75, 76
Otitis media
  advisability for implantation in children with, 190
  and sensorineural hearing loss, 75, 76
Otosclerosis, 76–79
  capsular, 78
  clinical diagnosis of, 76–77
  cochlear implantation and, 78–79
  histologic, 77–78
  location of, 77
  medical treatment of, 79

pathologic physiology of, 77
surgical treatment of, 77
Otospongiosis, 77
Ototoxicity, and hearing loss, 70–72
Outcome(s), of cochlear implantation, 4, 225 (*see also* Rehabilitation)
in adults, 234–243
cost-utility of, 272–275
in children, 243–253, 275–277
cost-benefit of, 283–285
cost-effectiveness of, 285–286
cost-utility of, 275–286
educational placement and, 280, 281–283 (*see also* Educational placement)
Educational Resource Matrix and, 277–280
maternal adjustment and, 183–186
rehabilitative services and, 278–279, 280–281
special education and, 277–278
clinical investigation of, 225–226
cost effectiveness of, 269–272
adults, 272–275
children, 275–286
implant research and, 226–227
measures of
individual variability in, 233–234
selecting appropriate, 227
speech perception, 227–228, 275–277
adult, 228–229
child, 229–233
speech intelligibility, child, 252–253
speech perception, adult, 234–242
auditory brain stem implants and, 242–243
factors influencing, 241–242
multichannel cochlear implant systems, 234–241
single channel cochlear implant systems, 234
speech perception, child, 243–247
comparisons of sensory aid use in, 248–249
factors influencing, 246–247, 249–251
multichannel cochlear implant systems, 244–246

single channel cochlear implant systems, 243–244
speech production, child, 251–252
Outer ear, *12*
collection of sound waves by, 11
Oval window, *12*, 13

P

Parental authority, 377
and choice of communication mode, 379–381
Parental response
and adjustment, 183–186
of deaf parents, 185
to hearing loss diagnosis, 181–183
of hearing parents, 184–186
Pediatric cochlear implantation (*see* Implantation, cochlear, in children; Outcomes)
Pendred's syndrome, 66, 67
Perception, auditory
anatomy of ear and, 11–14
fluids of inner ear and, 13
ascending auditory pathway in, 22–25
auditory nerve and brain input in, 14–18
cochlear nucleus and information processing in, 18–22
loss of, 25–28 (*see also* Sensorineural hearing loss)
Percutaneous connector, 109, *111*, 116–117
Periolivary belt, 23
Peristimulus time histograms (PSTHs), *21*
Permanent threshold shifts (PTS), 69–70
Phalangeal cells, damage to inner, 57–58
Phonologic language development, 303–304
Physiology, auditory, 14–30
ascending auditory pathway in, 22–25
auditory nerve in, 14–18
cochlear nucleus in, 18–22
pathology of, 25–30, 57–91 (*see also* Sensorineural hearing loss)
Pillar cells, damage to, 57–58
Pitch, of sound, 10
PMA (premarket approval application), 126

Posteroventral cochlear nucleus (PVCN), 19
Postprocessor, 139, *141*
Pragmatic language development, 303
Preemphasis filter, 145–146, *146*
Premarket approval application (PMA), 126
Presbycusis, 64–65, 68–69, 91
central auditory system in, 93
Primary (A1) auditory cortex, *47*
Primarylike responses, 21, *21*, *22*
Prosthesis (*see* Cochlear implant systems)
PSTHs (peristimulus time histograms), *21*
Psychosocial development, of children with hearing loss, 36–37, 319–321
PTAs (pure tone averages), 173–175, *174*
PTS (permanent threshold shifts), 69–70
PVCN (posteroventral cochlear nucleus), 19
Pyramidal cells, 22

Q

QALYs (quality-adjusted life years), 270

R

Radiologic imaging, before surgery, 191–193
Rate-level functions, of auditory neurons, 15–17, *16*
Rate response, of auditory neurons, 17–18
Reading and writing, in language development, 305–306
Reading development, and hearing loss, 315
assessment methods in, 317–318
cochlear implantation in, 318
educational programs in, 318
home environment in, 317
inferential and metacognitive factors in, 316–317
parent-child communication in, 316
school environment in, 317
sound and symbol correspondence in, 315–316
vocabulary and syntax in, 316
Receptive language, *334*

Recruitment
  definition of, 29
  and hearing aid use, 28–30
  mechanism underlying, 29
Refsum's disease, 66
Rehabilitation, aural
  after cochlear implantation, 5, 323
    adolescent, 355–357
      focus of, 357
    adult, 357–361
      postlingually deaf, 357–360
      prelingually deaf, 359–360
      resources for, 358–360
    child
      auditory capacity and performance in, 325
      curricula for, 326–331, 351–355
      didactic vs generalization approaches in, 339–341
      dimensions of, three, *330*
      educational placement and support in, 349–355 (*see also* Educational placement)
      formats and objectives of, *329*
      four components of, 323–325
      greenhousing in, 328–331
      hearing aided vs implant comparisons in, 325–326
      language development in, 331–341
      prelingually deaf, 323–325, 331–341
      services for, 278–281
      speech perception in, 325–331 (*see also* Outcomes; Speech perception)
      speech production in, 341–349 (*see also* Speech production)
  history of, 363–365
  profession of, beginning of, 364
  of World War II veterans, 363–364
Reimplantation surgery, 218
Research, on cochlear implants, 226–227, 253–254
Restored hearing, 4
Reverse telemetry, *117*
Right hemisphere, in language development, 307–308

Risks, of cochlear implantation, 4 (*see also* Implantation, cochlear, technique of; Outcomes)
Rubella, 72, *73*

S
SAS (simultaneous analog stimulation) processors, 149–152
  in Clarion cochlear implants, 240
  design strategies of, 163–164
Scala media, 13
Scala tympani (ST), *12, 13*
Scala vestibuli, *12, 13*
Screening Inventory for Educational Risk (SIFTER), 352
Selective listening, *19,* 21
Semantic language development, 304
Sensorineural hearing loss (SNHL), 25–28
  aging factors in, 64–65 (*see also* Presbycusis)
  amplification and loss of sensitivity in, 29–30, *30*
  auditory scene analysis and, 27
  autoimmune inner ear disease (AIED) in, 82–83
  basis of, ultrastructural, 26
  cochlear hair cells in, loss of, 25, 57–58
  cochlear implantation in, 30 (*see also* Cochlear implant systems)
  genetic, 63–68 (*see also* Genetic origins)
  infectious diseases and, 72–76
    bacterial meningitis, 74
    measles, 74
    mumps, 72, 74
    rubella, 72, *73*
    syphilis, 76
  Meniere's disease in, 79–82
  neuron population loss/damage in, 57–63, 93–96
  otitis interna and, *75,* 76
  otitis media and, *75,* 76
  otosclerosis in, 76–79
  ototoxicity in, 70–72
  physiologic consequences of (*see also* Hearing loss)
    in animals, 25–27, 42–44
  recruitment in, and hearing aid use, 28–30
  rehabilitation of, 52 (*see also* Rehabilitation)

  size of auditory neurons and, 93–96
  ultrastructural basis of, 26
Sensory cortex, adult, 46
Sensory development, 2
  auditory experience and, 34–36
  specialization in, 2
Sensory input, changes in, 2
Sensory plasticity, 2, 37–39 (*see also* Brain plasticity)
Set content, 228, 331–332
SIFTER (Screening Inventory for Educational Risk), 352
Signal processing, by hearing aids and cochlear implants, 27–28 (*see also* Speech processors)
Signed language, 374
  brain processing of, 309–310
    hemispheric specialization in, 310–312
  parental choice of communication mode, 379–381
  in rehabilitation of children with hearing loss, 336–339
Significant risk (SR) studies, 122
Simmons, FB, 106
Simultaneous analog stimulation processors (*see* SAS)
Single channel cochlear implant systems, 106
  speech perception outcomes in adults with, 234
  speech perception outcomes in children with, 243–244
SMSP (spectral maxima sound processor), 155–156, 161
Social development, auditory experience and, 36–37, 319–321 (*see also* Brain plasticity; Outcomes; Rehabilitation)
Somatosensory cortical plasticity, 46
Sound(s) (*see also* Sound waves)
  amplitude spectra of, 10, *11*
  consonant, 131–132, 131t
  levels of energy in, 10
  magnitude of, 10
  perception of (*see* Perception, auditory)
  pitch of, 10
  production of speech, 15, 17, *17,* 129–130 (*see also* Speech production; Speech representation)
  spectral and temporal properties of, 10–11

transduction of, 2
vowel, 10–11
   frequencies of, 11
Sound pressure units (dB SPL), 10
Sound representation, complex, 15, 17, *17*
Sound wave(s), 9–11
   collection of, by outer ear, 11
   conduction to cochlea, 11, 13
   frequencies of, 9–10, *11*
   intensity of, 9–10
   transformance of, to neural code, 13–14
   velocity of air molecules and pressure of, 9–10
   vibrations and, 9
Source-filter model, of speech, 129–130, *130*
Spatial mapping, 310
Spatial syntax, 310
SPEAK speech processors, 129, 141, 161
   CIS speech processors compared with, 160–161
   design strategy of, 156–157, *158,* 163
   MPEAK speech processors compared with, 157–160, *159*
   used in Nucleus cochlear implants, 235–237, 244–245
Special education, and outcomes of implantation in children, 277–278 (*see also* Outcomes; Rehabilitation)
Spectra 22 processor, 157
Spectral maxima sound processor (SMSP), 155–156, 161
Spectral peak (SPEAK), 129 (*see also* SPEAK speech processors)
Spectral splatter, 153
Speech intelligibility, after cochlear implantation in children, 252–253
Speech-language pathology, 364 (*see also* Language development; Rehabilitation; Speech perception)
Speech perception (*see also* Language development)
   adult, factors influencing, 241–242
   after implantation (*see also* Outcomes; Rehabilitation)
   adult outcomes of, 234–242
   auditory brain stem implants and, 242–243

factors influencing, 241–242
   multichannel cochlear implant systems, 234–241
   single channel cochlear implant systems, 234
   child outcomes of, 243–247, 325–331
   auditory capacity and performance in, 325
   comparisons of, 248–249, 325–326
   factors influencing, 246–247, 249–251
   multichannel cochlear implant systems, 244–246
   rehabilitative curricula in, 326–331
   single channel cochlear implant systems, 243–244
   measures of, 227–228, 331–341
   adult, 228–229
   child, 229–233, 275–277
   individual variability in, 233–234
   selecting appropriate, 227
   child, factors influencing, 246–247, 249–251
   evoked response potentials in, 308–309
   individual variation in, 233–234
   in infants, 184
   as intermodal event, 300
   multimodal, 228, 310–312
   neurobiologic basis of, 308–309
Speech Perception Instructional Curriculum and Evaluation, SPICE (Moog, et al), 328
Speech perception test batteries, for children, 230–231
Speech processing, neural mechanisms of, 52, 308–309 (*see also* Information processing)
Speech processors, 109, 110, 119–121, *120* (*see also* Speech representation)
   design strategies for, 138–139, 164–165
   compressed analog (CA), 149–152
   continuous interleaved sampling (CIS), 145–149

F0/F1/F2, *141,* 141–143, *142*
   feature extraction and multipeak, 141–145
   implementation of, 166
   interleaved pulses (IP), 138–141
   MPEAK, 143–145, *144*
   n-of-*m,* 161–163
   simultaneous analog stimulation (SAS), 163–164
   SPEAK, 156–157, *158*
   spectral maxima sound processor (SMSP), 155–156
   fitting, 165–166
   information processing by, 136–137
   purpose of, 129
   vocoders as, 133–136
      channel, 133–135, *134*
      formant, 135–136, *136*
Speech production
   after implantation in children, 251–252, 341–349
   communication mode effects in, 348–349
   phoneme perception and production in, 342–343
   research findings on, 342–343
   speech training procedures in, 343–349
   test batteries for, 231–233
   language development and, 300–301
   social influences in, 301–302
   vocal imitation in, 302–303
Speech reading, 363
Speech representation, 129–168
   elements of, 129–137
   model of, 129–130, *130*
   sounds in, 129–130
      classification of consonant and vowel, 131–132, 131t
      taxonomy of, 130–133
   speech processor strategies for, 138–165 (*see also* Speech processors)
   vocoder theory and models of, 133–136
Spike rate, of auditory neurons, 15–18, *16*
Spiral ganglion (SG) cells, 14
   electrical stimulation and effect on, 98
   and link to auditory brain stem, 23

Spiral ganglion (SG) cells
        (*contd.*)
    population of
        assessment of, before sur-
            gery, 191
        importance of, 58–59
        in various pathologies,
            61t
Spontaneous activity
    of cell types in cochlear nu-
        cleus, *22*
    and differences of sound con-
        duction, *17, 18*
Spontaneous language, in chil-
        dren with cochlear im-
        plants, 337
Spontaneous rate, and classifica-
        tion of auditory nerve re-
        sponses, 18
Stapes, *12, 13*
Stellate cells, 20–21, 22
    classification of, *22*
Stereocilia, of cochlea, 13
Stickler's syndrome, 63
Stimulus presentations, recorded
        and live-voice, 227–228
Streptococcus pneumoniae, 74
Support groups, for parents,
        182–183
Surgery (*see* Implantation, co-
        chlear, technique of)
Sustained choppers (ChS), *22*
Syphilis, 76

        T
Tactaid devices, 252
Temporal bones, histologic study
        of implanted, 218–219
Temporal channel interactions,
        152–153

Temporary threshold shifts
        (TTS), 69–70
Test batteries, for children
    speech perception, 230–231
    speech production, 231–233
Test formats, open-set and
        closed-set, 228
Therapy (*see* Rehabilitation)
3M/House device
    adult speech perception after
        implantation of, 234
    child speech perception after
        implantation of, 243–244
3M/Vienna device, speech percep-
        tion after implantation of,
        234
Tone
    sound waves and, 9–10
    waveform of, *10*
Tonotopy, 14
    in rehabilitative curriculum,
        352–355
Training effect
    adult brain plasticity and, 48
    neuronal tuning in, *49*
Transcutaneous link, 109, *111,*
        116–117
Transient choppers (ChT), *22*
TTS (temporary threshold shifts),
        69–70
Tuning curves, 15
    for low and high spike rate au-
        ditory neurons, *16–17*
Two-tone suppression, of audi-
        tory neurons, 15
Type I and II neurons, 14 (*see
        also* Auditory neurons)

        U
Units of sound pressure, 10
U.S. Food and Drug Administra-

tion (*see* Food and Drug
        Administration)
USCF/Storz speech processors,
        163–164
Usher's syndrome, 66, 67

        V
VAS (visual analog scale), 273
Ventilation tubes, advisability for
        implantation in children
        with, 190–191
Visual attention span, of children
        with cochlear implants,
        338
Vocabulary, familiarity of, 354
Vocal cords
    and frequencies of vowel
        sounds, 11
    transfer function of, 130
Vocal imitation, 302–303
Vocalization (*see* Sound(s);
        Speech representation)
Vocoder(s), 133–136
    channel, 133–135, *134*
    formant, 135–136, *136*
von Recklinghausen's disease, 64
Vowel sounds, 10–11
    classification of, 131–132, 131t
    frequencies of, 11

        W
Waardenburg's syndrome, 63
Wave forms, 9–11, *10, 11*
Wearable Speech Processor, 143
Wildervaank's syndrome, 68
Word Associations for Syllable
        Perception (WASP),
        343–349
Word learning, 300
World Federation of the Deaf,
        375